PREGNANCY AND INFANTS: MEDICAL, PSYCHOLOGICAL AND SOCIAL ISSUES

HANDBOOK FOR HIGH RISK PREGNANCY

CLINICAL MANAGEMENT

PREGNANCY AND INFANTS: MEDICAL, PSYCHOLOGICAL AND SOCIAL ISSUES

Additional books in this series can be found on Nova's website under the Series tab.

Additional e-books in this series can be found on Nova's website under the e-book tab.

PREGNANCY AND INFANTS: MEDICAL, PSYCHOLOGICAL AND SOCIAL ISSUES

HANDBOOK FOR HIGH RISK PREGNANCY

CLINICAL MANAGEMENT

ERNESTO GONZÁLEZ-MESA
AND
DANIEL ABEHSERA
EDITORS

New York

Library of Congress Cataloging-in-Publication Data

ISBN: 978-1-63482-299-2

Library of Congress Control Number: 2015932989

Published by Nova Science Publishers, Inc. † New York

CONTENTS

PREFACE

There is a group of women that have a greater chance of pregnancy complications due to pre-existing health conditions or the occurrence of a specific disease related to pregnancy. Although some of these conditions are common, others have a low prevalence and the management raises a number of concerns to health care providers. This book, whose chapters have a similar structure focused on the clinical, diagnostic and therapeutic features will become an important tool to display the most appropriate clinical management in high risk cases. The authors' have included sixteen chapters covering most obstetrics disorders.

Chapter 1 - The importance of obstetric risk assessment in every woman at childbearing age is that those considered high-risk pregnancies mark a significant increase or a serious likelihood of morbidity or mortality for the mother, fetus and newborn. The population considered at high risk corresponds to approximately 20 to 30% of all pregnant women and are responsible for 70-80% of perinatal mortality, and therefore these patients should be subjected to thorough checks with extensive scientific knowledge. Selecting population at risk is necessary to identify risk factors, defined as the biological, environmental or social characteristics that when present are associated with an increased likelihood of harm to the mother, fetus, or both. The purpose of identifying risk factors and diseases that may affect the normal course of pregnancy and / or newborn health is to advance preventive and therapeutic actions that benefit maternal and fetal health, allowing for a prenatal care plan. Risk factors identification is thus a fundamental objective to reduce perinatal and maternal morbidity and mortality. Although there is a good relationship between the existence of risk factors during pregnancy and the development of complications, problems can occur in pregnant women without risk factors. Risk factors selected by different authors are neither the same, nor are their relative importance in the different assessment systems.

Chapter 2 - Hyperemesis gravidarum is a serious condition whose management can achieve high levels of complexity. It is difficult to establish a specific aetiology, and its management often includes a psychological approach to the patient.

Chapter 3 - Gestational diabetes mellitus (GDM) is one of the most common complications in pregnancy. Normal pregnancy is a condition characterized by a series of complex hormonal adaptations that occur to ensure that sufficient glucose is available to meet the nutritional requirements of the growing fetus without causing maternal hypoglycemia. As normal pregnancy progresses, there is an increase in insulin resistance that may result in some cases in gestational diabetes. However, pregnancy can also occur in women with preexisting diabetes. Gestational diabetes mellitus is a disease characterized by underlying defects in maternal insulin sensitivity and secretion, which are unmasked in the response to the metabolic stressors of pregnancy. Later in this chapter the authors will sort out the different types of diabetes that can arise during pregnancy and before it. They will try to describe the maternal implications and fetal repercussions of gestational diabetes.

Women with GDM are at greater risk for prenatal complications than women without GDM. Maternal complications include obesity, overweight, polyhydramnios, premature broken membranes, preterm delivery, preeclampsia, instrumental delivery and primary cesarean section; and neonatal complications include greater infant birth weight, larger fetus for its gestational age, shoulder dystocia, neonatal hypoglycemia and necessity of phototherapy for hyperbilirubinemia. Alterations in other metabolic parameters besides glucose are associated with macrosomia, underlining the fact that protein and lipid abnormalities accompany glucose intolerance. Maternal free fatty acid levels and triglyceride levels at delivery correlate with neonatal weight and fat mass, suggesting that maternal lipid profiles influence neonatal weight. Maternal pre-pregnancy body mass index is a risk factor for macrosomia in women with GDM.

In pre-existing diabetes the most common anomalies involve the cardiovascular system (such as transposition of the great vessels, ventricular septal defect, situs inversus, single ventricle and hypoplastic left ventricle), the central nervous system (such as anencephaly, encephalocele, meningomyelocele, spina bifida, and holoprosencephaly), and the face and extremities. Rates of fetal malformation appear to be similar for maternal type 1 and type 2 pre-existing diabetes. Fortunately these complications are much lower than the others, according to Marco et al. 2012. Long term complications in the offspring were related with obesity, diabetes mellitus type II and behavior disturbances. The infants of women with GDM had excessive fetal growth and hyperinsulinemia as indicated by cord C-peptide and insulin concentrations. Diabetes recurrence, diabetes mellitus type II and the appearance of other cardiovascular risk factors associated with the metabolic syndrome (dyslipidemia, obesity and arterial hypertension) are more common to occur in mothers who have suffered from GDM.,

A dose-response effect was demonstrated, regarding the relation between congenital anomalies and glycemic control: the poorer the glucose control before conception or during an early stage of pregnancy is, the greater the risk for congenital anomalies. Equally important is the pregestational counseling in women with diabetes mellitus or insulin resistance, when they plan their pregnancy and before. In a recent review of Nandy et al. 2013, they explain this connection. The insulin/insulin-like growth factor (IGF) pathways and glucose metabolism act as mediators of human ovarian function and female fertility. In normal insulin action, insulin binds to its own receptors in the ovary to mediate steroidogenesis and acts as a co-gonadotropin. Insulin with other factors may influence ovarian growth and cyst formation. The IGF pathway also seems to influence normal ovarian function. Insulin signaling affects reproductive function. Dysregulation of this pathway leads to altered puberty, ovulation, and fertility.

Chapter 4 - Hypertensive disorders of pregnancy are an important cause of severe morbidity, long-term disability and death among both mothers and their babies. Among the hypertensive disorders that complicate pregnancy, pre-eclampsia and eclampsia stand out as major causes of maternal and perinatal mortality and morbidity. Hypertensive disorders during pregnancy occur in women with pre-existing primary or secondary chronic hypertension, and in women who develop new-onset hypertension in the second half of pregnancy. Hypertensive disorders during pregnancy carry risks for the woman and the baby.

Women with early-onset pre-eclampsia require admission to a tertiary care facility for treatment and one-third experience complications that may necessitate intensive care. Infants are often delivered preterm, need prolonged intensive care and develop complications, including lifelong disability, giving rise to large healthcare costs. Early identification of women at risk is a key aim of antenatal care.

Chapter 5 - Perinatal infections are transmitted in utero or during the postnatal period that immediately follows, and they play a major role in newborn mortality and morbidity rates. In the 1970s, the term TORCH was created to group the agents that could cause perinatal infections: Cytomegalovirus, rubeolla, toxoplasma, syphilis and herpes. However, in recent years, the following have been added as causes of these types of infections in fetuses and newborns: hepatitis, varicella-zoster, tuberculosis, HIV, enterovirus, parvovirus B19, Listeria monocytogenes, and in certain geographic regions, Plasmodium, Trypanosoma cruzi and Borrelia burgdorferi (Lyme disease). As a result, the TORCH acronym falls short, and the term perinatal infections is preferred. These infections may be bacterial, viral or parasitic, and they can be transmitted from the mother to the fetus or newborn in a number of ways: Intrauterine: This includes transplacentary transmission or vertical transmission through the vagina, which occurs primarily when the membranes rupture prematurely. During delivery or immediately after birth. Infectious agents that affect newborns may be present in the birth canal. Immediately after birth, certain infections present in mothers can be transmitted to newborns through contact between the two or through breastfeeding. The process of diagnosing perinatal infections is complex because each agent must be analyzed individually. Maternal IgG are transported through the placenta, so their detection in newborns does not imply infection. The detection of IgM and IgA antibodies is a diagnosis, but its sensitivity is not always high. Certain agents must be searched using direct methods, so searching for antibodies is of limited use.

The aim of this chapter is to highlight the most important aspects of perinatal infections caused by toxoplasma, Listeria monocytogenes, herpes simplex virus, cytomegalovirus and HIV. Chapter 6 - Pregnancy affects both the kidney and the remainder of the urinary tract.

1. Increased renal size: Both kidneys increase in size by 1 to 1.5 cm during pregnancy. Kidney volume increases by up to 30 percent, primarily due to an increase in renal vascular and interstitial volume. There are no histological changes or changes in number of nephrons, but the glomerular filtration rate is also increased. The renal pelvises and caliceal systems may be dilated as a result of progesterone effects and mechanical compression of the ureters at the pelvic brim.
2. Ureters: Dilatation of the ureters and renal pelvis is more prominent on the right than the left and is seen in up to 80 percent of pregnant women. These changes can be visualized on ultrasound examination by the second trimester, and may not resolve until 6 to 12 weeks postpartum.
3. Bladder: The bladder mucosa is edematous and hyperemic in pregnancy. Although progesterone-induced bladder wall relaxation may lead to increased capacity, the enlarging uterus displaces the bladder superiorly and anteriorly, and flattens it, which can decrease capacity.
4. Renal hemodynamic: Normal pregnancy is characterized by widespread vasodilatations, with increased arterial compliance and decreased systemic vascular resistance. These global hemodynamic changes are accompanied by increases in renal perfusion and glomerular filtration rate. In late gestation, assumption of the left

lateral position is associated with increases in glomerular filtration rate and sodium excretion.

Chapter 7 - The risk of venous thromboembolic events is high during pregnancy. Fifty percent of the patients with thrombosis during pregnancy will be found to have an underlying thrombofilia. Pulmonary thromboembolism (PTE) remains a major cause of direct maternal mortality, with many deaths associated with a failure to obtain objective diagnoses (often because of unfounded concerns such as radiation exposure for the fetus) and lack of adequate treatment.. Effective primary prevention and acute management of venous thromboembolism in pregnancy are important to reduce maternal mortality and morbidity. Venous thromboembolism complicates approximately 1 in 1600 births and is a leading cause of maternal morbidity in the United States. There is a strong association between inherited thrombophilias and venous thromboembolism, which makes detection of these mutations a logical target for prevention strategies.

Chapter 8 - Most systemic autoimmune diseases preferentially affect women, usually in the period covering the childbearing age. It is therefore not uncommon coexistence of pregnancy and systemic autoimmune disease with all the (diagnostic, therapeutic and prognostic) implications that entails both, pregnancy and underlying disease. The prognosis of these diseases has improved in recent decades, from being almost impossible for these women to have offspring, becoming it similar to that of the general population; although close monitoring of these patients is required due the maternal-fetal morbidity and mortality. Systemic lupus erythematosus (SLE) is the most representative autoimmune disease in which the connection with pregnancy and disease is known. Almost 90% of these patients are women and almost 70% of them are of childbearing age. Moreover the authors know the favorable role of hormones in the development and activity of disease.

Chapter 9 - Liver disease may complicate 3-5% of gestations. Liver disorders during pregnancy include: anodyne liver enzyme abnormalities and severe liver failure. Liver disease during pregnancy may become life threatening for the mother and/or the fetus.

Chapter 10 - Pregnant women are particularly susceptible to a group of changes in their skin that can be divided into physiological and pathological changes. These changes are due to vascular, endocrinological, metabolic and immunological modifications. Placental substances increase activity in endocrine system and alter the purification system, causing more availability of estrogens in plasma and generating a clinical impact. In addition to physiological changes in the skin and pre-existing skin disease, it can develop specific skin diseases that are seen only during pregnancy or postpartum period. The importance of detection of these disorders lies in the possible adverse maternal and fetal outcomes. Classification of skin diseases during pregnancy is highly controversial. Many different names have been used to define similar clinical disorders. It is very important to differentiate in a practical way the common changes from those that could have an effect on the mother and fetus. In order to differentiate the types of skin lesions the authors will summarize its nomenclature and semiological definition.

Chapter 11 - Thrombotic thrombocytopenic purpura (TTP) is one of the microangiopathic disorders that can be diagnosed during pregnancy. These alterations are characterized by the formation of microthrombi in small vessels, leading to thrombocytopenia, microangiopathic hemolytic anemia, and multiorgan damage. The hypercoagulability state observed during pregnancy conditions the incidence of such disorders in pregnant women compared with the general population. Specifically, these disorders comprise TTP, uremic hemolytic syndrome

(HUS), preeclampsia-HELLP syndrome, and some other autoimmune diseases like catastrophic antiphospholipid syndrome (CAPS). TTP is clinically characterized by a group of five symptoms: thrombocytopenia, microangiopathic hemolytic anemia, fever, neurological alterations and renal failure. It can exhibit a familial trait, though idiopathic TTP is the most common presentation. HUS in turn is characterized by renal failure, and although it is typically observed in children with a history of infection due to toxin-producing bacteria in the previous days or weeks, the disease occasionally has also been reported during pregnancy. On the other hand, both preeclampsia and HELLP syndrome belong to a range of disorders in which arterial hypertension is the fundamental clinical feature - HELLP syndrome being one of the most serious conditions. On the other hand, CAPS is a serious and rapidly progressive form of antiphospholipid syndrome leading to multiorgan failure. CAPS may be the first manifestation of the disease, although previous history of antiphospholipid syndrome, systemic lupus erythematosus, or in a small number of cases, Sjogren's syndrome or Systemic Sclerosis, could guide the doctor. In CAPS the activation of coagulation is caused by the presence of autoantibodies that bind to membrane phospholipids. Although the underlying physiopathological mechanisms differ, the clinical consequences are very similar. This makes it very difficult to establish a differential diagnosis. Each disease has its own treatment particularities, and maternal and perinatal morbidity and mortality is high when treatment is not appropriate. It is therefore necessary for gynecologists to have a thorough understanding of differentiating characteristics of these disorders.

Chapter 12 - Neurological symptoms and conditions are frequently observed in women in reproductive age. Most of them are caused by exacerbation of pre-existing disorders, others are pregnancy related disorders. Understanding the physiological changes during pregnancy is mandatory for the management of these conditions. Currently almost all of these neurological diseases are compatible with successful pregnancy outcome. However, neurological diseases contribute to maternal mortality, with stroke and epilepsy accounting for the majority of deaths from neurologic causes. Several other disabling neurologic conditions, ranging from multiple sclerosis to migraine, present both medical and obstetric challenges to clinicians unfamiliar with their management within the context of pregnancy. All these patients have specific therapies and risks that the physician should know.

Chapter 13 - Preterm Labor (PTL) is one of the leading cause of perinatal morbidity and mortality (70%-85%). The incidence rate of premature birth has not declined but increased over the last years, due to the use of assisted reproductive technology associated to the rise of multiple pregnancies, obstetric interventions and a better record of premature infants at lower gestational ages than in previous decades. New challenges are emerging with the definition of *fetal viability* as its gestational age is being discussed, but it is currently accepted to be around 24 weeks. However, either in a short or long term period the morbidity and mortality as well as the economic and emotional cost for the families increase in extremely premature infants. The specific trigger of PTL is largely unknown and its prevention is difficult due to different reasons like medical conditions affecting the mother or fetus in which continuation of pregnancy is hazardous.

Chapter 14 - Thrombocytopenia is the most common blood disorder during the pregnancy after anemia. Thrombocytopenia defined as a platelet count $<150 \times 10^9$ /L has a prevalence at the end of the pregnancy between 6.6% and 11%. However, counts $<100 \times 10^9$ /L, which is the definition for thrombocytopenia adopted by an International Working Group, are observed in only 1% of the pregnancy.

Chapter 15 - Pregnancy involves several changes in the pregnant's cardio respiratory system that lead to changes in the clinical expression as well as in proper therapeutic approach of each respiratory disease. Overall, these changes involve a decrease in the respiratory reserve, which normally doesn't involve any pathological implication, but might be crucial in patients with previous respiratory diseases or if a new one is developed during pregnancy. Respiratory diseases are an important cause of maternal morbidity and mortality, so it is essential to know their proper management during pregnancy for the best maternal and fetal prognosis to be granted.

Chapter 16 - Multiple pregnancies are commonly associated with maternal-fetal complications; that is the reason why these cases have always been a highlight in classic perinatal medicine studies. Nevertheless, this area of knowledge has currently gained popularity because of an increase of its incidence and the further investigations on multiple pregnancies. Factors that have predetermined an increase of the rate of twin gestation during the last years are quite diverse; however, it seems important to point out two of them that are also related. Advanced maternal age: as for older women the probability of double ovulation increases by an increase in the secretion of follicle stimulating hormone (FSH). Increased use of artificial reproductive technologies and fertility drugs. Approximately 30-35% of fertility treatments develop in a multiple pregnancy.

In: Handbook for High Risk Pregnancy: Clinical Management ISBN: 978-1-63482-299-2
Editors: E. González-Mesa and D. Abehsera

Chapter 1

OBSTETRIC RISK EVALUATION

Celia Cuenca Marín, PhD, and Marta García Sánchez, MD*

Obstetrics and Gynecology Department, University Quiron Hospital, Málaga, Spain

INTRODUCTION

The importance of obstetric risk assessment in every woman at childbearing age is that those considered high-risk pregnancies mark a significant increase or a serious likelihood of morbidity or mortality for the mother, fetus and newborn.

The population considered at high risk corresponds to approximately 20 to 30% of all pregnant women and are responsible for 70-80% of perinatal mortality, and therefore these patients should be subjected to thorough checks with extensive scientific knowledge (Aubry and Pennington, 1973).

Selecting population at risk is necessary to identify risk factors, defined as the biological, environmental or social characteristics that when present are associated with an increased likelihood of harm to the mother, fetus, or both.

The purpose of identifying risk factors and diseases that may affect the normal course of pregnancy and / or newborn health is to advance preventive and therapeutic actions that benefit maternal and fetal health, allowing for a prenatal care plan.

Risk factors identification is thus a fundamental objective to reduce perinatal and maternal morbidity and mortality. Although there is a good relationship between the existence of risk factors during pregnancy and the development of complications, problems can occur in pregnant women without risk factors. Risk factors selected by different authors are neither the same, nor are their relative importance in the different assessment systems. Pregnant women can be grouped in two subpopulations:

- Low-risk subpopulation whose pregnancy can be treated in primary health care.
- High-risk subpopulation should be referred to specialized care and or to other professionals in the monitoring of pregnancy.

* Corresponding author: Marta García Sánchez, MD. E-mail: martagarciasanchez.gine@gmail.com.

Obstetric risk degree should be assessed comprehensively in the first visit and reconsidered again in subsequent controls (Table 1).

Table 1. Obstetric risk factors

SOCIODEMOGRAPHIC RISK FACTORS
Maternal age <15 years or> 35 years
Obesity
Smoking> 10 cigarettes / day
Alcoholism
Drug Addiction
Low socioeconomic status
Occupational risk
MEDICAL HISTORY
Hypertension
Heart Disease
Kidney Disease
Diabetes mellitus
Endocrinopathies
Chronic respiratory disease
Hematologic disease
Epilepsy and other neurological diseases
Psychiatric illnesses
Liver disease with failure
Autoimmune disease with systemic involvement
Thromboembolism
Major Medico surgical pathology
REPRODUCTIVE HISTORY
Recurrent miscarriage
Preterm delivery history
Intrauterine growth restricted history
Perinatal death history
New born with residual neurologic injury
Congenital defects
Thromboembolism
Uterine surgery
Uterine malformation
Cervical incompetence
CURRENT PREGNANCY
Pregnancy-induced hypertension
Severe anaemia
Gestational diabetes
Urinary infections repeat
Infection of perinatal transmission
Rh isoimmunisation
Multiple pregnancy
Polyhydramnios. Oligohydramnios
Genital bleeding
Placenta previa (diagnostic ultrasound> 32 weeks)
Intrauterine growth retardation
Fetal congenital defect
Threatened preterm labour
Premature rupture membranes
Uterine tumour
Surgical procedures

1. Risk Assessment at the Preconceptional Visit

A good pregnancy outcome is partly determined by a women's preconception health and healthy lifestyle. The American College of Obstetricians and Gynaecologists (ACOG Committee Opinion nº 313, 2005) states that optimizing a woman's health before and between pregnancies must be an on-going process. Routinely addressing preconception issues in women of childbearing potential is important because, although many women intend to obtain preconception evaluation and counselling before attempting pregnancy, almost 50 per cent of pregnancies are unintended (Finer and Zolna, 2006). The most vulnerable period for fetal defects is between 4 and 10 weeks of gestation, the period of embryogenesis, meaning that counselling for a healthy life style and reducing high-risk conditions should start preferably before conception (Witters, Bogaerts and Fryns, 2010).

The main goals of obstetric risk evaluation are (ACOG Technical bulletin 205, 1995):

- Identify potential risks to the mother, fetus, and pregnancy.
- Educate women about these risks, options for intervention and management, and reproductive alternatives.
- Initiate interventions to provide optimum maternal, fetal, and pregnancy outcomes. Interventions include motivational counselling, education, disease optimization, and specialist referral.

1.1. Medical History

A thorough medical history is a good starting point for discussing how pregnancy can affect maternal health and the effect of maternal health and behaviours on the fetus and pregnancy. Guidelines generally target the following areas for preconception risk assessment (Johnson, Posner, Biermann, Cordero, Atrash, Parker, Boulet and Curtis, 2006):

1.1.1. Social and Demographic Factors

- *Age.* As maternal age increases, the risk of infertility, fetal aneuploidy, miscarriage, gestational diabetes, preeclampsia, and stillbirth also increases (Leuzzi and Scoles, 1996). Women should be aware of these risks and the consequences of delaying conception.
- *Psychosocial screening* of all women seeking pregnancy evaluation or pre-natal care should be performed, at the initial visit and at each trimester during pregnancy, regardless of social status, educational level, or race and ethnicity. Screening should include assessment of barriers to care, unstable housing, family planning, unintended pregnancy, communication barriers, nutrition, tobacco use, substance use, depression, safety, intimate partner violence, and stress (ACOG Committee Opinion No. 343, 2006).

1.1.2. Medical History

- *Chronic diseases.* The optimal time to start attending a future pregnancy in a woman with a chronic illness is the preconception period, allowing the study of the disease without the limitations imposed by pregnancy, placing women in the best of health before starting gestation and selecting the most appropriate time for conception, taking measures to protect the fetus against exposure to drugs and therapeutic actions during the critical period of the first weeks of development, provide information about the risks of pregnancy for disease progression and risks that can lead to disease on the development of pregnancy.

- *Genetic conditions and family history*. Counselling and genetic testing need should be assessed, if appropriate, in cases of family history or children with neurological, metabolic, genetic and chromosomal structural abnormalities, mental retardation, cystic fibrosis, etc.
- *Infectious diseases, immune status* and update vaccines.
- *Nutritional* deficiency states, dietary restrictions (folic acid intake), obesity and weight management.

1.1.3. Reproductive History

The gynaecologic and obstetric histories are important for identifying factors that may contribute to infertility or complications in a future pregnancy and initiating appropriate intervention to reduce or eliminate these risks, if possible (Stubblefield, Coonrod, Reddy, Sayegh, Nicholson, Rychlik and Jack, 2008).

All history should collect the antecedent of (Jack, Atrash, Moos, O´Donnell and Johnson, 2008):

- *Preterm delivery*. Given the possibility of recurrence, possible causes of preterm labour should be investigated and specific monitoring should be planned (Ib-A)
- *Recurrent miscarriage*. In case the patient has had repeated abortions, adequate study and treatment evaluation should be made (Ib-A)
- *Stillbirths*. The patient must be informed about the possibility of recurrence. The study of the causes must be completed and risk habits, such as tobacco consumption, should be modified (IIb)
- *Previous Caesarean*. A time interval between births of at least 18 months must be advised (IIb-B)

1.1.4. Environmental and Biomedical Risks

- *Medications known to be teratogens*. Consult guide FDA for pregnancy to avoid use of teratogens. Identifying use of teratogenic medications is the key component in medical assessment to establish medications that may be stopped, should be stopped, or can be changed to a safer one.
- *Substance use*, including tobacco, alcohol, and non-prescribed drugs. Women should be informed about the specific risks of smoking during pregnancy (such as the risk of having a baby with low birth weight and preterm birth). The benefits of quitting at any stage should be emphasised. Personalised information, advice and support on how to stop smoking can be offered (NICE Guideline, 2008).
- *Environmental exposure*. Questions about the woman's work, hobbies, pets, and home environment can identify potentially toxic exposures, such as mercury, lead,

pesticides, and endocrine disrupting chemicals (phthalates, bisphenol A, polybrominated diethyl ethers) (McDiarmid, Gardiner and Jack, 2008).

1.2. Physical Examination

General physical examination must be performed, being important blood pressure, body mass index (BMI) and gynaecological evaluation. Specific examinations will be performed in case of pre-existing pathologies.

1.3. Laboratory Assessment

Screening of certain infections within preconception counselling can identify potential risks to reproductive health and pregnancy outcome.

1.3.1. Universal Screening

- *Human immunodeficiency virus (HIV)* counselling and screening is recommended for all women planning pregnancy.
- *Rubella immunity.* Susceptibility screening should be offered early in prenatal care to identify women at risk of contracting rubella infection and to enable prenatal vaccination for future pregnancies protection.
- *Toxoplasmosis and cytomegalovirus* infection screening is controversial. Meanwhile, behavioural changes to reduce the risk of acquiring this and others infections are recommended.

1.3.2. Selective Screening

The following should be considered in appropriate high-risk groups:

- *Sexually transmitted infections* according to standard guidelines (gonorrhoea, chlamydia, syphilis, hepatitis, and other). Depending on the disease, these infections can cause subfertility/infertility, as well as congenital infection and medical and pregnancy complications.
- *Genetic carrier testing* when medical record - either own, partner, family or ethnic origin- indicate a higher probability of heritable disease, or upon request of patients. This information allows patients planning pregnancy to make informed reproductive decisions about adoption, surrogacy, use of donor sperm, in vitro fertilization after preimplantation genetic diagnosis, avoidance of pregnancy, and prenatal diagnosis (Solomon, Jack and Feero, 2008).
- *Glycated hemoglobin (A1C), fasting plasma glucose (FPG)* in women with a prior history of diabetes. Good glucose control in early pregnancy reduces the risk of miscarriage and congenital anomalies, and can take time to achieve.
- *Others.* Specific analytical tests can be done if pathologies are suspected: endocrinopathies (e.g., phenylketonuria), infectious contact (e.g., tuberculosis) or exposure to toxic (e.g., serum determination of lead level)

Preconception interventions include: health promotion, education and counselling related to reproductive health risks, optimizing the control of medical disorders, and referral for specialized care when appropriate. If pregnancy avoidance is desired, contraceptive options should be discussed and offered. Evidence observational data supports an association between preconception counselling and positive changes in maternal behaviour before pregnancy, particularly with respect to folic acid intake, improved glycemic control, and reduction in alcohol intake and cigarettes smoked (Williams, Zapata, D'Angelo, Harrison and Morrow, 2012). There is also evidence, from randomized trials, that the prevalence of congenital anomalies was reduced by preconception care of women with diabetes (Ray, O´Brien and Chan, 2001) or epilepsy (Winterbottom, Smyth, Jacoby and Baker, 2009).

2. Prenatal Care: On-Going Risk Evaluation

After the initial prenatal assessment, prenatal care is directed at continuous evaluation of mother and fetus health status, problems anticipated, and intervention, if possible, to prevent or minimize morbidity. The major goal of prenatal care is to ensure the birth of a healthy baby with minimal risk for the mother. There are several components involved in achieving this objective:

- Early accurate estimation of gestational age
- Patients risk identification
- Fetus and mothers on-going health status evaluation
- Preventive interventions
- Patient education and communication

Ideally, prenatal care is initiated in the 10th week of gestation. The percentage of pregnant women who initiate prenatal care in the first trimester is one of the standard clinical performance measures used to assess maternal healthcare quality.

Prenatal visits: frequency and guidelines. Observational studies (WHO Antenatal Care Trial Research Group, 2001) comparing pregnancy outcomes in women who receive and do not receive prenatal care are consistently confounded by socioeconomic and other factors that influence access to prenatal care and maternal/perinatal outcome. Data suggest that prenatal care saves lives compared to no prenatal care, (Martin, Hamilton, Sutton, Ventura, Mathews and Osterman, 2010). However, there are limited data as to what constitutes the optimal number and frequency of prenatal visits, or the optimal content of those visits. The National Institute of Health and Clinical Excellence suggests, for a woman with an uncomplicated pregnancy, a reduced frequency of visits: 10 appointments for nulliparous women and 7 appointments for parous women, and each visit should have a specific purpose. Although there is no precise definition for high-risk pregnancy, there is consensus that these women need additional care during pregnancy (NICE Antenatal Care, 2012).

National organizations in each country – ACOG, NICE- publish guidelines for routine prenatal care with some differences depending on the prevalence for some disorders and the available resources.

2.1. Initial Visit

In case the patient has not had a 'preconception obstetrical risks evaluation' everything described in the section above - preconception visit- should be added to the next:

Medical history.

- Current pregnancy history and estimated date of delivery.
- Psychosocial information: whether the pregnancy was planned or unintended, potential barriers to care (e.g., communication, transportation, child care issues, economic constraints, work schedule), whether the patient has stable housing, and her mental health and level of stress (ACOG Committee Opinion No. 343, 2006). The American College of Obstetricians and Gynaecologists guidelines on intimate partner violence (ACOG Committee Opinion No. 518, 2012) and reproductive and sexual coercion (ACOG Committee Opinion No. 554, 2013) recommend that physicians routinely assess all pregnant women for past or current exposure to these behaviours.

The first prenatal visit is an appropriate time to discuss the patient's responsibilities and when to call the provider (See 2.3 section).

Physical examination.

- *Uterine size and shape and evaluation of the adnexa.* Sonography is useful to evaluate the different causes for a discrepancy between uterine size and that expected by last menstrual period (LMP) –uterine fibroids, malposition, multiple gestation, incorrect date of LMP – and for evaluating suspected adnexal masses.

Laboratory tests (Table 2).

- *Pregnancy test.* Suspected pregnancy should be confirmed by laboratory evaluation, in the absence of diagnostic physical findings (confirmation of pregnancy by ultrasound examination or identification of fetal cardiac activity). The standard test is the detection of the beta-subunit of human chorionic gonadotropin (hCG) in blood or urine.
- *Routine tests.* A standard panel of laboratory tests should be obtained on every pregnant woman at the first prenatal visit. Considerations:
    - An early *screening for anaemia,* at the booking appointment, and each time other blood screening tests are being performed, allows enough time for treatment if anaemia is detected.
    - *Infections Screening:* Screening for *syphilis* and for *hepatitis B* should be offered to all pregnant women at an early stage in antenatal care because, in the first case, treatment is beneficial to the mother and baby, and in the second one, effective postnatal interventions can be offered to infected women to decrease the risk of mother-to-child transmission.

The available evidence does not support routine screening in pregnant women for *cytomegalovirus, toxoplasma and hepatitis C virus* and it should not be offered because screening risks may outweigh potential benefits, and they are not cost effective. Pregnant women should be informed of primary prevention measures to avoid those infections.

- *At-risk woman laboratory tests.* Additional testing for specific conditions can augment the panel above. Considerations:
  - *Screening for infections. Chlamydia* test and other screening for sexually transmitted infections should not be offered as part of routine antenatal care. At the booking appointment, healthcare professionals should inform pregnant women younger than 25 years about the high prevalence of chlamydia infection in their age group, in order to decide doing or not those tests depending on patient medical history. The possibility of other infection diseases (Chagas, Tuberculosis, and others) should be thought and tested depending on endemic prevalence in each country, patient exposures, habits and travels.
  - *Urine protein dipstick* and more frequent blood pressure measurements should be considered for pregnant women who have any of the following risk factors for preeclampsia (NICE Guideline, 2008):
    - Age: 40 years or older
    - nulliparity
    - more than 10 years pregnancy interval
    - preeclampsia family history
    - preeclampsia previous history
    - body mass index 30kg/m2 or above
    - pre-existing vascular disease such as hypertension
    - pre-existing renal disease
    - multiple pregnancy.
  - *Screening Thyroid function*: because of insufficient evidence to support universal TSH screening in the first trimester, most professional societies, including the American Thyroid Association (ATA), the Endocrine Society, and the American College of Obstetricians and Gynecologists, recommend targeted case finding rather than universal screening. The ATA recommend testing pregnant women for thyroid dysfunction if they have any of the following (American Thyroid Association Taskforce on Thyroid Disease During Pregnancy and Postpartum, 2011):
    - symptoms of thyroid disease
    - from an area of known moderate to severe iodine insufficiency
    - thyroid disease personal or family history
    - thyroid peroxidase antibodies (TPOAb)
    - type 1 diabetes
    - preterm delivery or miscarriage history
    - head or neck radiation history
    - morbid obesity (BMD ≥40 kg/m2)
    - infertility
    - age >30 years

In women who meet the screening criteria, we should measure serum TSH during the first trimester as the screening test for hypothyroidism. If the serum TSH is normal, no further testing should be performed. If the TSH is >2.5 mU/L, free T4 should be measured to determine the degree of hypothyroidism.

- *Screening for gestational diabetes* using risk factors is recommended in a healthy population. At the booking appointment, the following risk factors for gestational diabetes should be determined (NICE Guideline, 2008):
  - body mass index above 30 kg/m^2
  - previous macrosomic baby weighing 4.5 kg or above
  - previous gestational diabetes
  - diabetes family history (first-degree relative with diabetes)
  - family origin with a high prevalence of diabetes: South Asian, black Caribbean, Middle Eastern

Women with any one of these risk factors should be offered testing for gestational diabetes.

Ultrasound examination. Randomized trials have shown that routine early ultrasound examination is beneficial in an unselected population to get a better estimation of gestational age, resulting in significantly reduced frequency of labour induction for post term pregnancy and use of tocolysis for suspected preterm labour, an earlier detection of clinically unsuspected fetal malformations and aneuploidies, and an earlier detection of multiple pregnancy.

2.2. Follow-Up Visits

In order to control the clinical pregnancy evolution, the healthcare provider should actualize at each visit:

- Medical history and current pregnancy evolution since last meeting.
- Test and scans recommended. Following own countries guidelines.
- Perinatal risk classification (See Table 1).
- Patient information and education.
- Promote specific interventions, if necessary.

2.2.1. Routine Assessments

- Maternal blood pressure* and weight measurement
- Uterine size or fundal height measurement, to assess fetal growth
- Fetal cardiac activity documentation
- Maternal perception of fetal activity (in the second and third trimesters)
- Fetal presentation (in the third trimester)

Table 2. Laboratory test

ROUTINE LABORATORY TEST
Rhesus type and antibody screen
Haematocrit or haemoglobin and mean corpuscular volume
Cervical cytology cancer screening
Rubella immunity
Varicella immunity
Urine culture
Syphilis testing
Hepatitis B antigen testing
Human immunodeficiency virus
AT RISK WOMAN LABORATORY TESTS
Urine protein
Thyroid function
Type 2 diabetes
Testing for infection Chlamydia testing N. Gonorrhoea Bacterial vaginosis Trichomonas vaginalis Herpes simplex virus Tuberculosis Toxoplasmosis Hepatitis C antibodies CMV Chagas disease
Inherited disorders evaluation Cystic fibrosis Fragile X Hemoglobinopathies
Spinal muscular atrophy
Phenylketonuria
Lead level screening

*The presence of significant hypertension and/or proteinuria should alert the healthcare professional to the need for increased surveillance. Alternative screening methods for preeclampsia, have not demonstrated satisfactory sensitivity and specificity, and therefore they are not recommended. Routine *Urine dipstick test for protein* has a questionable value in women with normal blood pressure (Rhode, Shapiro and Jones, 2007).

2.2.2. Gestational Week-Specific Assessments

- *Screening for fetal aneuploidy*. Down syndrome (trisomy 21) is the most common chromosome abnormality among live born infants. All pregnant women should be offered

Down syndrome (trisomy 21) screening, this screening can be performed during the first or the second trimester, been preferably the combined test before 13 +6 of gestation week.

- Screening for neural tube defects: from 15 to 24 gestation week
- Ultrasound screening for fetal structural anomalies: Women should be given information

about the purpose and implications of the anomaly scan to enable them to make an informed choice about whether or not having the scan done. The purpose of the scan is to identify fetal anomalies and allow:

- Reproductive choice (termination of pregnancy).
- Managed birth in a specialised centre or provide intrauterine therapy.
- Parents' mental preparation for any treatment/disability/palliative care

Women should be informed about limitations of routine ultrasound screening and about detection rates varying depending on the type of fetal anomaly, the woman's body mass index and the position of the unborn baby at the time of the scan.

Although many congenital anomalies can be identified in the first trimester, sensitivity is higher in the second trimester and every pregnant must be offered a screening for fetal structural anomalies between 18 and 22 gestation week.

- o *Transvaginal ultrasound measurement* of short cervical length between 16 and 28 gestation week (g.w.), in order to screen increased risk of spontaneous preterm birth is controversial.
- o *Screening for gestational diabetes:* between 24 and 28 gestation weeks.
- o In Rh(D)-negative women, *red cell (RBC) antibody screening* is repeated at 28 gestation weeks, and anti-D immune globulin is administered
- o *Sexually transmitted disease.* The CDC recommends testing for sexually transmitted diseases (STDs, e.g, HIV, syphilis, hepatitis B surface antigen, chlamydia, gonorrhoea) in the third trimester (from 28 to 36 g.w.) in women who: have risk factors for acquiring a STD. In addition, the CDC recommends that all women ≤25 years of age should be retested for Chlamydia trachomatis late in pregnancy (Workowski and Berman, 2010).
- o *Group B beta-hemolytic streptococcus* testing: All pregnant women should be screened, at restation week 35 to 37, for group B beta-hemolytic streptococcus (GBS) colonization with swabs of both the lower vagina and rectum. The only patients who are excluded from this screening are those with GBS bacteriuria earlier in the current pregnancy or those who gave birth to a previous infant with invasive GBS disease.
- o *Monitoring fetal wellbeing.* Women with uncomplicated pregnancies should be offered labour induction beyond 41 g.w. From 42 g.w. women who decline induction of labour should be offered increased antenatal monitoring consisting of, at least twice weekly, cardiotocography and ultrasound estimation of maximum amniotic pool depth.

2.3. Warning Signs and Symptoms

Signs and symptoms that may indicate pathological conditions - abortion risk, placental abruption, placenta praevia, premature rupture of membranes, premature delivery, preeclampsia, and others - should be reported to the health care provider promptly. Patients should be educated about it.

These include, but are not limited to:

- Vaginal bleeding, spotting
- Leakage of fluid per vagina
- Increased uterine activity, menstrual-like cramps, increased pelvic pressure, low backache, and contractions.
- Decreased fetal activity
- Severe headache, blurred vision, epigastria pain, vomiting.

References

American College of Obstetricians and Gynecologists. (2006). The importance of preconception care in the continuum of women´s health care. ACOG Committee Opinion number 313. *Obstetrics and Gynecology,* 106:665-6.

American College of Obstetricians and Gynecologists. (2005). Psychosocial risk factors: perinatal screening and intervention. ACOG Committee Opinion number 343. *Obstetrics and Gynecology,* 108(2):469.

American College of Obstetricians and Gynecologists. (1995). Preconceptional care. *ACOG technical bulletin 205.*

Aubry, R. H., Pennington, J. C. (1973). Identification and evaluation of high-risk pregnancy: The perinatal concept. *Clinical Obstetrics and Gynecology*, 16:3.

Finer, L. B., Zolna, M. R. (2011). Unintended pregnancy in the United States: incidence and disparities, 2006. *Contraception*, 84:478.

Jack, B. W., Atrash, H., Conrood, D. V., Moos, M. K., O´Donnell, J., Johnson, K. (2008) The clinical content of preconception care: an overview and preparation of this supplement. *American Journal of Obstetrics and Gynecology,* 199: 266-78.

Johnson, K., Posner, S. F., Biermann, J., Cordero, J. F., Atrash, H. K., Parker, C. S., Boulet, S., Curtis, M. G. (2006). Recommendations to improve preconception health and health care-United States. Areport of the CDC/ATSDR Preconception Care Work Group and the Select Panel on Preconception Care. *MMWR Recommendations and Reports,* 55:1.

Leuzzi, R. A., Scoles, K. S. (1996). Preconception counseling for the primary care physician. *Medical Clinics of North America,* 80:337.

Martin, J. A., Hamilton, B. E., Sutton, P. D., Ventura, S. J., Mathews, T. J., Osterman, M. J. (2010). Births: Final data for 2008. *National vital statistics reports,* 59(1):3-71.

McDiarmid, M. A., Gardiner, P. M., Jack, B. W. (2008). The clinical content of preconception care: environmental exposures. *American Journal of Obstetrics and Gynecology,* 199:357.

National Institute for Health and Clinical Excellence. (2012). Antenatal Care: Routine care for the Healthy Pregnant Woman.

NICE guideline. (2008). Antenatal Care. CG62.

Ray, J. G., O´Brien, T. E., Chan, W. S. (2001). Preconception care and the risk of congenital anomalies in the offspring of women with diabetes mellitus: a meta-analysis. *An International Journal of Medicine.* 94:435.

Rhode, M. A., Shapiro, H., Jones, O. W. (2007). Indicated vs. routine prenatal urine chemical reagent strip testing. *The Journal of Reproductive Medicine,* 52:214.

Solomon, B. D., Jack, B. W., Feero, W. G. (2008). The clinical content of preconception care: genetics and genomics. *American Journal of Obstetrics and Gynecology,* 199:340.

Stagnaro-Green, A., Abalovich, M., Alexander, E., Azizi, F., Mestman, J., Negro, R., Nixon, A., Pearce, E. N., Soldin, O. P., Sullivan, S., Wiersinga, W., American Thyroid Association Taskforce on Thyroid Disease During Pregnancy and Postpartum (2011). Guidelines of the American Thyroid Association for the diagnosis and management of thyroid disease during pregnancy and postpartum. *Thyroid,* 21(10):1081.

Stubblefield, P. G., Coonrod, D. V., Reddy, U. M., Sayegh, R., Nicholson, W., Rychlik, D. F., Jack, B. W. (2008). The clinical content of preconception care: reproductive history. *American Journal of Obstetrics and Gynecology,* 199 (6 Suppl. 2):373.

Villar, J., Ba'aqeel, H., Piaggio, G., Lumbiganon, P., Belizán, J., Farnot, U., WHO Antenatal Care Trial Research Group. (2001). WHO antenatal care randomised trial for the evaluation of a new model of routine antenatal care. *Lancet,* 357(9268):1551.

Williams, L., Zapata, L. B., D'Angelo, D. V., Harrison, L., Morrow, B. (2012). Associations between preconception counseling and maternal behaviors before and during pregnancy. *Matern Child Health Journal,* 16(9):1854-61.

Winterbottom, J., Smyth, R., Jacoby, A., Baker, G. (2009). The effectiveness of preconception counseling to reduce adverse pregnancy outcome in women with epilepsy: what´s the evidence? *Epilepsy and Behavior*, 14:273.

Witters, I., Bogaerts, A., Fryns, J. P. (2010). Preconception care. *Genetic Counseling,* 21 (2): 169-82.

Workowski, K. A., Berman, S., Centers for Disease Control and Prevention (CDC) (2010). Sexually transmitted diseases treatment guidelines. *MMWR Recommendations and Reports,* 59:1.

In: Handbook for High Risk Pregnancy: Clinical Management ISBN: 978-1-63482-299-2
Editors: E. González-Mesa and D. Abehsera

Chapter 2

SPECIFIC FIRST TRIMESTER HIGH MATERNAL RISK: HYPEREMESIS GRAVIDARUM. PREVIOUS RECURRENT PREGNANCY LOSS. FIRST TRIMESTER BLEEDING

Daniel Abehsera Davó, MD, PhD[1,*],
Rocío Alcedo Olea, MD[2], and Mair Abehsera Bensabat, MD, PhD[1]
[1]Obstetrics and Gynecology Department, Quirón Hospital, Málaga, Spain
[2]Pediatrics Department, Las Albarizas Health Center, Málaga, Spain

INTRODUCTION

1. Hyperemesis Gravidarum

Hyperemesis gravidarum is a serious condition whose management can achieve high levels of complexity. It is difficult to establish a specific aetiology, and its management often includes a psychological approach to the patient.

1.1. Concept

Nausea and vomiting are very common in pregnancy from very early stages; 50-80% of pregnant women experience nausea and occasional vomiting daily during the first half of gestation (Jarnfelt-Samsioe, 1987). In contrast with simple nausea and vomiting in pregnancy, hyperemesis gravidarum is defined as nausea and uncontrollable vomiting during pregnancy, often (but not always) accompanied by alterations of fluid and electrolyte balance, and moderate ketonuria, requiring hospitalization (Niebyl, 2010). Hyperemesis gravidarum is the most frequent cause of hospitalization in the first half of pregnancy, which generates significant annual health care costs (Goodwin, 2008). Although maternal deaths due to hyperemesis gravidarum are now unusual, the lack of appropriate interventions can be fatal.

* Corresponding author: Daniel Abehsera Davó, MD, PhD. E-mail: danielabehsera@hotmail.com.

The reduction in maternal deaths probably reflects a better understanding of the hyperemesis gravidarum, and the acceptance of abortion in critical cases (Sanu et al., 2011).

1.2. Risk Factors and Pathogenesis

The real cause of hyperemesis is unknown. We have identified several risk factors such as the maternal age (<20 years), nulliparity, multiple pregnancy, low educational level, female fetal sex, and genetic factors. Women with a family history of hyperemesis are more prone to the disease as well as those that presented the disease in the previous pregnancy. In addition, women who experienced hyperemesis in their first pregnancy are at significant risk of recurrence compared with women who did not experience the disease in their first pregnancy. It is controversial to determine whether the change in parenting influences the recurrence of the disease in future pregnancies (Sanu et al., 2011).

- Response of the central nervous system to emetic stimuli has been observed in women with hyperemesis that have an aversion to certain smells and tastes, and the vision of certain types of foods can induce the gagging feeling. Increased olfactory sensitivity has not been proved to be associated with nausea and vomiting in pregnancy (Hummel et al., 2002). Pregnant women with a history of dizziness are more likely to experience hyperemesis than women without such a history (Whitehead et al., 1992). Pregnant women with hyperemesis have increased abnormalities in the vestibular-ocular reflex, but it has not been proven whether these abnormalities are induced by the gagging feeling (Goodwin et al., 2008).
- Placental factors: in pregnant women with hyperemesis, the proportion of IL-4 produced by Th2 cells in the placenta, and plasma levels of human chorionic gonadotropin, estradiol and progesterone are higher than in pregnant women without hyperemesis (Yoneyama et al., 2002). Cytokines have proved to induce hyperemesis through peripheral and central stimulation of the vomiting reflex arc (Woolf, 1991).
- Hormonal factors: three hormones involved in the pathogenesis of hyperemesis gravidarum are produced in the placenta; progesterone, estradiol, and human chorionic gonadotropin. Chorionic gonadotropin levels increase during the first quarter and first half of the second quarter, and are later kept in plateau the same as the hyperemesis gravidarum clinic, while the levels of progesterone and estradiol increase during pregnancy (Lagiou et al., 2003). An increase in the proportion of acidic isoforms of human chorionic gonadotropin, and not the total serum chorionic gonadotropin, seems to be involved in the development of hyperemesis gravidarum, and this is correlated to the levels of estradiol, free T4 and thyroid stimulating hormone (Jordan et al., 1999).
- Gastrointestinal factors: the gastrointestinal stimulus probably plays a role in the pathogenesis of hyperemesis. This is evidenced by the fact that when a patient is admitted to hospital for hyperemesis, total intake restriction stops vomiting. Progesterone has an inhibitory effect on the smooth muscle of the digestive tract, leading to slower intestinal transit, which could favor nausea and vomiting in pregnancy (Sanu et al., 2011). Several studies have shown an association between the presence of hyperemesis and gastric infection by Helicobacter pylori (Aytac et al., 2007; Larraz et al., 2002; Shirin et al., 2004; Weyermann et al., 2003), but there is no

sufficient scientific evidence yet to systematically investigate the presence of this bacterium in all patients with hyperemesis (Niemeijer et al., 2014).

- Psychological factors: the child's personality, hysteria and conversion disorder have been associated with hyperemesis gravidarum. There is neither enough scientific evidence to involve psychological factors in the pathogenesis of hyperemesis nor to think that hyperemesis is the expression of a rejection of the pregnancy. It is possible that psychological disorders associated with hyperemesis are a consequence of it, but not due to the illness itself (Simpson et al., 2001).

1.3. Clinical Manifestations. Differential Diagnosis. Investigations

Classically, hyperemesis is diagnosed when the mother has prolonged vomiting over time, associated with an inability to tolerate solid foods and liquids, and ketonuria (Sonkusare, 2011). However, several studies have shown no association of hyperemesis with ketonuria; however, an association has been found in a specific group of patients between Helicobacter pylori infection and hyperemesis (Niemeijer et al., 2014). Questionnaires were used to give a score to predict the severity of the disease (Koren et al., 2002), but have not shown to have any clinical utility (Sonkusare, 2011). The duration of vomiting is important from the point of view of the complications that may develop, like Wernicke encephalopathy as a result of thiamine deficiency (Chiossi et al., 2006).

Differential diagnosis is necessary in order to exclude other digestive entities such as hepatitis, pancreatitis, and gastrointestinal ulcer. In addition to this, we must consider the urological system diseases and endocrine disorders such as diabetic ketoacidosis and hyperthyroidism. Neurological diseases such as brain tumors and migraine should also be taken into account as well as typical complications of pregnancy such as acute fatty liver in pregnancy and preeclampsia (Sonkusare, 2011) although these two diseases are developed later on during gestation.

The physical examination will determine the heart rate and blood pressure, along with the evaluation of mucosal hydration and firmness of the skin, and abdominal examination to assess the epigastric tenderness, presence of organomegaly, pain in the renal angle, and the size of the uterus.

Blood and urine analysis should be evaluated for electrolytes, liver function, thyroid function, creatinine, blood urea nitrogen, cytochemical urinalysis and a complete blood count (Sonkusare, 2011).

Obstetric Ultrasound has traditionally been associated with the presence of molar pregnancy and multiple gestation (Fellet al., 2006). However, a recent study shows the same rates of the disease in both single and multiple gestations (Kirk et al., 2006).

Physiological effects of hyperemesis gravidarum: the vomiting, nausea, and decreased appetite interfere with fluid and caloric intake, resulting in weight loss, dehydration, deterioration of nutritional status, acid-base and electrolyte imbalance. One can observe a slight ketonuria, which reflects the metabolism of fatty acids, due to the decreased intake of calories and protein. These patients are prone to thiamine deficiency due to increased demand for glucose metabolism, and the inability to tolerate food supplements Temporary suppression of thyroid-stimulating hormone is common, but most patients have a euthyroid state.

An increase in liver enzymes (up to four times as much) is reversible when hyperemesis is treated successfully; and the same can be noticed in blood amylase values of salivary origin (Sonkusare, 2011).

1.4. Clinical Management

Hyperemesis of pregnancy is a self-limited situation whose treatment is supportive; based on achieving the cessation of vomiting and nausea as well as the correction of the fluid and electrolyte balance (Sonkusare, 2011).

On admission, the patient will be fed with oral intake at least for 24 hours, having as a top priority the restoration of the fluid and electrolyte balance.

a) Restoration of the water and electrolyte balance (Bottomley et al., 2009):
   - During the first 24 hours the fluid therapy is administered stepwise as follows: 1 liter of 0.9% saline for 2 hours with 20 mmol of potassium chloride. Repeated treatment within 4 hours. Subsequently, 1 liter of saline is administered to 0.9% every 6 hours to complete 24 hours of fluid therapy.
   - Then 1 liter of 0.9% saline is administered every 8 hours as care regimen. Potassium levels will be recovered depending on the serum ones; dextrose solutions and high concentrations of sodium chloride are avoided.

b) Antiemetic treatment:
   - Thiamine: depletion of thiamine (vitamin B12) may occur after 3 weeks of persistent vomiting, so thiamine supplementation in patients admitted for hyperemesis is essential to prevent Wernicke - Korsakoff encephalopathy (Singleton et al., 2001).
   - Antihistamines are the drugs most commonly used to treat nausea and vomiting during pregnancy, but currently there are neither placebo-controlled studies on the use of parenteral or oral antihistamines for patients hospitalized with hyperemesis nor prospective studies comparing the antihistamine with another antiemetic drug. These drugs are not commonly used by a patient admitted for hyperemesis gravidarum (Sanu et al., 2011).

c) Phenothiazines: these drugs have proved to be useful in the treatment of nausea and vomiting during pregnancy, but it has not proved to be useful compared to placebo in patients admitted for hyperemesis gravidarum. It is possible that the usefulness of phenothiazines in patients admitted has not been properly evaluated, since several authors advocate a similar utility as the serotonin antagonist receptors (ondansetron). They are safe drugs from the standpoint of teratogenicity. However, they are frequently extrapyramidal symptoms as side effects (Sanu et al., 2011).

d) Serotonin antagonist receptor (ondansetron): there is little information on the possible teratogenic effects of ondansetron. However, the data available suggest that it is a safe drug. No trials compared to placebo for the treatment of hyperemesis in pregnancy. However, it is considered as the most effective drug because of the remission of the symptoms reported by the patients after its administration (Sanu et al., 2011).

e) Benzamides: the metoclopramide is a drug widely used for the treatment of hyperemesis gravidarum, and it has been shown that it has no teratogenic effects. The most common side effects are extrapyramidal reactions, but this occurs in a minority of cases. It has proved useful both for treatment of nausea and vomiting in pregnancy and in cases of patients hospitalized for hyperemesis (Sanu et al., 2011).

f) Butyrophenones: the most characteristic drug within this group is domperidone. There are neither published data on possible teratogenic effects nor controlled clinical trials.
g) Ginger: ginger has shown to reduce nausea and vomiting in patients admitted for hyperemesis when the treatment was compared with placebo (Fischer-Rasmussen et al., 1991).
h) Corticosteroids: their use is restricted because during the first trimester of pregnancy they have been associated with the development of cleft lip in the fetus (Carmichael et al., 2007).
i) Supplementary feeding: enteral feeding allows the infusion of fluids and nutrients without the associated cephalic phase (visual signals, food aroma and flavor) which stimulates the production of saliva and gastric secretions, and may influence the nausea and vomiting produced in these patients. If a patient has not responded to the aforementioned treatments, enteral feeding should be considered. Enteral feeding, ideally through the gastric route, is an approach that has proven to provide significant relief of nausea and vomiting, preventing hospitalization, and leading to fetal positive results. For those patients who did not respond to enteral feeding, the feeding must be parenteral (Sonkusare, 2011).
j) Emotional support: as mentioned earlier in the chapter, it is common for patients with hyperemesis in pregnancy to suffer from psychological disorders, so it is important to identify these patients in order to provide adequate support.

1.5. Consequences of Hyperemesis in the Fetus and the Mother

Several studies have associated the fetuses of mothers with hyperemesis, with the following complications: low birth weight, lower gestational age at birth, and a tendency to prematurity. They are also frequently female fetuses and one study showed an association between hyperemesis and testicular cancer in the offspring (Veenendaal et al., 2011).

Besides Wernicke encephalopathy, no long-term effects on the mother have been reported. There are doubts about the long-term psychological effects, such as a lack of bond with the newborn or fear of future pregnancies (Sonkusare, 2011).

2. Recurrent Pregnancy Loss

The clinical management of a patient who presented miscarriages repeatedly in the past is always difficult. The ideal situation is the one where we identify a responsible cause and get the patient to undergo a treatment that prevents pregnancy loss again; however, the cause of repeated miscarriages is not established in a lot of cases.

2.1. Definition and Epidemiology

Recurrent pregnancy loss is defined as the loss of three or more consecutive pregnancies before the 20th week of pregnancy, and a fetal weight of $\leq$ 500 g (ACOG, 2002; Lee et al., 2000; Regan et al., 2000). However, there is no consensus and some accept that losses cannot be consecutive, for the fact of having a live birth before or between miscarriages does not seem to decrease the likelihood of returning to miscarry (Brigham et al., 1999, Li et al., 2002).

Nor is there consensus on the number of miscarriages to justify the initiation of a study. It is reasonable to individualize each case and consider the age of the woman, the circumstances surrounding the early pregnancy loss, personal and family background, and anxiety of the couple. Ideally, the study should start after two miscarriages, because the probability of recurrent miscarriage is similar after three miscarriages (24-30% vs. 30-33%) (ACOG, 2002).

About 50% of recurrent pregnancy loss will remain undiagnosed; however, couples that try to have another pregnancy will obtain 70% of live births (Lee et al., 2000). This situation is conditioned by maternal age, so that the likelihood of a new miscarriage in women <30 years is below 25%, whereas in women $\geq$ 40 years would be 50-60% (Clifford et al., 1997).

2.2. Etiology

The following summarizes the possible causes that may lead to recurrent pregnancy loss (Tang et al., 2010):

a) Genetic structural factors: Chromosomal abnormalities are the most common early miscarriages, especially in older women. We can find 70% of chromosomal abnormalities in early miscarriages compared to 20% miscarriages between 13 and 20 weeks of gestation.
b) Anatomical factors: the prevalence of congenital uterine anomalies as septate uterus, bicornuate uterus or arcuate uterus; among the general population it is 6.7% and in the case of patients with recurrent pregnancy loss it rises to 16.7%. Besides, the presences of fibroids, endometrial polyps, and uterine synechiae syndrome have also been related to the recurrent miscarriage.
c) Prothrombotic factors: thrombophilia (factor V Leiden, resistance to activated protein C gene mutation G20210A prothrombin, protein S deficiency, etc.) have been associated with recurrent pregnancy loss.
d) Endocrine factors: these factors represent 10% of cases of recurrent pregnancy loss.
    - Polycystic ovary syndrome: there is a link between this syndrome and recurrent pregnancy loss, probably related to hyperandrogenism, obesity, and insulin resistance.
    - Hyperprolactinemia: high levels of prolactin can inhibit the secretion of progesterone, which influences the endometrial quality.
    - Abnormalities in glucose metabolism and thyroid metabolism: these patients benefit from a proper fit pre-pregnancy shape.
    - Luteal phase deficiency: the mechanism by which the luteal phase deficiency leads to a pernicious effect on the endometrium is unclear, but it has been linked to a decrease in progesterone production by the corpus luteum, abnormal hormone secretion of LH, or to a poor endometrial response to the progesterone which is available.
e) Immunological factors: immunological mechanisms play an important role in the success of pregnancy in which the mother's immune system interacts with allogeneic embryonic differences. These mechanisms include autoimmunity, inflammation, and the relationship of various immune cells and cytokines. The association between autoantibodies and recurrent pregnancy loss is weak, except in the case of antiphospholipid syndrome.

- Antiphospholipid syndrome: This syndrome is present in 15% of cases of recurrent pregnancy loss.
- Thyroid antibodies: the presence of these antibodies is associated with recurrent pregnancy loss, even in cases of normal thyroid function.
- Natural Killer Cells: these cells of the immune system are mainly in the endometrium during implantation by regulating trophoblast invasion and angiogenesis. The role of these cells is controversial in patients with recurrent pregnancy loss.
- Endometrial cytokines: it is believed that endometrial cytokines play an important role in endometrial receptivity for a proper introduction.

2.3. Unexplained Recurrent Pregnancy Loss

We will not find a reason to justify the miscarriages in approximately 50% of cases after a successful evaluation of patients. However, the healthy newborn rate is around 50% in these patients, even though we do not carry out any intervention (Scott, 1994). The following summarizes the different interventions that can be performed in these patients:

- Emotional support: patients who have had recurrent pregnancy loss may be anxious, depressed and frustrated due to poor obstetric history. It is therefore important to address their concerns and preferences regarding prenatal care in subsequent pregnancies. Several authors have demonstrated the benefits in terms of obstetric outcome of conducting a special care for these patients, including a psycho-therapeutic approach (Whitley et al., 2014).
- Lifestyle modification: the elimination of consumption of snuff, alcohol, drugs, toxins, etc.; seems to increase the chances of getting pregnant. It is also advisable to get a normal body mass index (ASRM, 2013).
- Progesterone: progesterone use in cases of patients with unexplained recurrent pregnancy loss has proven to be useful (Coomarasamy et al., 2011; Haas et al., 2013). It is not clear what is the mechanism by which progesterone prevent miscarriages, although it has been proposed to be due to an immunomodulatory effect (Choi et al., 2000). Both oral and vaginal Progesterone can be used, and the dose varies in different studies from 100 to 200 micrograms / day.
- Use of aspirin and heparin: the usefulness of aspirin alone or in combination with heparin to reduce the rate of recurrent unexplained pregnancy loss (Kaandorp et al., 2010) has not been proved. Despite the fact that its use in this patient profile is widespread, there is no scientific evidence to recommend its use in the absence of thrombophilia.
- HCG: The same as Progesterone, the use of this hormone has been proposed for reducing unexplained recurrent pregnancy loss. You may especially benefit those patients who presented oligomenorrhea. The scientific evidence available to date is equivocal, so randomized studies are needed to elucidate whether the use of this hormone is useful in patients with recurrent pregnancy loss (Morley et al., 2013).
- Immunotherapy: maternal immune dysfunction or imbalance between the production of cytotoxic cytokines and cytokines that promote immunosuppression is one of the many mechanisms that have been proposed as a cause of unexplained recurrent

pregnancy loss. The use of granulocyte colony stimulating factor treatment with promising preliminary results has been proposed, yet their use should be restricted to the field of research (Whitley et al., 2014).

Intravenous immunoglobulin has proved beneficial in patients with underlying autoimmune and alloimmune factors, including a high frequency of thyroid autoantibodies and high levels of natural killer cells in peripheral blood. However, its utility in patients with unexplained recurrent miscarriage has not been tested.

3. First Trimester Bleeding

The first-trimester metrorrhagia is one of the most frequent causes of consultation in the emergency department, and one of the key warning signs during the first trimester of pregnancy. Encompasses a broad spectrum of patients ranging from trivial to severe emergency situations. Spontaneous first-trimester abortion and ectopic pregnancy are the two main diseases that manifest with bleeding in the first quarter.

3.1. Spontaneous First Trimester Miscarriage

a) Concept and epidemiology:

Miscarriage is defined as a spontaneous loss of an intrauterine pregnancy, which occurs before the fetus can survive outside the uterus. Miscarriages are described as early (≤12 weeks' gestation) or late (13-24 weeks' gestation). Miscarriage is the most common complication of pregnancy. The reported rate of pregnancy loss in women with a missed menstrual period and positive urine pregnancy test is 12-24%. The true rate of miscarriage is probably higher because many losses occur preclinically, before a menstrual period is missed. About 125000 miscarriages occur annually in the United Kingdom, resulting in 42000 hospital admissions. Reported UK maternal mortality rates after miscarriage in the period 1985 to 2008 range from 0.05 to 0.22 per 100000 maternities.4 The most common causes of death were haemorrhage and sepsis, which tended to occur more often after second trimester losses (Jurkovic et al., 2013).

A large prospective epidemiological study from Demark found that the risk of miscarriage is 15% or less up to the age of 34 years but increases to 25% at 35-39 years, 51% at 40-44 years, and greater than 90% in women aged 45 years or more (Nybo Andersen et al., 2000).

b) Etiology

Chromosomal abnormalities are the most common cause of first trimester miscarriage (Ohno et al., 1991). Other less common causes of miscarriage include antiphospholipid syndrome, inherited thrombophilias (antithrombin deficiency, deficiency of protein C and protein S, factor V Leiden mutation, and mild hyperhomocysteinaemia), and congenital structural abnormalities of the uterus. The risk of miscarriage is also increased in women with poorly controlled type 1 diabetes or disease of the thyroid gland. Obese women who become pregnant after successful fertility treatment are also more likely to experience miscarriage, but the risk is not increased in those who conceive spontaneously.

Studies have shown no clear association of socioeconomic circumstances, caffeine consumption, smoking, or low to moderate alcohol consumption with the risk of miscarriage (Jurkovic et al., 2013).

c) Clinical findings

Vaginal bleeding and loss of pregnancy symptoms are suggestive of miscarriage. Miscarriage is traditionally classified as threatened, inevitable, incomplete, or complete on the basis of clinical history and findings on speculum and digital pelvic examination (Howie, 1986). Although the value of the physical examination has been questioned (Jurkovic et al., 2013), it is essential to establish the source of bleeding, eliminating the possibility that genital bleeding is due to urological, cervical or vaginal lesions.

d) Role of ultrasound

Transvaginal ultrasonography has become the accepted standard for examining women with suspected complications of early pregnancy. Ultrasound classification of miscarriage is based solely on the morphological appearances of pregnancy and does not take into account the amount of vaginal bleeding or cervical findings (Tierney et al., 2006).

Early fetal demise (also described as empty sac; blighted ovum; missed, delayed, or silent miscarriage) refers to the early stage in the course of a miscarriage when an intact gestational sac is still present within the uterine cavity. The diagnosis of early fetal demise is based either on the absence of an embryo within a gestational sac or on the absence of cardiac activity in a visible embryo. The main difficulty when diagnosing early embryonic demise is to avoid confusing a healthy, early, normal intrauterine pregnancy with a miscarriage. Because the ultrasound diagnosis of early fetal demise is based on negative findings, the risk of diagnostic error is high. This is particularly so in women who are unsure of their dates, have irregular cycles, conceived while taking hormonal contraception, or have had fewer than three menstrual periods since their last pregnancy. The risk of misdiagnosis is also increased in women with a retroverted uterus, congenital uterine anomaly, uterine fibroids, intra-abdominal adhesions after previous caesarean sections, or other pelvic surgery affecting uterine position. Misdiagnosis of a normal pregnancy as a miscarriage could result in inadvertent termination of a wanted normal pregnancy (Jurkovic et al., 2013). Recent National Institute for Health and Care Excellence (NICE) guidelines recommend that the diagnosis is confirmed at a follow-up visit seven to 14 days later or by a second observer in all women with suspected early fetal demise on ultrasound (National Collaborating Centre for Women's and Children's Health, 2012).

Incomplete miscarriage is defined by the presence of retained products of conception without a well defined gestation sac. The ultrasound diagnosis of incomplete miscarriage is difficult and no consensus exists regarding the best diagnostic criteria. Endometrial thickness (measured as the anterior-posterior diameter of the uterine cavity) has been used to aid this diagnosis (Jurkovic et al., 2013).

The diagnosis of complete miscarriage is made in women in whom ultrasound fails to identify any signs of pregnancy tissue within the uterine cavity. This diagnosis can be made with confidence only in women who had clear evidence of intrauterine pregnancy on previous ultrasound examinations. If no scan has previously been done, the pregnancy should be described as a “pregnancy of unknown location” and followed up with biochemical markers (National Collaborating Centre for Women's and Children's Health, 2012).

e) Role of biochemical markers

Biochemical markers are not routinely used in the diagnosis of miscarriage. They are useful, however, to confirm the diagnosis of early pregnancy failure in women in whom ultrasound findings are non-diagnostic. Human chorionic gonadotrophin concentrations in maternal serum double over 1.4-1.6 days from the time of first detection to the 35th day of pregnancy and then double every 2.0-2.7 days from the 35th day to 42nd day. It has been well documented that slower doubling times are associated with miscarriage. However, absolute concentrations of the hormone cannot be used to discriminate between viable and non-viable pregnancies. In women with non-diagnostic ultrasound scan findings, declining chorionic gonadotrophin values can diagnose a complete miscarriage with a sensitivity of 93-97% (Jurkovic et al., 2013).

f) Treatment

Prevention: there is no evidence that miscarriage can be prevented by bed rest (Aleman et al., 2005) or by administration of vitamin supplements (Rumbold et al., 2011). A meta-analysis of four trials showed that treatment with progesterone in women with threatened miscarriage was associated with significantly lower risk of miscarriage compared with placebo. The quality of evidence, however, was poor, the dose and route of administration of progesterone varied between the studies, and the final outcome measures varied. Routine progesterone supplements should not be offered to women with threatened miscarriage until the results of a well conducted prospective multicentre randomised trial are available (National Collaborating Centre for Women's and Children's Health, 2012).

Treatment of incomplete abortion: depending on the amount of intrauterine remains we can offer the patient the possibility of medical treatment with either misoprostol or methylergometrine, or surgical treatment by curettage.

In the treatment of early fetal demise we can offer three possibilities: expectation, abortion medical treatment or surgical treatment.

- Expectant management is often chosen by women because of a desire for a natural approach. A meta-analysis of published studies comparing expectant management with active management (medical or surgical) showed a higher rate of unplanned emergency interventions (35% v 18%; relative risk 2.28, 95% confidence interval 1.93 to 2.7). It also found higher rates of blood transfusions (1.6% v 0.4%; 3.39, 1.08 to 10.61) in women randomised to expectant management, but no significant difference in infection rates. Women are usually advised to wait for two weeks for miscarriage to complete, but it is safe to continue with expectant management for longer if there are no signs of infection (Jurkovic et al., 2013).
- Medical treatment: Medical management is chosen as the primary treatment option in 20-30% of women. The drug most commonly used is a prostaglandin analogue misoprostol, which can be given in single or divided doses. It is licensed for oral use only, but can also be given vaginally, sublingually, or rectally. The success of medical management depends on the type of miscarriage, the drug dosage, the route of administration, and the time allowed for products to be passed. Medical treatment may be arranged on an outpatient or inpatient basis. Side effects include nausea in 22-35% of women, fever in 15%, diarrhoea in 6-21.2%, and vomiting in 7%. Bleeding usually starts within hours of administration of the drug and may continue

for up to three weeks. Heavy bleeding requiring emergency surgery occurs in 1% of women treated with misoprostol. Review women who do not start bleeding within 24 hours after initiation of treatment to decide on further management. Women who bleed for longer than three weeks should also attend for clinical review to rule out persistent retained products of conception or molar pregnancy. The treatment of choice is usually single dose misoprostol 800 μg transvaginally (Jurkovic et al., 2013).

- Surgical treatment: Emergency surgery remains the primary treatment of choice for women who present with excessive bleeding, are haemodynamically unstable, have signs of infected retained products of conception, or have a provisional diagnosis of gestational trophoblastic disease. In clinically stable women, surgery can be offered as a semi-elective procedure for those who prefer surgical intervention and for those in whom conservative management has been unsuccessful. Surgical management is more successful than medical treatment of miscarriage that has higher unplanned intervention rates, it's more likely to experience gastrointestinal side effects, and it has significantly longer duration of bleeding. Surgical complications (2–8%) include uterine perforation, cervical laceration, haemorrhage, and intrauterine synechiae. In recent years, surgery has also been carried out using manual vacuum aspiration under systemic analgesia (including patient controlled analgesia) in operating theatres. This procedure can also be carried out in the outpatient setting, under local anaesthetic. The benefits of outpatient procedures are increased safety due to reduced anaesthetic risks, minimal social disruption, and reduced costs (Jurkovic et al., 2013).
- Uterine curettings are routinely sent for histological examination to confirm the diagnosis of intrauterine pregnancy and to exclude a molar pregnancy. Chromosome testing should be performed on products of conception of the third and subsequent consecutive miscarriage only and not after sporadic pregnancy loss (Jurkovic et al., 2013).

Antibiotic prophylaxis and anti-D for Rhesus negative women are not needed with expectant or medical treatment but should be offered to women undergoing surgical treatment. Normal menstrual periods usually resume within a month or two after miscarriage. It is safe for women to resume sexual activity once the bleeding has stopped. Women need not delay trying for a new pregnancy for medical reasons. Because most miscarriages are caused by chromosomal abnormalities, women need not be routinely investigated for other less common causes of miscarriage unless they experience recurrent losses. Some women may develop anxiety and depression after a pregnancy loss and they may benefit from receiving additional counselling and psychological support (Jurkovic et al., 2013).

3.2. Ectopic Pregnancy

a) Epidemiology

Ectopic pregnancy or extra uterine pregnancy refers to the blastocyst implantation outside the uterine cavity endometrium with over 95.5% implanting in the fallopian tube; where fetus or embryo is often absent or stops growing. The other most common implantation sites are ovarian (3.2%) and abdominal (1.3%) sites. This is a major track and significant cause of morbidity and mortality with associated risks of tubal rupture and intra abdominal hemorrhage in women and can lead to substantial future reproductive morbidity, including subsequent ectopic pregnancy and infertility. It is a medical emergency that requires immediate treatment.

The annual incidence has increased over the past 30 years. In the western world 4-10% of pregnancy related deaths have been observed, from this issue and now it is a growing problem in developing countries also. Although advances in diagnostic methods have allowed for earlier diagnosis, it still remains a life threatening condition. Approximately, 75% of deaths in the first trimester and 9% of all pregnancy-related deaths are due to an ectopic pregnancy.

b) Risk factors

Risk factors for ectopic pregnancy (Ankum et al., 1996) can be divided into those that confer high, moderate, or low risk (Table 1). However, the characteristics that place a woman at risk for ectopic pregnancy are not completely independent of one another.

c) Pathology

The fallopian tube is the dominant site in the majority of cases of ectopic pregnancy. 75–80% occur in the ampullary portion, 10–15% in the isthmic portion and about 5% in the fimbrial end of the fallopian tube (Rana et al., 2013). Several factors may be involved in the pathogenesis of tubal pregnancies, but they are generally believed to be the result of conditions that delay or prevent passage of the fertilized oocyte into the uterine cavity or factors inherent in the embryo that result in premature implantation.

Cervical ectopic pregnancy is rare form of ectopic pregnancy in which the trophoblast implants in the cervical tissue of the endocervical canal. It represents only 0.15% of all ectopic pregnancy (Rana et al., 2013).

Ovarian ectopic pregnancy is one of the rarest variants, and it incidence is estimated to be 0.15-3% of all diagnosed ectopic pregnancy (Rana et al., 2013).

Cesarean scar ectopic pregnancy is another rare form of the disease with an incidence of 1:1,800 pregnancies due to increased number of cesarean deliveries over the last 30 years (Rana et al., 2013). The pregnancy is located in the scar outside of the uterine cavity and surrounded by myometrium and connective tissue.

Ilustración 1 Table 1. Risk factors for ectopic pregnancy

Degree of risk	Risk factors	Odds ratio
High	Previous ectopic pregnancy	9.3-47
	Previous tubal surgery	6.0-11.5
	Tubal ligation	3.0-139
	Tubal pathology	3.5-25
	In utero DES exposure	2.4-13
	Current IUD use	1.1-45
Moderate	Infertility	1.1-28
	Previous cervicitis (gonorrhea, chlamydia)	2.8-3.7
	History of pelvic inflammatory disease	2.1-3.0
	Multiple sexual partners	1.4-4.8
	Smoking	2.3-3.9
Low	Previous pelvic/abdominal surgery	0.93-3.8
	Vaginal douching	1.1-3.1
	Early age of intercourse (<18 years)	1.1-2.5

Adapted from data in: Ankum WM, Mol BW, Van der Veen F, Bossuyt PM. (1996). Risk factors for ectopic pregnancy: a meta-analysis. *Fertility and Sterility*; 65(6):1093.

Implantation in this location is believed to occur because the embryo migrates through a defect within the scar (Ash et al., 2007).

Interstitial or cornual pregnancy is a pregnancy implanted at the interstitial portion of the fallopian tube. Originally, the term cornual pregnancy referred only to pregnancies implanted in either the horn of a bicornuate uterus, a rudimentary horn of a unicornuate uterus, or in the lateral half of a septated or partially septated uterus. Interstitial pregnancies may be misdiagnosed as intrauterine because they are partially implanted in the endometrium. A clue to correct diagnosis is its eccentric location and thin (less than 5 mm) myometrial mantle. These pregnancies are uncommon, comprising about 2 to 3 percent of all ectopic pregnancies. The risk factors are similar to those for other tubal pregnancies, except for ipsilateral salpingectomy that is a risk factor that is specific to interstitial pregnancy (Tulandi, 2013).

Angular pregnancy is an intrauterine pregnancy with a clinical course distinct from interstitial pregnancy. The pregnancy is implanted medial to the uterotubal junction in the lateral angle of the uterine cavity, close to the proximal ostium of the fallopian tube. In contrast with an interstitial pregnancy, an angular pregnancy is located medial to the round ligament. When viewed from the exterior of the uterus during laparoscopy or laparotomy, the uterine enlargement caused by an angular pregnancy displaces the round ligament superiorly and laterally, while remaining medial to the ligament itself. On the other hand, an interstitial pregnancy causes an enlargement of the uterus that is lateral to the round ligament. Angular pregnancy appears to be rare and there are few current reports regarding its diagnosis or management (Tulandi, 2013).

Abdominal ectopic pregnancy with 1.3% of cases is diagnosed at a rate of 1:10,000 births and is an extremely rare and serious form of extrauterine gestation. It is described as primary or secondary abdominal ectopic pregnancy and usually results from an implantation following tubal rupture or abortion through the fimbricated end of the fallopian tube. The fetus continues to grow following attachment to an abdominal structure, using its blood source, which may be extensive. It usually attaches to the surface of the uterus, broad ligaments, or ovaries, but may also attach to the liver, spleen, or intestines (Rana et al., 2013).

Heterotopic pregnancy refers to the combination of an intrauterine pregnancy and a concurrent pregnancy at an ectopic location. The estimated incidence of heterotopic pregnancy is dependent upon the rates of ectopic pregnancy and dizygotic twinning. The incidence has been rising, mainly due to the increasing number of pregnancies derived from assisted reproductive technology (Tulandi, 2013).

d) Diagnosis

- Clinical manifestations: The triad of pain, vaginal bleeding and amenorrhoea was historically used to suspect a diagnosis of ectopic pregnancy. These symptoms, with or without syncope, shoulder tip pain and shock, generally led to surgical intervention. Now, history and physical examination alone rarely leads to the diagnosis or exclusion of an ectopic pregnancy, with most diagnosed earlier in the course of the disease. One-third of women with an ectopic pregnancy have no clinical signs and up to 10% have no symptoms. The symptoms of ectopic pregnancy are often non-specific and difficult to differentiate from those of other gynaecological, gastrointestinal and urological disorders, including appendicitis, salpingitis, corpus luteum cyst rupture, miscarriage, adnexal torsion or urinary tract infection. The amount of bleeding associated with ectopic pregnancy varies, although classically the patient will complain of 'spotting'. Heavy bleeding, in the absence of further transvaginal ultrasonography and human chorionic gonadotrophin assessment, may lead to a clinical misdiagnosis of miscarriage. Abdominal pain is often absent or a late finding, probably due to earlier recognition of pregnancy from the use of highly sensitive commercially available urinary pregnancy tests and to easy access to transvaginal ultrasonography. The majority of women with abdominal pain in early pregnancy do not have an ectopic pregnancy. Less common features of ectopic pregnancy include nausea, vomiting and diarrhoea. In ruptured ectopic pregnancy, there may be abdominal distension and tenderness, peritonism and haemorrhagic shock. A diagnosis of ectopic pregnancy should be considered in all women of reproductive age with a sudden onset of abdominal pain or gastrointestinal symptoms (Kirk et al., 2014).

- Ultrasound diagnosis: the use of transvaginal ultrasonography has changed the diagnostic approach to one based on visualizing the ectopic mass. Transvaginal ultrasonography has been demonstrated to be superior to transabdominal ultrasound. It is important to appreciate that not all ectopic pregnancy will be seen using transvaginal ultrasonography and certainly not on one visit (Kirk et al., 2014).

There is no specific endometrial appearance or thickness that reliably supports a diagnosis of ectopic pregnancy. In up to 20% cases a collection of fluid may be seen within the endometrial cavity classically referred to as a 'pseudosac' (Kirk et al., 2014).

A small amount of anechoic free fluid in the Pouch of Douglas is commonly found with both intrauterine and ectopic gestations. The presence of echogenic fluid has been reported in 28–56% of women with an ectopic pregnancy. This correlates well with the surgical findings of haemoperitoneum, but does not confirm tubal rupture, as blood commonly leaks from the fimbrial tube. The amount of echogenic fluid visualized in the pelvis correlates closely with findings at surgery. As a rule of thumb, if fluid reaches the fundus of the uterus or is present in the utero-vesical pouch, it is significant. A further marker of serious intra-abdominal bleeding is the presence of fluid in Morrison's pouch between the liver and the kidney (Kirk et al., 2014).

Tubal ectopic pregnancies are usually positively diagnosed using ultrasound by visualizing an adnexal mass that moves separate to the ovary. The most common finding, in around 60% of cases, is an inhomogeneous or a non cystic adnexal mass sometimes known as the 'blob' sign. The mass is generally spherical, but amore tubular appearance may be seen if bleeding creates a haematosalpinx. In around 20% of cases it may be possible to visualize an empty extrauterine gestational sac or 'bagel sign'.

In another 20%, this sac may contain a yolk sac and/or an embryonic pole that may or may not have cardiac activity. The term 'viable ectopic' is applied when embryonic cardiac activity is visualized. A recent consensus on nomenclature proposed that the term 'definite ectopic pregnancy' be used if a yolk sac and/or embryo (with or without cardiac activity) is seen. The term 'probable ectopic pregnancy' is suggested if an inhomogeneous mass or an extrauterine sac-like structure is visualized. Using this classification, the specificity of ultrasound to detect ectopic pregnancy is very high, but the sensitivity is lower as the inhomogeneous and empty sac masses are not counted as definitive ectopic pregnancies (Kirk et al., 2014).

Pulsed doppler ultrasound has been examined as a tool for diagnosing ectopic pregnancy.

Table 2. Sonopgraphic criteria for the diagnosis of an ectopic pregnancy

TYPE OF ECTOPIC PREGNANCY	SONOGRAPHIC CRITERIA
Tubal	Empty uterine cavity
	An inhomogeneous adnexal mass or, an empty extra-uterine gestation sac or a yolk sac or fetal pole + cardiac activity in an extra-uterine sac
Interstitial	Empty uterine cavity
	Products of conception/gestation sac located in the interstitial (intramyometrial) portion of the tuve surrounded by a continuous rim of myometrium
	Interstitial line sign (thin echogenic line extending from a central uterine cavity echo to the periphery of the interstitial sac)
Cornual	A single interstitial portion of the Fallopian tube in the main uterine body
	Products of conception/gestation sac mobile and separate from the uterus surrounded by the myometrium
	Vascular pedicle joining the gestational sac to the unicornuate uterus
Cervical	Empty uterine cavity
	Barrel shaped cervix
	Products of conception/gestation sac below the level of the internal cervical orifice
	Negative sliding organ sign
Caesarean section scar	Empty uterine cavity
	Products of conception/gestation sac located anteriorly at the level of the internal cervical orifice covering the presumed site of the previous lower segment Caesarean section scar
	Negative sliding organ sign
	Evidence of peritrophoblastic flow on color Doppler examination
Ovarian	Empty uterine cavity
	Cystic structure with a wide echogenic ring on or within the ovary, generally seen surrounded by ovarian cortex and separate from the corpus luteum
Intramural	Empty uterine cavity
	Products of conception/gestation sac completely surrounded by myometrium and separate from the endometrial cavity
Abdominal	Empty uterine cavity
	No evidence of a dilated Fallopian tube or complex adnexal mass
	Gestation sac surrounded by loops of bowel and separated by peritoneum
	Wide mobility similar to fluctuation of the sac

Adapted from data in: Kirk E, Bottomley C, Bourne T. (2014). Diagnosing ectopic pregnancy and current concepts in the management of pregnancy of unknown location. *Human Reproduction Update*; 20(2):250-61.

However, the range of values for vascular indices associated with an ectopic pregnancy means that there is significant overlap with those associated with angiogenesis within a corpus luteum. Currently doppler is not considered to significantly contribute to the diagnosis of ectopic pregnancy (Kirk et al., 2014).

Using 3D ultrasound, a coronal view of the uterus can be obtained. This view means that invariably a connection can be seen between the endometrial cavity and interstitial portion of the Fallopian tube. In the future it seems highly likely that the use of 3D ultrasound in this context will be an integral part of diagnostic guidance (Kirk et al., 2014).

In table 2 are shown the sonographic criteria for the diagnosis or ectopic pregnancies.

- Laboratory test: in all those patients in whom suspected ectopic pregnancy is necessary to obtain a complete blood count, blood group determination, and coagulation tests. For women treated with methotrexate, pre-treatment testing typically includes renal and liver function tests.
- Serum biochemistry:

Human chorionic gonadotrophin: single measurements of this hormone are not used to predict the outcome of suspected ectopic pregnancy. There is a common misconception that a single level, for example, 1000 IU/l, means an ectopic pregnancy is unlikely. This is a false assumption as the majority of ectopic pregnancies detected in modern practice have initial serum human chorionic gonadotrophin values below this level. Similarly, a high value does not necessarily exclude the presence of a viable intrauterine pregnancy, although it makes it less likely. In contrast serial measurement of serum human chorionic gonadotrophin offers good test performance for predicting viability and is certainly better at predicting location than measurements of serum progesterone. But it should also be remembered that some ectopic pregnancy also demonstrate a 'normal' rise in this hormone. The majority though, will have serial serum human chorionic gonadotrophin levels that increase more slowly than would be expected with an intrauterine pregnancy ('suboptimal rise') or decrease more slowly than would be expected with a failing pregnancy of unknown location (Kirk et al., 2014).

Progesterone: the serum progesterone level is a good indicator of early pregnancy viability, but a poor predictor of location. Finding a novel marker to better discriminate ectopic pregnancy from the rest of the pregnancy of unknown location population nevertheless remains an important area of research. Recent attention has focused on metalloprotease 12 and fibronectin as potentially promising candidate markers (Kirk et al., 2014).

- Other procedures: uterine curettage and laparoscopy are rarely necessary to confirm the diagnosis of ectopic pregnancy. For laparoscopy, should remember that it remains the reference method for the diagnosis of ectopic pregnancy in cases of doubt, even if they are used for this purpose it must be known that the false negative rate is 3-4% and the false positive rate is 5% (Sowter et al., 2004).
- Pregnancy of unknown location: pregnancy of unknown location is a descriptive term used to classify a pregnancy when a transvaginal ultrasound has shown no signs of either an intrauterine or extrauterine pregnancy or retained products of conception. In order to avoid errors in these situations, it is essential to have a reliable date of last

menstrual period of the patient. In these situations it is very useful to obtain serum human chorionic gonadotrophin. In general we recommend that if human chorionic gonadotrophin values are lower than 1000 IU / l, we reevaluate the patients within 48 hours, in order to establish whether it is an intrauterine pregnancy, ectopic pregnancy or spontaneous abortion. When hormone levels are above 1000 IU / l in the absence of signs of spontaneous abortion, ectopic pregnancy risk is high, so the patient should be carefully evaluated.

e) Differencial diagnosis: the differential diagnosis of bleeding or pain early in pregnancy also includes: physiologic (i.e., believed to be related to implantation), spontaneous abortion, gestational trophoblastic disease, pathology of the genital tract, subchorionic hematoma (Tulandi 2014).

f) Treatment:

- Expectant treatment: according to the most recent guideline, published by the American College of Obstetricians and Gynecologists, there may be a role for expectant management when the human chorionic gonadotrophin level is < 200 IU/l and which is further in decline phase. It should only be offered when transvaginal ultrasound remains non-diagnostic and human chorionic gonadotrophin levels continue to decline. Tubal rupture has occurred with low or declining human chorionic gonadotrophin levels. However, almost all ectopic pregnancies resolve spontaneously when the human chorionic gonadotrophin level reaches 15 IU/l (ACOG, 1999).
- Medical treatment: medical treatment of ectopic pregnancy is quite less expensive than surgery. Many different agents have been used to treat ectopic pregnancies including systemic and local methotrexate, local potassium chloride, hyperosmolar glucose, prostaglandins, danazol, etoposide, and mifepristone (RU486). Current therapies focus primarily on methotrexate treatments. Patients treated with methotrexate should be monitored closely because; it causes severe abdominal pain and side effect too. The serum human chorionic gonadotrophin concentration should be measured weekly. If it serum concentration has not declined by at least 25% in first week after methotrexate administration, a second dose should be given. Two common regimens are available for methotrexate, multidose (1 mg/kg i.m daily; days 0, 2, 4, and 6 alternated with folinic acid 0.1 mg/kg orally on days 1, 3, 5, 7) and single dose (0.4 to 1 mg/kg or 50 mg/m2 intramuscular without folinic acid). The multidose regimen alternates an every other day dose of intramuscular methotrexate 1 mg/kg with an every other day dose of intramuscular leucovorin calcium 0.1 mg/kg, a folic acid antagonist antidote, up to four doses of each until the human chorionic gonadotrophin level decreases by 15% on two consecutive days. The single-dose regimen is an intramuscular injection of methotrexate, 50 mg/m2, based on the patient's body surface, and does not include leucovorin rescue. If human chorionic gonadotrophin levels do not decline by 15% on days 4 and 7 after treatment, a second dose of methotrexate may be given after 1 week. About 20% of women will need a second treatment cycle. Many side effects associated with methotrexate treatment are nausea and vomiting, stomatitis, diarrhea, abdominal discomfort, pneumonitis, photosensitivity skin reaction, impaired liver function, reversible, severe neutropenia (rare), reversible alopecia (rare) (Rana et al., 2013).

- Surgical treatment: surgical treatment is the preferred treatment for ectopic pregnancy when there is rupture, hypotension, anemia, diameter of the gestational sac greater than 4cm on ultrasonography, or pain persisting beyond 24 hours. Surgical treatment of ectopic pregnancy should be reserved for those patients who have contraindications to medical treatment or to whom medical treatment has failed and those who are hemodynamically unstable. Two techniques are described to remove the EP from the fallopian tube: salpingectomy (the pregnancy is removed en bloc with the tube), and salpingostomy (an incision is made on the fallopian tube over the swelling, the ectopic pregnancy carefully removed with forceps or irrigation and the incision should be either closed or left to heal by secondary intention). The preferred method of surgical treatment of ectopic pregnancy today is diagnostic laparoscopy with salpingostomy and tubal conservation. Laparotomy is indicated in the case of hemodynamic instability because it allows rapid access to pelvic structures. Sometimes a prophylactic dose of methotrexate is given with salpingosotomy. Persistent ectopic pregnancy occurs as a result of incomplete removal of trophoblastic tissue, the most common complication of laparoscopic salpingostomy, occurs at a frequency of 5-20%. It is diagnosed during follow-up when human chorionic gonadotrophin concentrations measured once a week plateau or rise. Factors increasing risk are small ectopic pregnancies (<2cm diameter), early therapy (<42 days from last menstrual period), high concentrations of human chorionic gonadotrophin (>3000 IU/L) preoperatively, and implantation medial to the salpingostomy site. In high-risk cases, a single dose of methotrexate (1 mg/kg) can be administered postoperatively for prophylaxis (Rana et al., 2013).

REFERENCES

ACOG practice Bulletin. (2002). Management of recurrent early pregnancy loss. *International journal of gynaecology and obstetrics: the official organ of the International Federation of Gynaecology and Obstetrics;* 78(2):179-90.

ACOG practice bulletin. (1999). Medical management of tubal pregnancy. *International journal of gynaecology and obstetrics: the official organ of the International Federation of Gynaecology and Obstetrics*; 65(1):97-103.

Aleman, A., Althabe, F., Belizán, J., Bergel, E. (2005). Bed rest during pregnancy for preventing miscarriage. *The Cochrane Database of Systematic Reviews*; 18;(2):CD0035 76.

Ankum, W. M., Mol, B. W., Van der Veen, F., Bossuyt, P. M. (1996). Risk factors for ectopic pregnancy: a meta-analysis. *Fertility and Sterility*; 65(6):1093.

Ash, A., Smith, A., Maxwell, D. (2007). Caesarean scar pregnancy. *Britich Journal of Obstetrics and Gynecology*; 114(3):253-63.

ASRM. (2013). Optimizing natural fertility: a committee opinion. *Fertility and Sterility*; 100 (3):631-7.

Aytac, S., Türkay, C., Kanbay, M. (2007). Helicobacter pylori stool antigen assay in hyperemesis gravidarum: a risk factor for hyperemesis gravidarum or not?. *Digestive Diseases and Sciences*; 52(10):2840-3.

Bottomley, C., Bourne, T. (2009). Management strategies for hyperemesis. *Best Practice and Research Clinical Obstetrics and Gynaecology*; 23(4):549-64.

Brigham, S. A., Conlon, C., Farquharson, R. G. (1999). A longitudinal study of pregnancy outcome following idiopathic recurrent miscarriage. *Human reproduction*; 14(11):2868-71.

Carmichael, S. L., Shaw, G. M., Ma, C., Werler, M. M., Rasmussen, S. A., et al. (2007). Maternal corticosteroid use and orofacial clefts. *American Journal of Obstetrics and Gynecology*; 197(6):585.e1-7; discussion 683-4, e1-7.

Chiossi, G., Neri, I., Cavazzuti, M., et al. (2006). Hyperemesis gravidarum complicated by Wernicke encephalopathy: background, case report, and review of the literature. *Obstetrical and Gynecological Survey*; 61(4):255-68.

Choi, B. C., Polgar, K., Xiao, L., Hill, J. A. (2000). Progesterone inhibits in-vitro embryotoxic Th1 cytokine production to trophoblast in women with recurrent pregnancy loss. *Human Reproduction*; 15 Suppl. 1:46-59.

Clifford, K., Rai, R., Regan, L. (1997). Future pregnancy outcome in unexplained recurrent first trimester miscarriage. *Human reproduction*; 12(2):387-9.

Coomarasamy, A., Truchanowicz, E. G., Rai, R. (2011). Does first trimester progesterone prophylaxis increase the live birth rate in women with unexplained recurrent miscarriages?. *British Medical Journal*; 18;342:d1914.

Fell, D. B., Dodds, L., Joseph, K. S., Allen, V. M., Butler, B. (2006). Risk factors for hyperemesis gravidarum requiring hospital admission during pregnancy. *Obstetrics and Gynecology*; 107(2 Pt 1):277-84.

Fischer-Rasmussen, W., Kjaer, S. K., Dahl, C., Asping, U. (1991). Ginger treatment of hyperemesis gravidarum. *European Journal of Obstetrics, Gynecology, and Reproductive Biology*; 4; 38(1):19-24.

Goodwin, T. M. (2008). Hyperemesis gravidarum. *Obstetrics and Gynecology Clinics of North America*; 35:401-7.

Goodwin, T. M., Nwankwo, O. A., O'Leary, L. D., O'Leary, D., Romero, R., et al. (2008). The first demonstration that a subset of women with hyperemesis gravidarum has abnormalities in the vestibuloocular reflex pathway. *American Journal of Obstetrics and Gynecology*; 199(4):417.e1-9.

Haas, D. M., Ramsey, P. S. (2013). Progestogen for preventing miscarriage. *The Cochrane Database of Systematic Reviews*; 31;10:CD003511.

Howie, H. J. (1986). Spontaneous abortion. In: *Dewhurst's textbook of obstetrics and gynaecology*. 4th ed. Blackwell Science, 1986:176-87.

Hummel, T., Von Mering, R., Huch, R., Kolble, N. (2002). Olfactory modulation of nausea during early pregnancy? *British Journal of Obstetrics and Gynaecology*; 109:1394-7.

Jarnfelt-Samsioe, A. (1987). Nausea and vomiting in pregnancy: a review. *Obstetrical and Gynecological Survey*; 42:422-7.

Jordan., Grebe, S. K., Cooke, R. R., Ford., Larsen, P. D., et al. (1999). Acidic isoforms of chorionic gonadotrophin in European and Samoan women are associated with hyperemesis gravidarum and may be thyrotrophic. *Clinical endocrinology*; 50(5): 619-27.

Jurkovic, D., Overton, C., Bender-Atik, R. (2013). Diagnosis and management of first trimester miscarriage. *British Medical Journal*; 19;346:f3676.

Kaandorp, S. P., Goddijn, M., van der Post, J. A., Hutten, B. A., Verhoeve, H. R., et al. (2010). Aspirin plus heparin or aspirin alone in women with recurrent miscarriage. *The New England Journal of Medicine*; 29;362(17):1586-96.

Kirk, E., Bottomley, C., Bourne, T. (2014). Diagnosing ectopic pregnancy and current concepts in the management of pregnancy of unknown location. *Human Reproduction Update*; 20(2):250-61.

Kirk, E., Papageorghiou, A. T., Condous, G., Bottomley, C., Bourne, T. (2006). Hyperemesis gravidarum: is an ultrasound scan necessary?. *Human reproduction*; 21(9):2440-2.

Koren, G., Boskovic, R., Hard, M., Maltepe, C., Navioz, Y., et al. (2002). Motherisk-PUQE (pregnancy-unique quantification of emesis and nausea) scoring system for nausea and vomiting of pregnancy. *American Journal of Obstetrics and Gynecology*; 186(5 Suppl. Understanding):S228-31.

Larraz, J., Marin, N., Piñeiro, L., Cilla, G., Pérez-Trallero, E. (2002). Lack of relationship between infection by Helicobacter pylori and vomiting that usually occurs during pregnancy, although possible relationship with severe forms of emesis. *Revista Española de Enfermedades Digestivas*; 94(7):417-22.

Lagiou, P., Tamimi, R., Mucci, L. A., Trichopoulos, D., Adami, H. O., et al. (2003). Nausea and vomiting in pregnancy in relation to prolactin, estrogens, and progesterone: a prospective study. *Obstetrics and Gynecology*; 101:639-44.

Lee, R. M., Silver, R. M. (2000). Recurrent pregnancy loss: summary and clinical recommendations. *Seminars in Reproductive Medicine*; 18(4):433-40.

Li, T. C., Makris, M., Tomsu, M., Tuckerman, E., Laird, S. (2002). Recurrent miscarriage: aetiology, management and prognosis. *Human Reproduction Update*; 8(5):463-81.

Morley, L. C., Simpson, N., Tang, T. (2013). Human chorionic gonadotrophin (hCG) for preventing miscarriage. *The Cochrane Database of Systematic Reviews*; 31;1:CD008611.

National Collaborating Centre for Women's and Children's Health (UK). (2012). Ectopic Pregnancy and Miscarriage: Diagnosis and Initial Management in Early Pregnancy of Ectopic Pregnancy and Miscarriage. *National Institute for Health and Clinical Excellence: Guidance*.

Niebyl, J. R. (2010). Clinical practice. Nausea and vomiting in pregnancy. *New England Journal of Medicine*; 363: 1544-50.

Niemeijer, M. N., Grooten, I. J., Vos, N., Bais, J. M., van der Post, J. A., et al. (2014). Diagnostic markers for hyperemesis gravidarum: a systematic review and metaanalysis. *American Journal of Obstetrics and Gynecology*; 211(2):150.e1-150.e15.

Nybo Andersen, A. M., Wohlfahrt, J., Christens, P., Olsen, J., Melbye, M. (2000). Maternal age and fetal loss: population based register linkage study. *British Medical Journal*; 24; 320(7251):1708-12.

Ohno, M., Maeda, T., Matsunobu, A. (1991). A cytogenetic study of spontaneous abortions with direct analysis of chorionic villi. *Obstetrics and Gynecology*; 77(3):394-8.

Rana, P., Kazmi, I., Singh, R., Afzal, M., Al-Abbasi, F. A. (2013). Ectopic pregnancy: a review. *Archives of Gynecology and Obstetrics*; 288(4):747-57.

Regan, L., Rai, R. (2000). Epidemiology and the medical causes of miscarriage. Baillière's best practice and research. *Clinical obstetrics and gynaecology*; 14(5):839-54.

Rumbold, A., Middleton, P., Pan, N., Crowther, C. A. (2011). Vitamin supplementation for preventing miscarriage. *The Cochrane Database of Systematic Reviews*; 19;(1):CD0040 73.

Sanu, O., Lamont, R. F. (2011). Hyperemesis gravidarum: pathogenesis and the use of antiemetic agents. *Expert Opinion on Pharmacotherapy*; 12(5):737-48.

Scott. (1994). Recurrent miscarriage: overview and recommendations. *Clinical Obstetrics and Gynecology*; 37(3):768.

Shirin, H., Sadan, O., Shevah, O., Bruck, R., Boaz, M., et al. (2004). Positive serology for Helicobacter pylori and vomiting in the pregnancy. *Archives of Gynecology and Obstetrics*; 270(1):10-4.

Simpson, S. W., Goodwin, T. M., Robins, S. B., Rizzo, A. A., Howes, R. A., et al. (2001). Psychological factors and hyperemesis gravidarum. *Journal of Women's Health and Gender-based Medicine*; 10(5):471-7.

Singleton, C. K. 1., Martin, P. R. (2001). Molecular mechanisms of thiamine utilization. *Current Molecular Medicine*; 1(2):197-207.

Sonkusare, S. (2011). The clinical management of hyperemesis gravidarum. *Archives of Gynecology and Obstetrics*; 283(6):1183-92.

Sowter, M. C., Farquhar, C. M. (2004). Ectopic pregnancy: an update. *Current Opinion in Obstetrics and Gynecology*; 16(4):289-93.

Tang, A. W., Quenby, S. (2010). Recent thoughts on management and prevention of recurrent early pregnancy loss. *Current Opinion in Obstetrics and Gynecology*; 22(6):446-51.

Tierney, J. P., Welsh, J., Owen, P. Effective Gynaecology in Glasgow Group. (2006). Management of early pregnancy loss--a complete audit cycle. *Journal of Obstetrics and gynaecology*; 26(3):229-32.

Tulandi, T. Clinical manifestations and diagnosis of ectopic pregnancy. In: *UpToDate*, Post, T. W. (Ed.), UpToDate, Waltham, MA. (Accessed on August 28, 2014).

Tulandi, T. Incidence, risk factors, and pathology of ectopic pregnancy. In: *UpToDate*, Post, T. W. (Ed.), UpToDate, Waltham, MA. (Accessed on August 25, 2014).

Veenendaal, M. V., van Abeelen, A. F., Painter, R. C., van der Post, J. A., Roseboom, T. J. (2011). Consequences of hyperemesis gravidarum for offspring: a systematic review and meta-analysis. *British Journal of Obstetrics and Gynaecology*; 118(11):1302-13.

Weyermann, M., Brenner, H., Adler, G., Yasar, Z., Handke-Vesely, A., et al. (2003). Helicobacter pylori infection and the occurrence and severity of gastrointestinal symptoms during pregnancy. *American Journal of Obstetrics and Gynecology*; 189(2): 526-31.

Whitehead, S. A., Andrews, P. L. R., Chamberlain, G. V. P. (1992). Characterisation of nausea and vomiting in early pregnancy: a survey of 1000 women. *Journal of Obstetrics and Gynaecology*; 12:364-9.

Whitley, K. A., Ural, S. H. (2014). Treatment modalities in recurrent miscarriages without diagnosis. *Seminars in Reproductive Medicine*; 32(4):319-22.

Woolf, C. J. (1991). *British Medical Bulletin*; 47:523-33.

Yoneyama, Y., Suzuki, S., Sawa, R., Yoneyama, K., Doi, D., et al. (2002). *American Journal of Obstetrics and Gynecology*; 187:1631-5.

In: Handbook for High Risk Pregnancy: Clinical Management ISBN: 978-1-63482-299-2
Editors: E. González-Mesa and D. Abehsera

Chapter 3

DIABETES AND GESTATION

Paula Chamocho Lloro, MD[1,*], and Omar Rahmouni, MD[2]
[1]Obstetrics and Gynecology Department, Quiron Hospital, Malaga, Spain
[2]Obstetrics and Gynecology Department, Clinical University Hospital, Malaga, Spain

INTRODUCTION

Gestational diabetes mellitus (GDM) is one of the most common complications in pregnancy. Normal pregnancy is a condition characterized by a series of complex hormonal adaptations that occur to ensure that sufficient glucose is available to meet the nutritional requirements of the growing fetus without causing maternal hypoglycemia. As normal pregnancy progresses, there is an increase in insulin resistance that may result in some cases in gestational diabetes. However, pregnancy can also occur in women with preexisting diabetes. Gestational diabetes mellitus is a disease characterized by underlying defects in maternal insulin sensitivity and secretion, which are unmasked in the response to the metabolic stressors of pregnancy. Later in this chapter we will sort out the different types of diabetes that can arise during pregnancy and before it. We will try to describe the maternal implications and fetal repercussions of gestational diabetes.

Women with GDM are at greater risk for prenatal complications than women without GDM. Maternal complications include obesity, overweight, polyhydramnios, premature broken membranes, preterm delivery, preeclampsia, instrumental delivery and primary cesarean section; and neonatal complications include greater infant birth weight, larger fetus for its gestational age, shoulder dystocia, neonatal hypoglycemia and necessity of phototherapy for hyperbilirubinemia. Alterations in other metabolic parameters besides glucose are associated with macrosomia, underlining the fact that protein and lipid abnormalities accompany glucose intolerance (Nuremberg et al. 2014). Maternal free fatty acid levels and triglyceride levels at delivery correlate with neonatal weight and fat mass, suggesting that maternal lipid profiles influence neonatal weight. Maternal pre-pregnancy body mass index is a risk factor for macrosomia in women with GDM.

* Corresponding author: paulaoscense@hotmail.com

In pre-existing diabetes the most common anomalies involve the cardiovascular system (such as transposition of the great vessels, ventricular septal defect, situs inversus, single ventricle and hypoplastic left ventricle), the central nervous system (such as anencephaly, encephalocele, meningomyelocele, spina bifida, and holoprosencephaly), and the face and extremities (Yessoufou et al. 2011). Rates of fetal malformation appear to be similar for maternal type 1 and type 2 pre-existing diabetes. Fortunately these complications are much lower than the others, according to Marco et al. 2012.

Long term complications in the offspring were related with obesity, diabetes mellitus type II and behavior disturbances. The infants of women with GDM had excessive fetal growth and hyperinsulinemia as indicated by cord C-peptide and insulin concentrations. Diabetes recurrence, diabetes mellitus type II and the appearance of other cardiovascular risk factors associated with the metabolic syndrome (dyslipidemia, obesity and arterial hypertension) are more common to occur in mothers who have suffered from GDM.,

A dose-response effect was demonstrated, regarding the relation between congenital anomalies and glycemic control: the poorer the glucose control before conception or during an early stage of pregnancy is, the greater the risk for congenital anomalies (Kim et al. 2012).

Equally important is the pregestational counseling in women with diabetes mellitus or insulin resistance, when they plan their pregnancy and before. In a recent review of Nandy et al. 2013, they explain this connection. The insulin/insulin-like growth factor (IGF) pathways and glucose metabolism act as mediators of human ovarian function and female fertility. In normal insulin action, insulin binds to its own receptors in the ovary to mediate steroidogenesis and acts as a co-gonadotropin. Insulin with other factors may influence ovarian growth and cyst formation. The IGF pathway also seems to influence normal ovarian function. Insulin signaling affects reproductive function. Dysregulation of this pathway leads to altered puberty, ovulation, and fertility.

Definition

Gestational diabetes is a glucose tolerance alteration, of varying severity, that is recognized for the first time during pregnancy, regardless of preexisting diabetes, the gestational weeks at the diagnosis, the requirements of insulin for its control and persistence after delivery (Putsky et al. 2013).

The GDM will be reclassified definitively postpartum. Damasceno et al. explain in their review how diabetes develops in pregnancy.

Prevalence

The incidence and prevalence of GDM is increasing worldwide. Approximately 7% of pregnancies are complicated by GDM (ranging from 1 to 14%), depending on the population studied (GDM is higher in Hispanic and Afroamerican women) and the diagnostic tests employed. The proportion of pregnancies complicated by type II diabetes mellitus and GDM is likely to continue to rise due to an increase in obesity rates. In a multicentric study in Spain the GDM prevalence reported was 8,2% (Gaudineau et al. 2013). In the last decades this important increase was caused by body mass index rise, type of alimentation, lifestyle and pregnancy average age (Flores Le-Roux et al. 2012).

DIAGNOSIS

There are no specific symptoms of GDM that we can detect early in pregnancy, that is why a lot of pregnant women debut with GDM complications. In women without preexisting diabetes mellitus a universal screening test needs to be passed in order to detect as many GDM cases as possible to decrease the impact of negative effects at short and long term (Gallo et al. 2013). Professional organizations continue to have different recommendations concerning the best screening strategy for GDM. The US National Institute of Health has recently recommended continuing with the O'Sullivan test.

The most commonly used screening test is the O'Sullivan one, and it consists in the intake of 50 grams of glucose and determinate venous levels of glycemia one hour after the intake, at any moment of day and regardless if the patient has taken some food before or not. The cutoff universally accepted are levels of glycemia exceeding 140 mg/dl. That cutoff demonstrates a high sensibility (80%) and specificity (87%). The results of this test were statistically associated with fetal-maternal outcomes ($p < 0{,}001$). However, not all the women screened with that test, developed GDM, only 11% of individuals with a positive test developed GDM (Benhalima et al. 2013). Nonetheless, positive screening tests were also associated with macrosomia and gestational hypertension.

There is a lot of controversy among the researchers about when women without preexisting diabetes mellitus should be screened (Gheorman et al. 2011). In many countries the screening is made during the first quarter of pregnancy (between 10 and 14 weeks of pregnancy).

By common consent the test will be done to all pregnant women who are between 24 and 28 weeks of pregnancy and without known diabetes mellitus.

We will start screening in the first trimester of pregnancy in case we have some of the following risk factors:

- GDM in previous pregnancies
- Negative outcomes that suggest GDM in previous pregnancies
- Obesity (it is defined as body mass index exceeding 30 kg/m2)
- Personal background of diabetes mellitus or other metabolic glucose disturbances.
- First-degree relative with GDM.
- Age > 35 years.

If we have a positive screening test we have to carry out a diagnosis test.

To confirm the diagnosis in a pregnant women with positive O'Sullivan test, we have to do an overload oral glucose. Before the intake of glucose we have to determine basal venous glycemia levels.

The patients will take a normal diet during the previous days (non restrictive carbohydrates diet). Then they will intake 100 grams of glucose and the glycemia will me measured after one hour, then after two hours and finally after three hours. The pregnant woman has to remain sitting and without smoking during the entire test. Commonly we use the cutoff criteria of the US National Health Institute, which are the most extended and useful worldwide.

It will be positive some values that surpass the following cutoffs:

- Basal glycemia values exceeding 105 mg/dl
- First hour glycemia exceeding 190 mg/dl
- Second hour glycemia exceeding 165 mg/dl
- Third hour glycemia exceeding 145 mg/dl

To confirm the diagnosis we need to have two positive values in that test. If only one value is positive there is considered to be a glucose intolerance. However, we will consider diabetic any pregnant woman that has two basal glycemia determinations higher than 126 mg/dl measured in two different days or any pregnant women that have a single value of glycemia that overmatches 200 mg/dl measured at any time and regardless of the fact that she had eaten before.

In the last years there has been a lot of controversy about which are the most appropriate cutoffs to use in order to detect a greater number of GDM pregnant with the aim to decrease the impact of negative obstetrics outcomes.

The Spanish Group of Diabetes and Pregnancy (GEDE) recommends using those criteria for our population features.

The use of a determination of glycated hemoglobin levels can be useful in the preconceptional counseling. The value accepted for an optimal control is less than 7 mg/dl. However that concept is not appropriate to detect GDM, but it can be used to control pregnant women with GDM and women with preexisting diabetes types I and II.

TREATMENT

Women with gestational diabetes generally start their treatment with diet and lifestyle changes (Hopkins et al. 2013); when these changes are not enough to reach optimal glycemic control, insulin therapy must be considered.

Women with diabetes type 2 using oral hypoglycemic agents are advised to change to insulin therapy.

Those with diabetes type 1 should start intensive glycemic controls (Negrato et al. 2012).

1. Lifestyle Changes

- Diet: The diet is the first treatment strategy in the gestational diabetes (recommendation grade B).

Eating habits of a diabetic pregnant woman should not be hypocaloric nor HC restrictive, and only refined sugar and products that contain it in big quantities should be avoided.

The caloric input and the weight increase should be similar to non-diabetic pregnant women. (1800-2000 kcal/day)

- Exercise: Aerobic exercise should be recommended during 30-60 minutes per day, the insulin resistance improves with the exercise.

2. Pharmacological Treatment

Insulin: is the gold standard treatment for any type of diabetes during pregnancy, most of insulin preparations that are used today have been shown to promote good glycemic control during pregnancy.

Their targets for glycemic control during pregnancy are fasting plasma glucose levels of 60-90 mg/dl, pre-prandial levels of 60-105mg/dl, one-hour postprandial levels< 140 mg/dl, two-hour postprandial levels < 120 mg/dl. All these levels should be obtained without the appearance of hypoglycemia.

Insulin requirements rise during pregnancy because there is a progressive increase in insulin resistance generally associated with weight gain and decreased physical activity.

In the last 10 years, biosynthetic insulin is the most commonly used.

Types of insulin

- Rapid-acting insulin analogues: Are generally necessary to control postprandial hyperglycemia, and to optimize the doses of intermediate-acting insulins in adequate insulin basal rate.

Compared with regular human insulin, their use is associated with lowering in postprandial glucose levels 0,3% to 0,5%, reduction in HbA1c and a 20% to 30% reduction in hypoglycemic episodes during the day, but especially during the night.

As it has already been evidenced in many studies, rapid-acting insulin analogues cannot cross the human placenta

- Insulin lispro: Its action begins in 15 minutes or less after the injection, and has its peak after 30-90 minutes, lasting from four to six hours. Insulin lispro can be used immediately before or after a meal.
- Insulin aspart: It starts to act 10-15 minutes after the injection, and the peak occurs after 30-60 minutes. Its action lasts 4-5 hours.
  Both analogues are safe and in several aspects, more efficient than human regular insulin in the treatment of pregnancy women with diabetes.
- Insulin glulisine: there are no clinical trials using glulisine during pregnancy so far, so it cannot be recommended in pregnancy.

- Short-acting insulin: Human regular insulin has almost entirely been replaced by rapid actions analogues.
- Intermediate-acting insulin (NPH/ NPL): Rapid acting associated with protamine (basic protein) to slow the absorption and prolong its effect.
- Long-acting insulin analogues:

- Insulin glargine has a glycine substitution that decreases the solubility in the subcutaneous tissue and confers greater stability while has longer action. It starts to act about 90 minutes after the injection, action lasts 24 hours, and has no peak of action. It does not cross the placenta and many studies have shown the safety and efficacy of its use in pregnancy. In fact, maternal complications were more frequently found in women with pregestational diabetes treated with NPH compared to those treated with glargine. In women with gestational diabetes treated with NPH it was observed an increased of new-onset pregnancy hypertension, micro and macroalbuminuria, hypoglycemia compared with glargine. Among neonatal outcomes, significantly higher rates of NICU admission and fetal death were observed in infants born to women with pregestational diabetes treated with NPH insulin. And congenital malformations were significantly more frequent in NPH treated patients. It has been concluded that the use of insulin glargine during pregnancy, from preconception to delivery, showed to be safe since it was associated with decreased maternal and neonatal adverse outcomes when compared with NPH insulin treated patients.

– Insulin detemir: It has a peakless action sustained for 18-20 hours. Both insulins reduce fasting as well as postprandial glucose levels and are associated with less hypoglycemic events and lower weight gain. There are less studies comparing detemir to NPH, however insulin detemir is not inferior compared with NPH. Both analogues, glargine and detemir seem to be safe and in, several aspects, more efficient than NPH insulin in the treatment of diabetes in pregnancy.

Finally, it must be known that the rapid acting analogues lispro and aspart, and the long acting insulin are assigned a use in pregnancy category B. Insulin glulisine and insulin glargine and detemir are assigned category C, should be used during pregnancy only if the potential benefits to the mother justify the potential risks to the fetus.

A valid regime of insulinitation is the next one: NPH 0,2 kg/day (2/3 of the dose in the morning, 1/3 of the dose in the night); fast insulin 0.05 U/kg/day (thirty minutes before meal); increases 10-20% of the dose according to glycemic later control.

Current developments: ORMD-0801 is an oral insulin that has completed its phase I trials, and its results are encouraging since it has proven to be safe, well tolerated, and insures consistent reduction in glucose and C-peptide. The other alternative routes of insulin delivery being developed are oral and inhaled, whereby insulin is taken directly into the mouth via a metered dose spray.

Oral antidiabetic: The use of ADO in the treatment of refractory DG to diet and exercise has been rejected by the medical community. It has based on a few studies with methodology deficits, that state that they cause more congenital malformation and fetal macrosomia. Insulin therapy can be inconvenient because of the need for multiple injections, its associated cost, pain at injection site, need for refrigeration, and skillful handling; all these has contributed to poor patient compliance. This has also led to search for oral hypoglycemic agents as an alternative option to insulin therapy.

For that reason there exist reviews about safety and advantages of the glyburide and metformin during pregnancy.

Types of ADO:

Insulin secretory or secretogogues:

- Sulfonylureas: (Glyburide (Category B), glibenclamida) they join the cells b pancreatic receptors, stimulating insulin secretion. It reduces the fasting blood glucose as well as glycosylated hemoglobin. Glyburide does not cross the placenta despite its low molecular weight and its high protein-binding capacity of 99.8%. The first adverse effect is maternal hypoglycemia. Langer et al. carried out a study that included 404 women who were randomly assigned to insulin and glyburide. The outcome was comparable since 82% of glyburide group and 88% insulin group achieved good glycemic control. In addition, the glyburide group experienced less maternal hypoglycemia (2%) compared to insulin group (20%). There was no difference in other maternal outcomes like preeclampsia, rate of cesarean delivery and neonatal hypoglycemia. This trial proved glyburide as a safe and effective alternative therapy.
- Meglitinides: (Nateglinide, repaglinide) Its mechanism of action is similar to sulfonylureas. But there is no data regarding the use of nateglinide during pregnancy. A randomized controlled trial with repaglinide and insulin demonstrated that the pre and postprandial glucose levels were the same in the treatment of the control groups and there was no difference in the fetal and neonatal outcome.

Insulin sensibilations:

- Biguanides: (Metformin-Categoria B) It improves the action of insulin on peripheral tissues and reduces hepatic glucose production, hepatic glycogenolysis, and increases the insulin stimulated uptake of glucose in skeletal muscles. The biguanides does not stimulate the fetal pancreatic cells to produce insulin and there is no association with neonatal hyperinsulinemia. Studies have identified that metformin crosses the placenta but has minimal effect on transplacental flux (Cassina et al. 2014). The transfer into human breast milk is minimal and they can be used safely during lactation.

The first advantage is that metformin does not stimulate insulin production so it does not cause hypoglycemia. Metformin appears to be effective and safe for the treatment of GDM particularly for overweight or obese women. Studies show that "no evidence that metformin is associated with an increased risk of major birth defects in women affected by pregestational diabetes type 2 and treated during the first trimester". The use of metformin throughout pregnancy in women with polycystic ovary syndrome reduces the rates of early pregnancy loss and preterm labor and protects against fetal growth restriction. Metformin can also delay the insulin therapy use, it can lower insulin doses, and its administration is more comfortable than insulin therapy.

- Thiazolidinediones: (Rosiglitazone and Pioglitazone). –They act on selective agonists of the insulin receptors located in the nucleus, and improve insulin sensitivity. We don't have enough data to use them in pregnancy.
- Alpha-glucosidase inhibitors: (Miglitol and acarbose): They inhibit glucose uptake in the upper gastrointestinal, so they reduce postprandial glycemic. The first adverse effect is flatulence and rumbling. Acarbose do not cross human placenta. It is less

effective than glyburide in reducing the glycemic levels and its use is restricted in combination with glyburide or metformin.

- Exenatide: It is a peptide similar to glucagon. Its mechanism of action is to enhance insulin secretion while inhibiting the secretion of glucagon, and slows gastric emptying and promotes satiety. This drug is administrated by subcutaneous injection with sulfonylurea or metformin. It reduces fasting and postprandial glucose. There is not enough data about its use.

INTRAPARTUM GLYCEMIC CONTROL

In women with pregestational type 1 and type 2 diabetes, hyperglycemia during labour and delivery is an important factor in the development of neonatal hypoglycaemia (neonatal glycemic less than 40mg/dl), so intrapartum management protocols have established the simultaneous use of intravenous infusions of insulin and glucose. The glycemic level during labor and delivery should be less than 140 mg/dl. But there is no consensus about glycemic control during labor and delivery in women with gestational diabetes. There are studies that recommend the management of intrapartum insulin depending on the treatment administered during pregnancy, so women who have been treated with insulin during the pregnancy could require treatment with insulin during labor and delivery and women treated with a diet during pregnancy are not recommended to undergo a specific control during delivery. But Basells et al. affirm that the need of insulin during delivery does not appear to correlate with the need of insulin during pregnancy. There are protocols that monitor maternal glycemia and ketonemia and allow an easy adjustment of insulin and glucose perfusion during delivery.

PREVENTION

Pregnancy in women with Mellitus Diabetes should be planned and pre-pregnancy counseling is essential. Strategies are needed in order to offer to pregnant women interventions associated with improved pregnancy outcomes, such as maintaining periconceptional euglycemic (glycosylated hemoglobin < 7) and folic acid use (supplementation of 1 to 5 mg per day) beginning before conception and continuing during pregnancy.

Supplementation with vitamin D beyond what is contained in routine prenatal vitamins will prevent GDM or improve glucose tolerance for women with GD (Gunderson et al. 2013).

Higher dietary vitamin E intake is associated with lower fasting glucose, lower insulin resistance and higher insulin sensitivity.

Omega 3 fatty acids that are contained in prenatal vitamins improve the hyperlipidemia induced by diabetic pregnancy.

In a lot of recent studies, lactation demonstrated to benefit insulin sensitivity and to reduce the risk of developing DM type 2 at a long term in women who have GDM, however, that results are not consistent, and we need to do more studies to clarify that.

Exercise has as well documented to have health benefits and to reduce peripheral insulin resistance in non pregnant women. Women who are more active before pregnancy are less insulin resistant in pregnancy and have lower rates of GDM.

Conclusion

1. Diabetes is a frequent pathology during pregnancy and its prevalence is increasing due to the increase of obesity and the fact that women are delaying pregnancy.
2. Diabetes has high rate of complications in mothers, fetuses, newborn and childhood.
3. To avoid adverse outcomes we have to carry out screening tests during pregnancy and pregnant women who are known previously to be diabetics must undergo periconceptional euglycemic controls.
4. The most common screening test to detect GDM is the O'Sullivan test, but not every women who have a positive test will develop a GDM, that is why the confirmation test is needed.
5. The first treatment of diabetes may be diet and exercise, but if it is not enough the best treatment during pregnancy is insulin.
6. Oral antidiabetics like metformin are safe and can be used during pregnancy alone or along with insulin treatment.
7. The intake of supplements during pregnancy like vitamin D, vitamin E, folic acid, and omega 3 fatty acids can prevent gestational diabetes or improve glucose tolerance.
8. Finally, lactating women exhibit more favorable blood glucose and insulin profiles than non lactating women due to the fact that they experiment an insulin sensitivity increase compared to non lactating women.

References

Benhalima K1, Mathieu C. 2013 Gestational diabetes: update of screening strategy and diagnostic criteria. *Current Opinion in Obstetrics and Gynecology,* 25(6):462-7.

Berggren EK1, Boggess KA. 2013 Oral agents for the management of gestational diabetes Clinical Obstetric and Gynecology, 2013 Dec;56(4): 827-36.

Burris HH1, Camargo CA Jr. 2014 Vitamin D and gestational diabetes mellitus. *Current Diabetes Report,* 14(1):451.

Cassina M, Donà M, Di Gianantonio E, Litta P, Clementi M. 2014 First-trimester exposure to metformin and risk of birth defects: a systematic review and meta-analysis. *Human Reproduction Update,* 2014 Sep;20(5): 656-669.

Damasceno D.C, Sinzato Y.K, Bueno A, Netto A.O, Dallaqua B, Gallego F.Q, Lessi I.L, et al 2013 Mild Diabetes Models and Their Maternal-Fetal Repercussions. *Journal of Diabetes Research,* 473575.

Flores JA Le-Roux, Benaiges Boix D, Botet JP. 2013 Diabetes mellitus gestacional: importancia del control glucémico intraparto. Arterioesclerosis. Vol. 25. Núm. 04.

Gallo M. 2013. Diabetes gestacional: Nuevos tratamientos, Situaciones de difícil manejo en el embarazo. (15) 177 Herrera Peral JA, Gallo JL. Amolca. Caracas.

Gaudineau A et al. 2013 Prevalence, risk factors, maternal and fetal morbidity and mortality of intrauterine growth restriction and small-for-gestational age. Journal de gynecologie, *obstetrique et biologie de la reproduction,* 42(8):895-910.

Gheorman L, Iliescu D, Ceauşu I, Paulescu D, Pleşea I.E, Gheorman V Importance of early complex evaluation in high-risk pregnancy associated to diabetes mellitus. Case presentation and review of the literature. *2011 Romanian Journal of Morphology and Embryology,* 52(3 Suppl):1127–1132.

Gunderson EP. 2013. The role of lactation in GDM women. *Clinical Obstetric and Gynecology,* 2013;56(4):844-52.

Hopkins SA1, Artal R. 2013. The role of exercise in reducing the risks of gestational diabetes mellitus. *Womens Health,* 9(6):569-81.

Kavitha N, Somsubhra De, Kanagasabai S 2013 Oral Hypoglycemic Agents in pregnancy: *An Update Journal of Obstetric and Gynaecology of India,* 63(2): 82–87.

Kim C et al. 2014 Gestational Diabetes Mellitus in Korean Women: Similarities and Differences from Other Racial/Ethnic Groups. *Diabetes and Metabolism Journal,* 38(1): 1–12.

Kim SY1, Sharma AJ, Callaghan WM. 2012 Gestational diabetes and childhood obesity: what is the link? Current Opinion in Obstetrics and gynecology. *Gynecol,* 24(6):376-81.

Ley SH1, Hanley AJ, Sermer M, Zinman B, O'Connor DL.2013 Lower dietary vitamin E intake during the second trimester is associated with insulin resistance and hyperglycemia later in pregnancy. *European Journal of Clinical Nutrition,* 67(11):1154-6.

Lautatzis ME, Goulis DG, Vrontakis M. 2013 Efficacy and safety of metformin during pregnancy in women with gestational diabetes mellitus or polycystic ovary syndrome: a systematic review. Metabolism: *clinical and experimental,* 62(11):1522-34.

Marco LJ, McCloskey K, Vuillermin PJ, Burgner D, Said J, Ponsonby A-L. 2012 Cardiovascular Disease Risk in the Offspring of Diabetic Women: The Impact of the Intrauterine Environment. Experimental Diabetes Research. 565160.

Nandi A1, Poretsky L. 2013 Diabetes and the female reproductive system. 2013. *Endocrinology and Metabolism Clinics of North America,* 42(4): 915-46.

Negrato A; Montenegro Junior RM; Von Kostrisch LM; Guedes MF; Mattar R; Gomes MB 2012 Insulin analogues in the treatment of diabetes in pregnancy. Arquivos Brasileiros de Endocrinologia & Metabologia vol.56.

Pellicer 2014. Diabetes y gestación. Obstetricia y Ginecología Guía de Actuación. Pellicer MA, Hidalgo JJ, Perales A, Diaz C. Editorial Médica Panamericana SA. Madrid. Pp 590.

Prutsky GJ, Domecq JP, Sundaresh V, Elraiyah T, Nabhan M, Prokop LJ et al. 2013. Screening for gestational diabetes: a systematic review and meta-analysis. *The Journal of Clinical endocrinology and metabolism,* 98(11): 4311-8.

Wahabi H A, Alzeidan R A, Esmaeil S A 2012 Pre-pregnancy care for women with pre-gestational diabetes mellitus: a systematic review and meta-analysis BMC Public Health. 12: 792.

Yessoufou A, Moutairou K 2011. Maternal Diabetes in Pregnancy: Early and Long-Term Outcomes on the Offspring and the Concept of "Metabolic Memory" Experimental Diabetes Research. 218598.

In: Handbook for High Risk Pregnancy: Clinical Management ISBN: 978-1-63482-299-2
Editors: E. González-Mesa and D. Abehsera

Chapter 4

HYPERTENSION AND PREECLAMPSIA

Laura Baños Cándenas[1*], Pedro Azumendi Gómez[2] and Daniel Abehsera Davó[1]
[1]Obstetrics and Gynecology Department, Quirón University Hospital, Málaga, Spain
[2]Obstetrics and Gynecology Department, Regional University Hospital of Málaga, Málaga, Spain

1. INTRODUCTION

Hypertensive disorders of pregnancy are an important cause of severe morbidity, long-term disability and death among both mothers and their babies. Among the hypertensive disorders that complicate pregnancy, pre-eclampsia and eclampsia stand out as major causes of maternal and perinatal mortality and morbidity. Hypertensive disorders during pregnancy occur in women with pre-existing primary or secondary chronic hypertension, and in women who develop new-onset hypertension in the second half of pregnancy. Hypertensive disorders during pregnancy carry risks for the woman and the baby. (Nice guideline 107, 2011). Women with early-onset pre-eclampsia require admission to a tertiary care facility for treatment and one-third experience complications that may necessitate intensive care. Infants are often delivered preterm, need prolonged intensive care and develop complications, including lifelong disability, giving rise to large healthcare costs. Early identification of women at risk is a key aim of antenatal care (Velauthar, Plana, Kalidindi, Zamora, Thilaganathan, Illanes, Khan et al., 2014).

2. DEFINITIONS

2.1. What Is Raised Blood Pressure?

Hypertension, also known as high or raised blood pressure, is a condition in which the blood vessels have persistently raised pressure. Blood is carried from the heart to all parts of

* Corresponding author: Email: laurabc84@hotmail.es.

the body in the vessels. Each time the heart beats, it pumps blood into the vessels. Blood pressure is created by the force of blood pushing against the walls of blood vessels (arteries) as it is pumped by the heart. The higher the pressure the harder the heart has to pump. Normal adult blood pressure is defined as a blood pressure of 120 mm Hg (millimeters of mercury) when the heart beats (systolic) and a blood pressure of 80 mm Hg when the heart relaxes (diastolic). When systolic blood pressure is equal to or above 140 mm Hg and/or a diastolic blood pressure equal to or above 90 mm Hg the blood pressure is considered to be raised or high (World Health Organization)

To complete the definition, the Guideline Development Group (GDG) has defined mild, moderate and severe hypertension:

- Mild hypertension diastolic blood pressure 90–99 mmHg, systolic blood pressure 140–149mmHg.
- Moderate hypertension diastolic blood pressure 100–109 mmHg, systolic blood pressure 150–159 mmHg.
- Severe hypertension diastolic blood pressure 110 mmHg or greater, systolic blood pressure 160 mmHg or greater.

2.2. Importance of an Optimal Measurement of Blood Pressure (BP)

The patient should be asked to remove all clothing that covers the location of cuff placement. The individual should be comfortably seated, with the legs uncrossed, and the back and arm supported, such that the middle of the cuff on the upper arm is at the level of the right atrium (the mid-point of the sternum). Measurements made while the patient is on an examining table do not fulfill these criteria and should preferably be made while the patient is seated in a chair. At the initial visit, blood pressure should be measured in both arms. The patient should be instructed to relax as much as possible and to not talk during the measurement procedure; ideally, 5 minutes should elapse before the first reading is taken. If elevated on initial assessment, the BP measurement should be repeated after several minutes to attempt to eliminate spuriously elevated BP determinations (Pickering, Hall, Appel, Flakner, Graves, & Hill et al., 2005)

2.3. Proteinuria: Presence of More than 300 mg (0.3 g) of Protein in a 24 Hours Urine Specimen in the Absence of Urinary Infection

Table1. Recommendations for BP measurement (Magee, Pels, Helewa, Rey, Dadelszen, 2014)

Blood pressure should be measured with the woman in the sitting position with the arm at the level of the heart. (II-2A)
An appropriately sized cuff (i.e., length 1.5 times the circumference of the arm) should be used. (II-2A)

Korotkoff phase V should be used to designate diastolic blood pressure. (I-A)
If blood pressure is consistently higher in one arm, the arm with the higher values should be used for all blood pressure measurements. (III-B)
Blood pressure can be measured using a mercury sphygmomanometer, a calibrated aneroid device, or an automated blood pressure machine that has been validated for use in preeclampsia. (II-2A)
Automated blood pressure machines that have not been validated for use in women with preeclampsia may underestimate or overestimate blood pressure in those women; a comparison of readings using mercury sphygmomanometry or a calibrated aneroid device is recommended. (II-2A)
In the office setting, when blood pressure elevation is non-severe and preeclampsia is not suspected, ambulatory blood pressure monitoring or home blood pressure monitoring is useful to confirm persistently elevated blood pressure. (II-2C)
When home blood pressure monitoring is used, maternity care providers should ensure that patients have adequate training in measuring their blood pressure and interpreting the readings. (III-C)
The accuracy of all blood pressure measurement devices used in hospitals or offices should be checked regularly against a calibrated device. (II-3C)
The accuracy of all automated devices used for home blood pressure monitoring should be checked regularly against a calibrated device. (III-C)

Table 2. Causes of proteinuria in pregnancy (Thadhani & Maynard 2014). UpToDate

Primary renal diseases
IgA nephropathy
Minimal change disease
Membranous nephropathy
Focal segmental glomerulosclerosis
Primary glomerulonephritis
Allergic interstitial nephritis
Polycystic kidney disease
Systemic causes
Preeclampsia
Diabetic nephropathy
Lupus nephritis (diffuse proliferative, focal proliferative, membranous)
Hypertensive nephrosclerosis
Thrombotic thrombocytopenic purpura (TTP)
Infection-associated glomerular disease (eg, HIV, hepatitis B/C)
Systemic vasculitis
Multiple myeloma
Chronic vesicoureteral reflux
Antiphospholipid syndrome
Symptomatic urinary tract obstruction

3. Definitions of Pregnancy-Related Hypertensive Disorders

3.1. Chronic or Preexisting Hypertension

Chronic or preexisting hypertension is defined as systolic pressure greater than or equal to (≥) 140 mmHg and/or diastolic pressure greater than or equal to 90 mmHg that antedates pregnancy or is present before the 20th week of pregnancy (on at least two occasions) or persists longer than 12 weeks postpartum. It can be primary (primary hypertension, formerly called "essential hypertension") or secondary to a variety of medical disorders (August & Sibai, 2014).

3.2. Gestational Hypertension

Gestational hypertension: systolic blood pressure ≥140 mmHg and/or diastolic blood pressure ≥90 mmHg in a previously normotensive pregnant woman who is ≥20 weeks of gestation and has no proteinuria or new signs of end-organ dysfunction (Roberts, Druzin, August, Gaiser, Bakris, Granger, Barton, et al. 2012)

3.3. Preeclampsia

Preeclampsia is a pregnancy-specific hypertensive disease with multisystem involvement is thought to be predominantly as the consequence of impaired placentation (Poon & Nicolaides, 2014). Is a syndrome that chiefly includes the development of new-onset hypertension in the second half of pregnancy. Although often accompanied by new-onset proteinuria, preeclampsia can be associated with many other signs and symptoms, including visual disturbances, headaches, epigastric pain, and the rapid development of edema. Diagnostic criteria include the development of hypertension, defined as a persistent systolic blood pressure (BP) of 140 mm Hg or higher, or a diastolic BP of 90 mm Hg or higher after 20 weeks of gestation in a women with previously normal blood pressure.

Table 3. Criteria for gestational hypertension. UptoDate 2014

Systolic blood pressure ≥140 mmHg
OR
Diastolic blood pressure ≥ 90 mmHg
AND no proteinuria
Developing AFTER the 20th week of gestation in women known to be normotensive before pregnancy. Blood pressure should be elevated on at least two occasions at least six hours apart.

3.3.1. Assessing the severity of preeclampsia

Some clinical findings increase the risk of morbidity and mortality in the setting of preeclampsia and, when present, segregate preeclampsia into a more severe category. The more severe forms of preeclampsia are characterized by the certain findings in women meeting the basic criteria for diagnosing the disorder. Additionally, women who have met the basic criteria for preeclampsia with systolic BP levels of 140–160 mm Hg or diastolic BP levels of 90–110 mm Hg, along with new evidence of thrombocytopenia, impaired liver dysfunction, renal insufficiency, pulmonary edema, or visual loss or cerebral disturbance, also should be considered as having severe disease.

Massive proteinuria, greater than 5 g, has been eliminated from the consideration of preeclampsia as severe, because of the minimal relationship between the quantity of urinary protein and pregnancy outcome in preeclampsia. Also, because fetal growth restriction is managed similarly in pregnant women with and without preeclampsia, it has been removed as a finding indicating severe preeclampsia (Roberts et al., 2012)

Table 4. Diagnostic criteria for preeclampsia. Hypertension in pregnancy: Report of the American College of Obstetricians and Gynecologists' Task Force on Hypertension in Pregnancy. Obstet Gynecol 2013; 122:1122

Blood pressure	Greater than or equal to 140 mm Hg systolic or greater than or equal to 90 mm Hg diastolic on two occasions at least 4 hours apart after 20 weeks of gestation in a woman with a previously normal blood pressure Greater than or equal to 160 mm Hg systolic or greater than or equal to 110 mm Hg diastolic, hypertension can be confirmed within a short interval (minutes) to facilitate timely antihypertensive therapy
AND	
Proteinuria	Greater than or equal to 300 mg per 24 hour urine collection (or this amount extrapolated from a timed collection) Protein/creatinine ratio greater than or equal to 0.3* Dipstick reading of 1+ (used only if other quantitative methods not available)
ORin the absence of proteinuria, new-onset hypertension with the new onset of any of the following:	
Thrombocytopenia	Platelet count less than 100,000/microliter
Renal insufficiency	Serum creatinine concentrations greater than 1.1 mg/dL or a doubling of the serum creatinine concentration in the absence of other renal disease
Impaired liver function	Elevated blood concentrations of liver transaminases to twice normal concentration
Pulmonary edema	
Cerebral or visual symptoms	

3.4. Eclampsia

Eclampsia refers to the development of grand mal seizures in a woman with preeclampsia, in the absence of other neurologic conditions that could account for the seizure (August, 2014). Eclampsia is defined as the presence of new-onset grand mal seizures in a woman with preeclampsia (Roberts et al., 2012). Other authors define eclampsia like the occurrence of one or more generalized convulsions and/or coma in the setting of preeclampsia and in the absence of other neurologic conditions. The clinical manifestations can appear anytime from the second trimester to the puerperium. In the past, eclampsia was thought to be the end result of preeclampsia (hence the nomenclature); however, it is now clear that seizures should be considered merely one of several clinical manifestations of severe preeclampsia (Table 5), rather than a separate disease. Despite advances in detection and management, preeclampsia/eclampsia remains a common cause of maternal death (Norwitz, 2014).

3.5. Chronic Hypertension

Chronic hypertension with superimposed preeclampsia refers to the new onset of either proteinuria or end-organ dysfunction after 20 weeks of gestation in a woman with chronic or preexisting hypertension. For women with chronic/preexisting hypertension who have proteinuria prior to or in early pregnancy, superimposed preeclampsia is defined by worsening or resistant hypertension in the last half of pregnancy or development of signs and symptoms of the severe spectrum of the disease (August, et al., 2014)

Table 5. Severe Features of preeclampsia. Hypertension in pregnancy: Report of the American College of Obstetricians and Gynecologists' Task Force on Hypertension in Pregnancy. Obstet Gynecol 2013; 122:1122

Symptoms of central nervous system dysfunction:
New onset cerebral or visual disturbance, such as: Photopsia, scotomata, cortical blindness, retinal vasospasm Severe headache (ie, incapacitating, "the worst headache I've ever had") or headache that persists and progresses despite analgesic therapy Altered mental status
Hepatic abnormality:
Severe persistent right upper quadrant or epigastric pain unresponsive to medication and not accounted for by an alternative diagnosis or serum transaminase concentration ≥ twice normal, or both
Severe blood pressure elevation:
Systolic blood pressure ≥160 mmHg or diastolic blood pressure ≥110 mmHg on two occasions at least four hours apart while the patient is on bedrest (unless the patient is on antihypertensive therapy)
Thrombocytopenia:
<100,000 platelets/microL
Renal abnormality:
Progressive renal insufficiency (serum creatinine >1.1 mg/dL or doubling of serum creatinine concentration in the absence of other renal disease)
Pulmonary edema

3.6. HELLP

HELLP is an acronym that refers to a syndrome characterized by Hemolysis with a microangiopathic blood smear, Elevated Liver enzymes, and a Low Platelet count. It probably represents a severe form of preeclampsia, but the relationship between the two disorders remains controversial. As many as 15 to 20 percent of patients with HELLP syndrome do not have antecedent hypertension or proteinuria, leading some authorities to believe that HELLP is a separate disorder from preeclampsia. Both severe preeclampsia and HELLP syndrome may be associated with serious hepatic manifestations, including infarction, hemorrhage, and rupture (Sibai, 2014). Variant of severe preeclampsia that is diagnosed when it appears: hemolysis with lactate dehydrogenase (LDH) more than 600UI/L, aspartate aminotransferase (AST) more than 62UI/L or platelets less than 100000/μl. The syndrome is considered incomplete when any of the criteria is missing.

HELLP develops in approximately 0.1 to 0.8 percent of pregnancies overall and in 10 to 20 percent of women with severe preeclampsia/eclampsia (Sibai, 2014).

3.7. Postpartum Hypertension

Postpartum hypertension refers to women with normotensive gestations who develop hypertension in a period that ranges from 2 weeks to 6 months postpartum. Blood pressure remains labile for months postpartum, usually normalizing by the end of the first year. Little is known of this entity, and, like gestational hypertension, it may be a predictor of future chronic hypertension (Roberts et al. 2012).

3.8. Atypical Preeclampsia

3.8.1. Gestational hypertension without proteinuria or proteinuria without hypertension

It must be considered a form of preeclampsia when coexisting symptoms of severe preeclampsia like headaches, visual disturbances, dyspnea, ascites or blood pressure greater or equal to 160/110, or analytical alterations compatible with microangiopathy (Creatinine > 1.2 mg/dl, abnormal levels of LDH, AST/ALT and thrombocytopenia).

3.8.2. Preeclampsia before 20 weeks of gestation

The presence of hypertension, proteinuria and laboratory abnormalities in pregnant women less than 20 weeks must be ruled out lupus nephritis, hemolytic uremic syndrome, antiphospholipid syndrome and thrombotic thrombocytopenic purpura. Although preeclampsia/HELLP is the most common cause of hypertension, thrombocytopenia, liver abnormalities, and renal abnormalities in pregnant women, the following conditions should be considered and excluded, if possible. Laboratory findings in these disorders are compared in the following tables (Tables 6 and 7) (August, 2014).

Table 6. Frequency of various signs and symptoms among imitators of preeclampsia-eclampsia. UptoDate

Signs and symptoms	HELLP syndrome, percent	AFLP, percent	TTP, percent	HUS, percent	Exacerbation of SLE, percent
Hypertension	85	50	20-75	80-90	82 with APA, nephritis
Proteinuria	90-95	30-50	With hematuria	80-90	100 with nephritis
Fever	Absent	25-32	20-50	NR	Common during flare
Jaundice	5-10	40-90	Rare	Rare	Absent
Nausea and vomiting	40	50-80	Common	Common	Only with APA
Abdominal pain	60-80	35-50	Common	Common	Only with APA
Central nervous system	40-60	30-40	60-70	NR	50 with APA

HELLP: hemolysis, elevated liver enzymes, low platelets; AFLP: acute fatty liver of pregnancy; TTP: thrombotic thrombocytopenic purpura; HUS: hemolytic uremic syndrome; SLE: systemic lupus erythematosus; APA: antiphospholipid antibodies with or without catastrophic antiphospholipid syndrome; NR: values not reported; Common: reported as the most common presentation.

Table 7. Frequency and severity of laboratory findings among imitators of preeclampsia-eclampsia. UpToDate

Laboratory findings	HELLP syndrome	AFLP	TTP	HUS	Exacerbation of SLE
Thrombocytopenia (less than 100,000/mm)	More than 20,000	More than 50,000	20,000 or less	More than 20,000	More than 20,000
Hemolysis (percent)	50-100	15-20	100	100	14-23 with APA
Anemia (percent)	Less than 50	Absent	100	100	14-23 with APA
DIC (percent)	Less than 20	50-100	Rare	Rare	Rare
Hypoglycemia (percent)	Absent	50-100	Absent	Absent	Absent
VW factor multimers (percent)	Absent	Absent	80-90	80	Less than 10
ADAMTS13 less than 5 percent (percent)	Absent	Absent	33-100	Rare	Rare
Impaired renal function (percent)	50	90-100	30	100	40-80
LDH (IU/L)	600 or more	Variable	More than 1000	More than 1000	With APA
Elevated ammonia (percent)	Rare	50	Absent	Absent	Absent

Laboratory findings	HELLP syndrome	AFLP	TTP	HUS	Exacerbation of SLE
Elevated bilirubin (percent)	50-60	100	100	NA	Less than 10
Elevated transaminases (percent)	100	100	Usually mild*	Usually mild*	With APA

HELLP: hemolysis, elevated liver enzymes, low platelets; AFLP: acute fatty liver of pregnancy; TTP: thrombotic thrombocytopenic purpura; HUS: hemolytic uremic syndrome; SLE: systemic lupus erythematosus; APA: antiphospholipid antibodies with or without catastrophic antiphospholipid syndrome; DIC; disseminated intravascular coagulopathy: VW: von Willebrand; ADAMTS: von Willebrand factor-cleaving metalloprotease; LDH: lactic dehydrogenase; NR: values are not available. * Levels less than 100 IU/L.

4. EPIDEMIOLOGY

4.1. Prevalence

Preeclampsia is a public health problem and a major cause of maternal death. The prevalence ranges from 1.8-16.7%, but the cause remains unknown and is associated with significant health problems.

Worldwide, the incidence of preeclampsia ranges between 2-10% of all pregnancies, which is a precursor to eclampsia and variations exist worldwide. The World Health Organization (WHO) estimates that the incidence of preeclampsia is seven times higher in developing countries than in developed (2.8% and 0.4% of live births respectively). (Vargas-Hernández, Acosta & Moreno. 2012) (Duckitt & Harrington, 2005)

4.2. Risk Factors

The following table (Table 8) shows the risk factors of preeclampsia.

Table 8. Factors associated with an increased risk of developing preeclampsia. UpToDate

Nulliparity
Preeclampsia in a previous pregnancy
Age >40 years or <18 years
Family history of preeclampsia
Chronic hypertension
Chronic renal disease
Antiphospholipid antibody syndrome or inherited thrombophilia
Vascular or connective tissue disease
Diabetes mellitus (pregestational and gestational)

Table 8. (Continued)

Multifetal gestation
High body mass index
Black race
Male partner whose mother or previous partner had preeclampsia
Hydrops fetalis
Unexplained fetal growth restriction
Woman herself was small for gestational age
Fetal growth restriction, abruptio placentae, or fetal demise in a previous pregnancy
Prolonged interpregnancy interval
Partner related factors (new partner, limted sperm exposure [eg, previous use of barrier contraception])
Hydatidiform mole
Susceptibility genes

The most significant risk factors for developing pre-eclampsia are a history of pre-eclampsia and the presence of antiphospholipid antibodies. Preexisting diabetes and body mass index (BMI)greater than or equal to 35 previous pregnancycan multiply the risk for four; nulliparity,a family history of preeclampsia, and twin pregnancycan be multiplied by three; and maternal age over 40, a booking BMI of ≥35, and a systolic blood pressure ≥130 at booking double the risk (Duckitt, et al. 2005).

5. Etiopathogenesis

The molecular pathogenesis of phenotypic preeclampsia was largely unknown, but recent observations support the hypothesis that altered expression of placental anti-angiogenic factors are responsible for the clinical manifestation of the disease. These anti-angiogenic factors produce systemic endothelial dysfunction, resulting in hypertension, proteinuria, and the other systemic manifestations of preeclampsia. The molecular basis for placental dysregulation of these pathogenic factors remains unknown, and the last studies investigate the role of angiogenic proteins in early placental vascular development (Maynard & Karumanchi, 2011). Although the etiology remains unknown the most accepted pathogenetic factors are explained below. The pathogenesis is incompletely understood, but the disorder is clearly initiated by the presence of trophoblast. Impaired remodeling of uterine spiral arteries, reduced placental perfusion, increased inflammation, increased production of anti-angiogenic factors, and maternal endothelial cell damage are hallmarks of the disorder (August, 2014).

5.1. Abnormal Development of the Placenta

Impaired placentation with abnormal blood-flow velocity and resistance in placental vessels is associated with pre-eclampsia and fetal growth restriction (Velauthar et al., 2014). The spiral arteries undergo a series of morphological changes during normal pregnancy. The vessels are firstly invaded by trophoblast, which then becomes incorporated into the vessel wall and replaces the endothelium and muscular layer. This results in the conversion of the small spiral arteries into vessels of greater diameter with low resistance and high compliance, in absence of maternal vasomotor control. This vascular transformation in the uterus is necessary to ensure a dramatic increase in blood supply to the intervillous space. The underlying mechanism for the development of preeclampsia is thought to be impaired trophoblastic invasion of the maternal spiral arteries and their conversion from narrow muscular vessels to wide nonmuscular channels (Poon & Nicolaides, 2014).

Abnormal remodeling of spiral arteries: In normal pregnancies, the cytotrophoblast cells of the developing placenta migrate through the decidua and part of the myometrium to invade both the endothelium and highly muscular tunica media of the maternal spiral arteries, the terminal branches of the uterine artery that supply blood to the developing fetus/placenta (Figure 1).

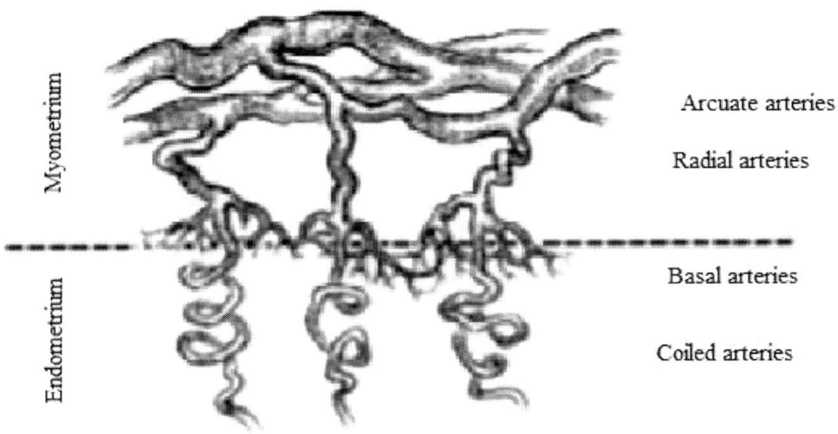

Figure 1. Stereographic representation of myometrial and endometrial arteries in the macaque. Above are shown parts of myometrial arcuate arteries from which myometrial radial arteries course toward the endometrium. There are found larger endometrial coiled arteries and smaller endometrial basal arteries. Modificated from UpToDate.

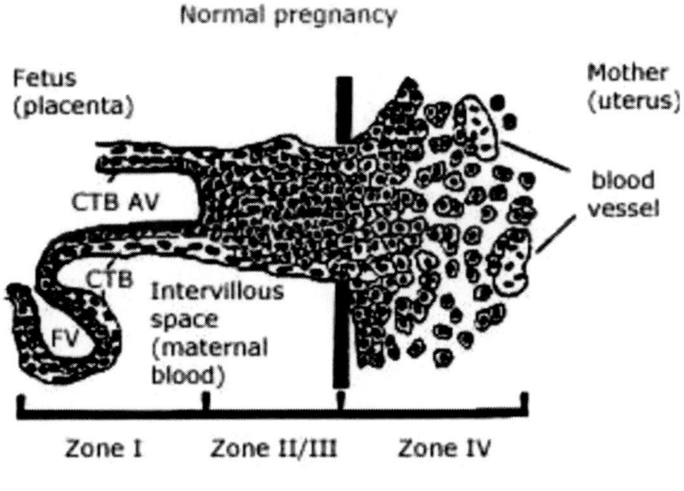

Figure 2. (Continued).

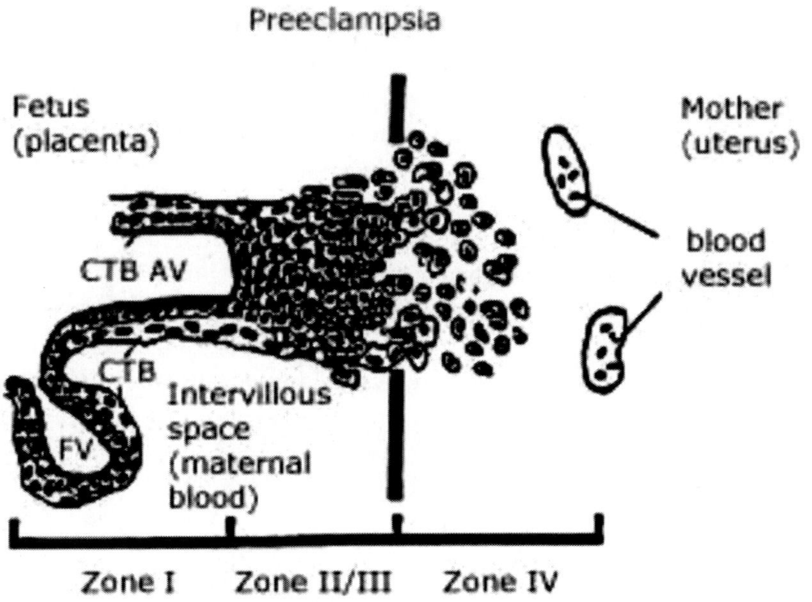

Figure 2. Diagram of anchoring villi (AV) at the maternalfetal interface in normal and preeclamptic pregnancy. The floating villi (FV) are in the intervillous space in direct contact with with the maternal blood. In normal pregnancy, invasive cytotrophoblasts (CTB) form cell columns (zone II/III) and invade maternal decidua and vasculature (zone IV). During the differentiation along the invasive path, the cytotrophoblasts dramatically alter their expression of various molecules, such as integrins. In preeclampsia, the invasive cytotrophoblasts fail to differentiate along the invasive pathway and do not gain access to spiral arteries. UpToDate.

By comparison, in preeclampsia, cytotrophoblast cells infiltrate the decidual portion of the spiral arteries, but fail to penetrate the myometrial segment. The spiral arteries fail to develop into large, tortuous vascular channels created by replacement of the musculoelastic wall with fibrinoid material; instead, the vessels remain narrow, resulting in placental hypoperfusion (Figure 2, Figure 3 and Figure 4).

Defective trophoblast differentiation: Is one possible mechanism responsible for defective trophoblast invasion of the spiral arteries. Trophoblast differentiation during endothelial invasion involves alteration in expression of a number of different classes of molecules. Hypoperfusion, hypoxia, ischemia: Hypoperfusion appears to be both a cause and a consequence of abnormal placental development and is also a result of abnormal placental development. The degree of hypoperfusion becomes more pronounced as pregnancy progresses since the abnormal uterine vasculature is unable to accommodate the normal rise in blood flow with increasing gestational age (Karumanchi, Lim & August, 2014).

5.2. Inmunologic Factors

Immune intolerance between maternal and fetal tissues.

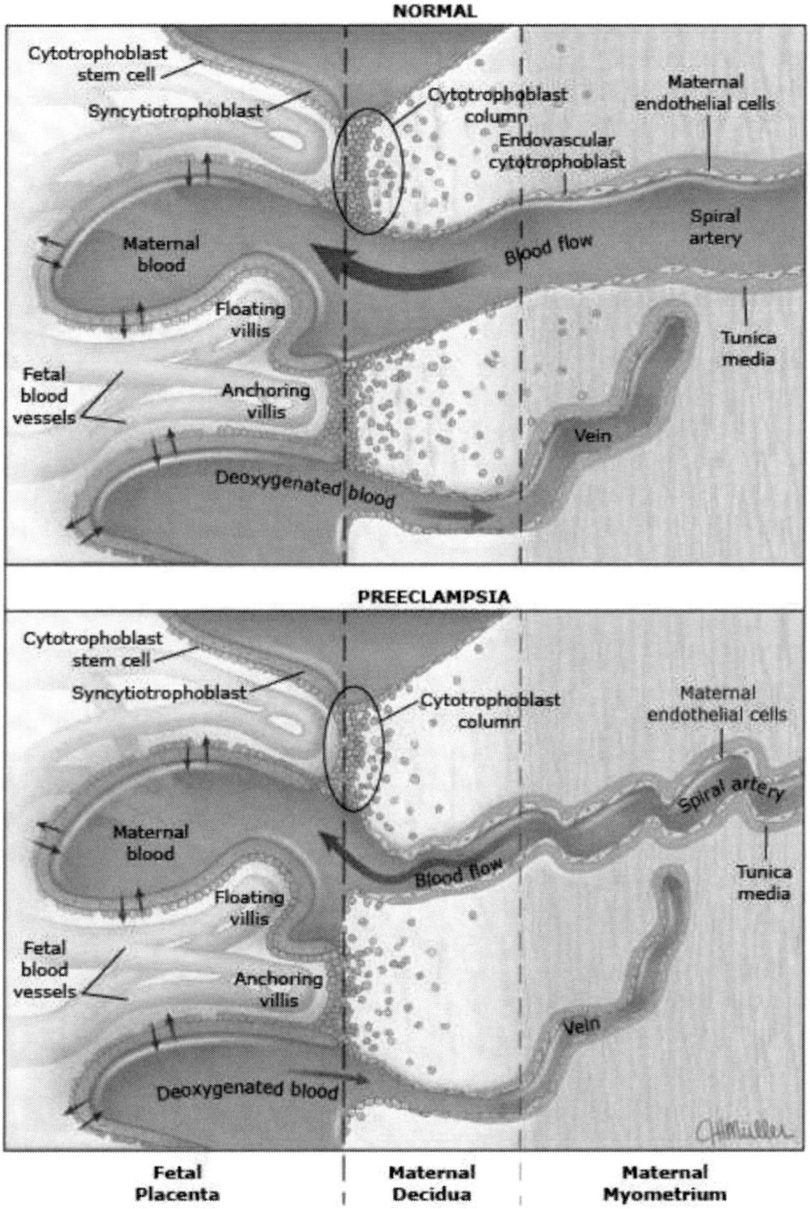

Figure 3. Abnormal placentation. Exchange of oxygen, nutrients, and waste products between the fetus and mother depends on adequate placental perfusion by maternal vessels. In normal placental development, invasive cytotrophoblasts of fetal origin invade the maternal spiral arteries, transforming them from small-caliber resistance vessels to high-caliber capacitance vessels capable of providing placental perfusion adequate to sustain the growing fetus. During the process of vascular invasion, the cytotrophoblasts differentiate from an epithelial phenotype to an endothelial phenotype, a process referred to as "pseudovasculogenesis" or "vascular mimicry" (Upper panel). In preeclampsia, cytotrophoblasts fail to adopt an invasive endothelial phenotype. Instead, invasion of the spiral arteries is shallow and they remain small caliber, resistance vessels (Lower panel). UpToDate.

5.3. Increased Sensivity to Angiotensin II

5.4. Genetic Factors

Although most cases of preeclampsia are sporadic, genetic factors are thought to play a role in disease susceptibility. Some studies suggest a possible genetic predisposition:

5.4.1. Primigravid women with a family history of preeclampsia are two tofive timeshigher risk of the disease than primigravid women without history.
5.4.2. The risk of preeclampsia is increased more than seven-fold in women who have had preeclampsia in a previous pregnancy.
5.4.3. Although not usually include the father figure in this disease has been observed that wives of men with a history of pregnancies with preeclampsia who were enrolled are more likely to develop preeclampsia compared with women without such a history in their husband.

5.5. Diet

The daily calcium intake may be related to the development of preeclampsia. The results are varied according to studies. It has shown no benefit in healthy nulliparous women with an adequate intake of calcium daily. The recommended daily dose during pregnancy is 1000 milligrams of calcium. Some clinical trials showed a reduced risk of developing preeclampsia with calcium supplementation in women with high risk factors. On the subject of calcium supplementation is important and dependent on the characteristics of the population (August, 2014).

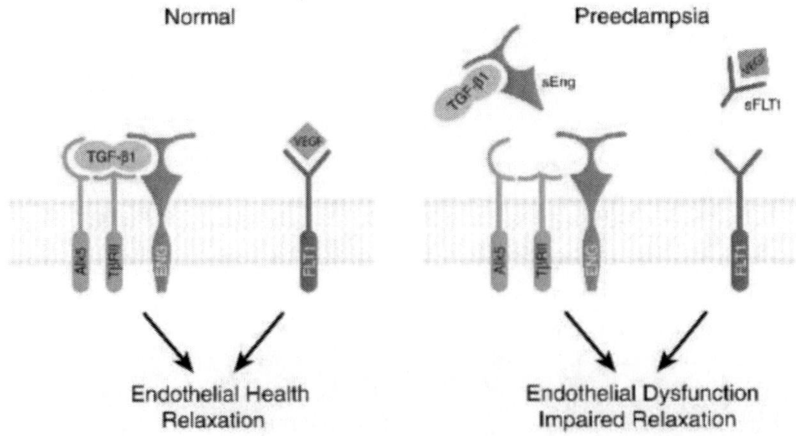

Figure 4. sFlt1 and sEng cause endothelial dysfunction by antagonizing VEGF and TGF-β1 signaling. Under physiologic conditions, and during normal pregnancy, VEGF and TGF-β1 maintain endothelial health by interacting with their endogenous endothelial receptors. In preeclampsia, excess placental secretion of sFlt1 and sEng inhibit VEGF and TGF-β1 signaling, respectively, in the vasculature. This results in endothelial cell dysfunction, including decreased prostacyclin, nitric oxide production, and release of procoagulant proteins. (Maynard et al., 2011).

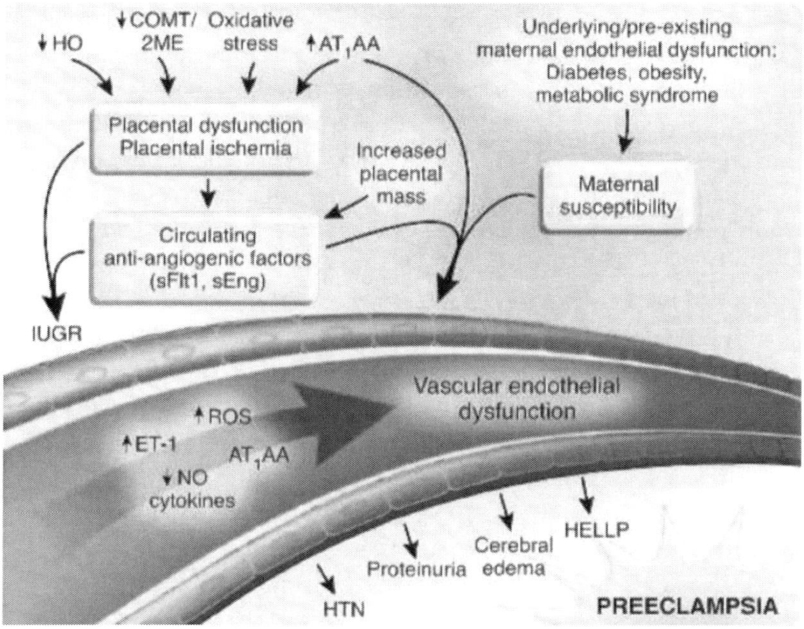

Figure 5. Hypothetical framework for the pathogenesis of preeclampsia. Placental dysfunction, triggered by poorly understood mechanisms—including genetic, immunologic, and environmental—plays an early and primary role in the development of preeclampsia. Alterations in regulatory factors including HO, catechol-o-methyltransferase (COMT)/2- methoxyestradiol (2ME), and angiotensin type 1 agonistic autoantibodies (AT1AA) lead to excess placental secretion of angiogenic factors into the maternal circulation. These factors lead to impaired VEGF/PlGF and TGF-β signaling, resulting in systemic endothelial cell dysfunction mediated by a variety of factors, as shown. Endothelial dysfunction, in turn, results in the systemic manifestations of preeclampsia (Maynard et al., 2011).

5.6. Systemic Endotelial Dysfunction

From a clinical point of view, the consequences of endothelial dysfunction associated with sustained elevated blood pressure, appear to be related to two fundamental aspects: one functional consequence of the imbalance in the regulation of vasomotor tone and that is the maintenance of elevated peripheral resistance, and a structural consequence of the growth of the vascular wall due to the imbalance between growth-promoting factors and inhibitors of this. Both alterations perpetuate and maintain hypertension and appear to be due to the development of organ damage associated with it; therefore can be considered that endothelial dysfunction is the link between hypertension and cardiovascular morbidity and mortality (Lahera, Cediel, de las Heras, Vázquez-Pérez, Sanz-Rosa, Vázquez-Cruz, & Cachofeiro, 2003).

6. Early Prediction

A good test for predicting women who will develop preeclampsia should be simple, rapid, noninvasive, inexpensive, easy to perform, and should not expose the patient to discomfort or risk. The technology should be widely available and the results reproducible and reliable, with a high likelihood ratio for a positive test and a low likelihood ratio for a negative result and good sensitivity and specificity. Ideally, it should provide an opportunity for intervention to prevent development of the disease, or at least result in better maternal and/or fetal outcomes (Norwitz, 2014). The likelihood ratio (LR) of a particular test result is the proportion of participants with the target condition who have a positive test result relative to the proportion without the target condition who have the same test result. Because the incidence of preeclampsia is relatively low, screening tests with positive test results require high LRs to adequately predict the disease's probability, and tests with negative results require low LRs to confidently exclude the disorder. Thus, useful prediction for preeclampsia would require a high LR (greater than 10) for a positive test as well as a low LR for a negative result (less than 0.2) (Roberts et al., 2012). The aim of such early identification of women at high-risk is to allow intensive maternal and fetal monitoring, leading to an earlier diagnosis of PE with the potential for mitigating an adverse outcome (Akolekar, Syngelaki, Sarquis, Zvanca & Nicolaides, 2011). Early-onset, rather than late-onset, preeclampsia is associated with an increased risk of perinatal morbidity and mortality, and both short-term and long-term maternal complications (Nicolaides, 2013).

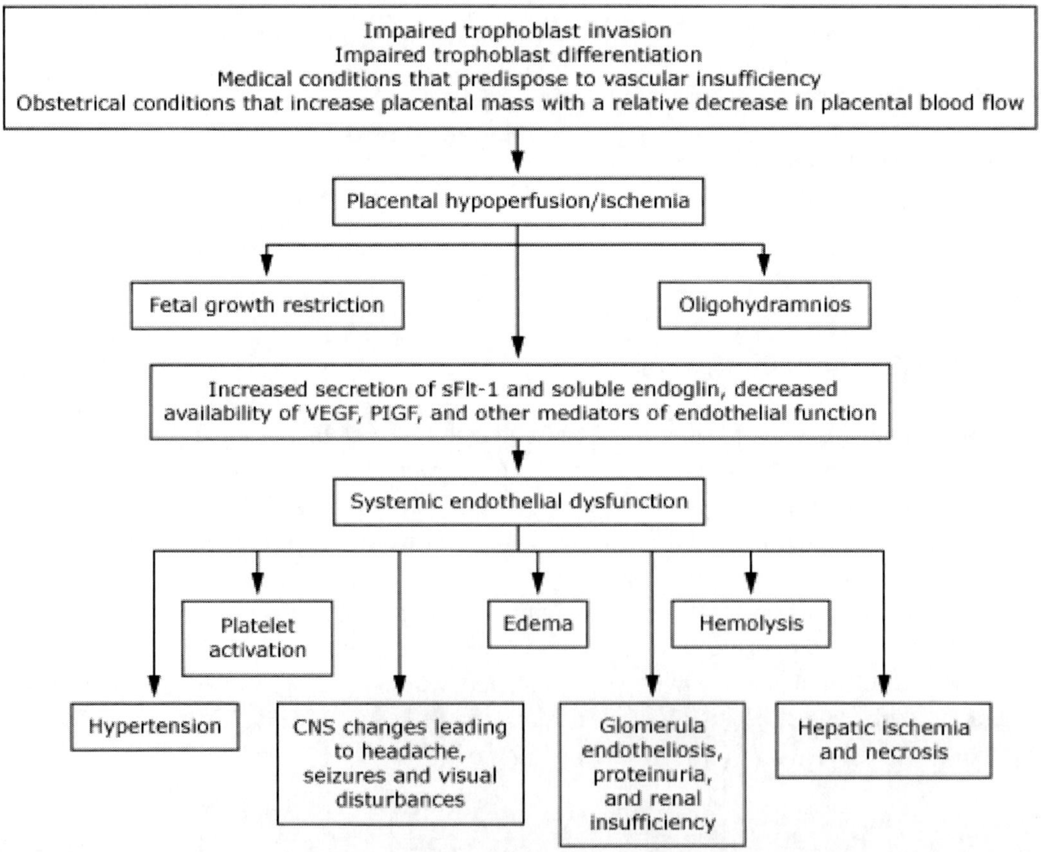

Figure 6. Model for pathogenesis of preeclampsia. UpToDate. sFlt-1: Soluble fms-like tyrosine kinase-1 VEGF: vascular endothelial growth factor, PIGF: placental growth factor, CNS: central nervous system.

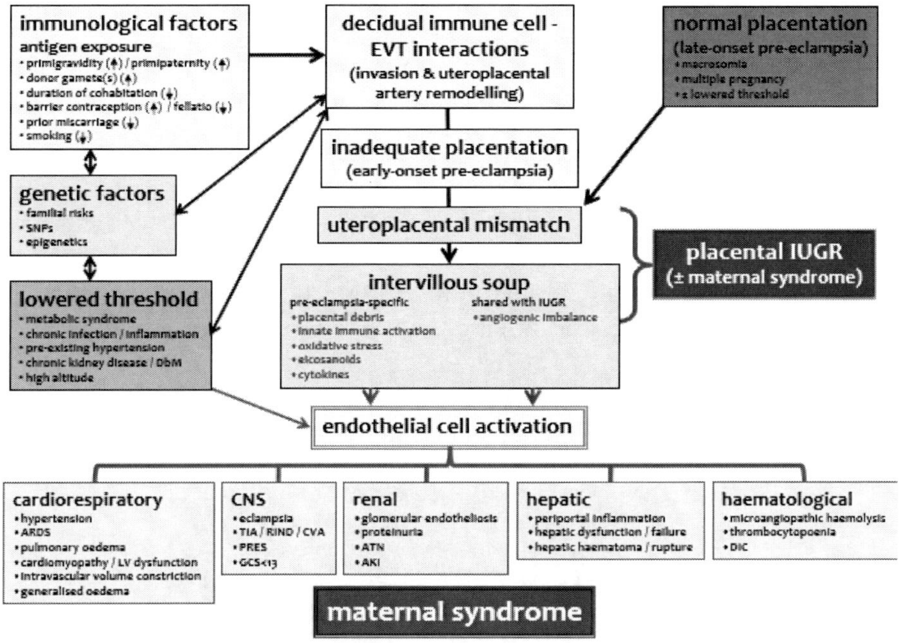

Figure 7. The origins and consequences of preeclampsia. EVT: extravillous trophoblast; SNP: single nucleotide polymorphism; ARDS: acute respiratory distress syndrome; CNS: central nervous system; TIA: transient ischemic attack; RIND: reversible ischemic neurological deficit; CVA: cerebrovascular accident; PRES: posterior reversible encephalopathy syndrome; GCS: Glasgow Coma Scale; ATN: acute tubular necrosis; AKI: acute kidney injury; DIC: disseminated intravascular coagulation; DbM: diabetes mellitus; LV: left ventricle. (Magee, et al., 2014)

6.1. Prediction of Preeclampsia Using Uterine Artery Doppler Velocimetry

A good screening for preeclampsia can be achieved by measurement of the uterine artery pulsatility index (PI) at 11–13weeks of gestation, used in combination with other markers like maternal history, blood pressure, serum pregnancy-associated plasma protein-A and placental growth factor (Nicolaides, 2011). For a false-positive rate of 5%, it has been estimated that the new combined method of screening can predict 90% of cases of preeclampsia requiring delivery before 34 weeks and 45% of cases of late-onset preeclampsia (Khalil & Nicolaides, 2013).

How to record uterine artery Doppler?

For uterine artery pulsatility index (PI measurement, the gestational age must be between 11 and 13+6 weeks. Transabdominal ultrasound should be used to obtain a midsagittal section of the uterus and cervical canal. The internal cervical os should be identified and the transducer tilted gently from side to side in each paracervical region, using color flow mapping, to identify the uterine arteries as aliasing vessels coursing along the side of the cervix and uterus (Figure 7). Pulsed wave Doppler should be used to obtain flow velocity waveforms from the ascending branch of the uterine artery at the point closest to the internal os. Pulsed wave Doppler is then used with the sampling gate set at 2mm to cover the whole vessel and care should be taken to ensure that the angle of insonation is less tan 30o. When three similar consecutive waveforms are obtained, the PI should be measured and the mean PI of the left and right arteries calculated (Figure 8) (Khalil, 2013) (Poon, 2014).

6.2. Prediction of Preeclampsia Using Biomarkers

A large number of biochemical markers have been investigated for the prediction of preeclampsia (Table 9). Biomarkers for the prediction of preeclampsia are integral to disease stratification and targeted therapy. Results from mechanistic studies not only have provided insights into the pathogenesis of the disease, but also have created opportunities to study circulating and urinary biomarkers to predict the disease. Maternal serum PAPP-A and PlGF are two biochemica lmarkers that have been investigated extensively and have shown promising results in the early prediction of preeclampsia (Roberts et al., 2012).

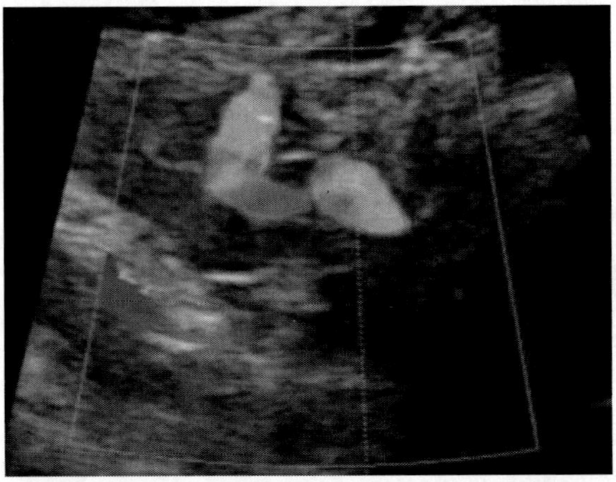

Figure 8. Parasagittal section of the uterus and cervix. Color flow mapping is used to identify the uterine arteries as aliasing vessels coursing along the side of the cervix and uterus (Khalil, 2013).

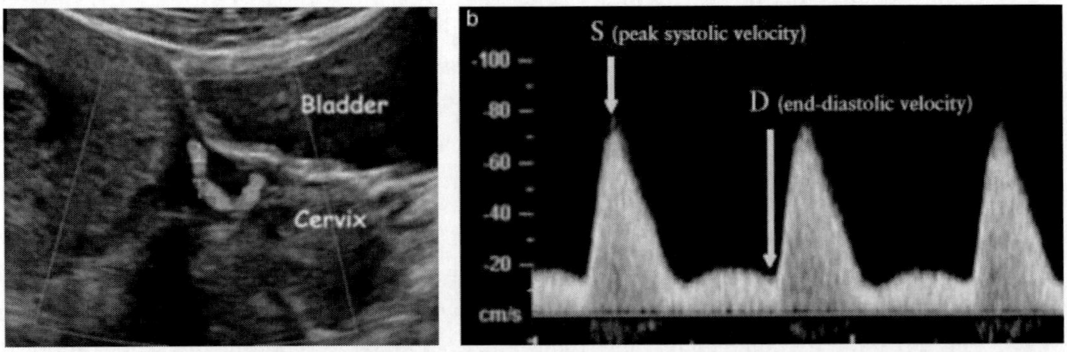

Figure 9. (a) The ascending branch of the uterine artery at its paracervical portion and at the point closest to the internal os is identified and pulsed wave Doppler is used to obtain flow velocity waveforms. (b) When three similar consecutive waveforms are obtained, the pulsatility index (PI) should be measured and the mean PI of the left and right arteries calculated. The PI is calculated as the difference between the peak systolic velocity (S) and the end-diastolic velocity (D), divided by the mean velocity (Vm): PI=(S−D)/Vm (Khalil, 2013).

PAPP-A is a syncytiotrophoblast-derived metalloproteinase, which enhances the mitogenic function of the insulin-like growth factors by cleaving the complex formed between such growth factors and their binding proteins. Low serum PAPP-A is associated with a higher incidence of preeclampsia. Increased level of maternal serum PAPP-A has been observed in established preeclapmsia.

PlGF, aglycosylated dimeric glycoprotein, is a member of the vascular endotelial growth factor subfamily. It binds to vascular endotelial growth factor receptor-1 which has been shown to rise in pregnancy. Preeclapmsia is associated with reduced placental production of PlGF and several studies reported that during the clínical phase the maternal serum PlGF concentration is reduced. These reduced levels precede the clinical onset of the disease and are evident from both the first and second-trimesters of pregnancy (Poon, 2014).

Table 9. Proposed maternal biochemical markers for the prediction of preeclampsia (Poon, 2014)

A disintegrin and metalloprotease 12(ADAM12)	L-Arginine
Activin-A	L-Homoarginine
Adiponectin	Leptin
Adrenomedullin	Magnesium
Alphafetoprotein	Matrix metalloproteinase-9
Alpha-1-microglobulin	Microalbuminuria
Ang-2angiopoietin-2 Antiphospholipidantibodies	Microtransferrinuria
AntithrombinIII	N-Acetyl-β-glucosaminidase
Atrial natriuretic peptide	Neurokinin B
Beta2-microglobulin	NeuropeptideY
C-reactive protein	Neutrophil gelatinase-associated lipocalin
Calcium	P-Selectin
Cellular adhesión molecules	Pentraxin 3
Circulating trophoblast	Placenta growth factor
Corticotropin release hormone	Placental protein 13
Cytokines	Plasminogen activator inhibitor-2
Dimethylarginine(ADMA)	Platelet activation
Endothelin	Platelet count
Estriol	Pregnancy associated plasma protein-A
Ferritin	Prostacyclin
FetalDNA	Relaxin
FetalRNA	Resistin
Free feta lhemoglobin	Serum lipids
Fibronectin	Soluble endoglin
Geneticmarkers	Soluble fms-like tyrosine kinase Thromboxane
Haptoglobin	Thyroidfunction
Hematocrit	Totalproteins
Homocysteine	Transferrin
Human chorionic gonadotropin	Tumor necrosis factor receptor-1
Human placental growth hormone InhibinA	Uric acid
Insulin-like growth factor	Urinary calcium to creatinine ratio
Insulin-like growth factor binding protein Insulin resistance	Urinary kallikrein
	Vascular endothelia lgrowth factor
Isoprostanes	Visfatin
	VitaminD

Alterations in concentrations of sFlt-1, PlGF, and soluble endoglin in the maternal circulation precede the clinical onset of preeclampsia by several weeks to months. The higher the sFlt-1 concentration, the more predictive it is of early-onset preeclampsia. However, because sFlt-1 is altered only 4–5 weeks before the onset of clinical symptoms, it is not useful when used alone as a screening test earlier in gestation. PlGF concentrations begin to decrease 9 to 11 weeks before the appearance of hypertension and proteinuria, which accelerates during the 5 weeks before the onset of disease.

First-trimester circulating levels of placental protein-13(PP13) are significantly lower in women who go on to develop early-onset preeclampsia and preterm birth. PP13 is predominantly expressed by the syncytiotrophoblast and released from the placenta into the maternal circulation. Indeed, PP13 turned to be a good early biomarker to assess maternal risk for the subsequent development of pregnancy complications caused by impaired placentation (Than et al., 2014). Combining first-trimester placental protein-13 with other predictive markers may further improve predictive performance.

Best results are obtained by combining individual markers: the logs of uterine pulsatility index, mean arterial pressure, pregnancy-associated plasma protein A (PAPP-A), serum-free PlGF, body mass index, and presence of nulliparity or previous preeclampsia (Roberts et al., 2012).

The table below (Table 10) shows the latest studies published with algorithms for the early detection of preeclampsia. The results are shown at a fixed false-positive rate (FPR) of 10%, exceptions are indicated.

The table shows that all sensitivity ranges are between 40 and 60% approximately. We can see an increased detection rates with the combination of more markers or in the detection of early onset preeclampsia.

7. TREATMENT

The first consideration in the management of women with mild gestational hypertension or preeclampsia without severe features is always safety of the woman and her fetus. The decision to treat hypertension during pregnancy should consider the risks and benefits for both mother and fetus. The level of blood pressure is the most important factor, as treatment of severe hypertension (systolic BP ≥160 mmHg and/or diastolic BP ≥110 mmHg) has a well-established maternal benefit of reduction in stroke risk (Roberts et al., 2012) (August, 2014).

7.1. Chronic Hypertension

The objective is to stabilize blood pressure and achieve levels less than or equal to 160/100. You can use different drugs, the choice of these depends on the experience and contraindications. The most used drugs are shown in Tables 11 and 12.

7.2. Gestational Hypertension

The indications for and choice of antihypertensive therapy in women with gestational hypertension are the same as for women with preeclampsia.

Table 10. Combined early screening of preeclampsia using various markers (Own desing). NR: Not reported. FPR: false-positive rates. PE: preeclampsia. PP13: Placental protein 13

Author	Markers	Results	Weeks of gestation
Di Lorenzo, 2012	Maternal history, utetine artery Doppler, serum biomarkers (PAPP-A, PlGF, PP-13, free β-hCG)	Sensitivity 60% (20%FPR) Specificity NR	11 - 13
Myatt, 2012	Maternal history, complete blood count, biochemical markers (ADAM-12, PAPP-A, PP13, PlGF, soluble fms-liketyrosine kinase-1, endoglin), systolic blood pressure	Sensitivity 46,1% Specificity 80%	9 - 12+6
Scazzocchio, 2013	Maternal history, biochemical markers (PAPP-A, free β-hCG), blood pressure, uterine artery Doppler	Sensitivity 39,6% (80,8% for early PE) Specificity NR	8 - 12 (laboratory markers) 11 - 13+6 (Doppler)
Akolekar, 2013	Maternal history, uterine artery pulsatility index, mean arterial pressure, biochemical markers (PAPP-A, PLGF)	Sensitivity 54% (96% before 34 weeks) Specificity NR	11 - 13
Myers, 2013	Maternal history, biochemical markers (PlGF, soluble endoglin and sFlt-1)	Sensitivity 45% (5% FPR) Specificity NR	14 - 16
Than, 2014	Maternal history, biochemical markers (PP-13), uterine artery pulsatility index	Sensitivity of PP13 52-59% (combination of all markers 93% early onset and 86% for all PE) Specificity NR	6 - 14
Giguére, 2014	Body mass index (BMI), mean arterial pressure (MAP), placental growth factor, soluble Fms-like tyrosine kinase-1, pregnancy-associated plasma protein A and inhibin A.	Sensitivity 39-50% Specificity NR	10 - 18

7.3. Preeclampsia

The definitive treatment of preeclampsia is delivery, which is always beneficial for the mother. As long as the pregnant remains undelivered, she is at increased risk of complications. The only benefit that has been demonstrated so far of antihypertensive therapy in pregnant women with mild hypertension is a reduction in risk of developing severe hypertension. The goal is to get a blood pressure between 140-155 systolic and diastolic between 90-105 with the minimum effective dose. Is important avoiding abrupt decreases in blood pressure because of the risk of placental hypoperfusion. Labetalol is considered the drug of first-line. The doses used in intravenous therapy to control blood pressure in acute cases are shown in table 9.

If blood pressure is not controlled should assess the need for pharmacological prevention of seizures. Prevention will be made in cases that have severity criteria (Table 5).

The first-line agent is magnesium sulfate. Magnesium sulfate is given intravenously to patients on the labor and delivery unit to prevent convulsions, and for fetal/neonatal neuroprotection in pregnancies between 24 and 32 weeks of gestation. Magnesium sulfate should be used in standard dosing, usually 4g intravenous loading dose followed by 1 g/hour (Magee et al., 2014). The goal is to maintain plasma levels between 4.2-8.4 mg/dl. The treatment of poisoning by magnesium sulfate is calcium glucamate, intravenous bolus of 1 gram administered in 3-4 minutes (Hernández, Gómez, Bellart, Domenech, Peguero, Mazarico, Plaza, Figueras, 2013). It is important to emphasize that seizure prophylaxis does not prevent progression of disease unrelated to convulsions. Approximately 10 to 15 percent of women in labor with nonsevere preeclampsia will develop signs of severe preeclampsia or abruptio placenta, whether or not they receive magnesium therapy (Norwitz & Repke, 2014).

7.4. HELLP Syndrome

After the diagnosis is confirmed, the initial steps in management are to stabilize the mother, assess the fetal condition, and decide whether prompt delivery is indicated. Antihypertensive drugs are used to treat severe hypertension. The approach to antihypertensive therapy is the same as that for preeclampsia (Tables 11 and 12). Actively bleeding patients with thrombocytopenia should be transfused with platelets. Platelet transfusion may be indicated to prevent excessive bleeding during delivery if the platelet count is less than 20,000 cells/microL, but the threshold for prophylactic platelet transfusion in this setting is controversial. The decision depends on patient specific factors; consultation with the hematology service may be helpful (Sibai, 2014). Antepartum treatment with high-dose corticosteroids. There are data demonstrating a clinical and laboratory improvement temporarily. Should be initiated if the platelet count is less than 100000 cells/microL (Hernández et al., 2013).

7.5. Timing of Delivery

It is important to know when is necessary to end the pregnancy, for it will be taken into account the risks and benefits for both mother and fetus.

Table 11. Common Oral Antihypertensive Agents in Pregnancy (Roberts et al., 2012)

Drug	Dosage	Comments
Labetalol	200-2400mg/d orally in two to three divided doses	Well tolerated Potencial bronchoconstricitve effects Avoid in patients with asthma and congestive heart failure
Nifedipine	30-120 mg/d orally of a slow- released preparation	Do not use sublingual
Methyldopa	0.5-3 g/d orally in two or three divided doses	Childhood safety data up to 7 years of age My not be as effective in control of severe hypertension
Thiazide diuretics	Depends on agent	Second-line agent
Angiotensin-converting enzyme inhibitors/ angiotensin receptor blockers		Associated with fetal anomalies Contraindicated in pregnancy and preconception period

Table 12. Antihypertensive Agents Used for Urgent Blood Pressure Control in Pregnancy (Roberts et al., 2012)

Drug	Dose	Comments
Labetalol	10–20 mg IV, then 20–80 mg every 20–30 min to a maximum dose of 300 mg or Constant infusion 1–2 mg/min IV	Considered a first-line agent Tachycardia is less common and fewer adverse effects Contraindicated in patients with asthma, heart disease, or congestive heart failure
Hydralazine	5mg IV or IM, then 5-10 mg IV every 20-40 min or constant infusión 0.5-10 mg/h	Higher or frecuente dosage associated with maternal hypotension, headaches, and fetal ditress- may be more common tan other agentes
Nifedipine	10-20 mg orally, reapeat in 30 minutes if needed; then 10-20 mg every 2-6 hours	May observe reflex tachycardia and headaches

7.5.1. Chronic/preexisting Hypertension

For women with uncomplicated preexisting hypertension who are otherwise well at ≥ 37 weeks of gestation, delivery should be considered at 38 to 39+6 weeks of gestation (Magee et al., 2014)

7.5.2. HELLP Syndrome

The key of therapy is delivery. This is curative and the only effective treatment. There is consensus among experts that prompt delivery is indicated after maternal stabilization for any of the following:

- Pregnancies ≥34 weeks of gestation
- Nonreassuring tests of fetal status
- Presence of severe maternal disease

When both the maternal and fetal status are reassuring, we administer a course of corticosteroids before delivering pregnancies complicated by HELLP syndrome at less than 34 weeks of gestation. Although a short delay in delivery for corticosteroid administration appears to be safe, we do not advise attempts to delay delivery beyond 48 hours because disease progression usually occurs, sometimes with rapid maternal deterioration (Sibai, 2014).

7.5.3. Gestational Hypertension or Preeclampsia

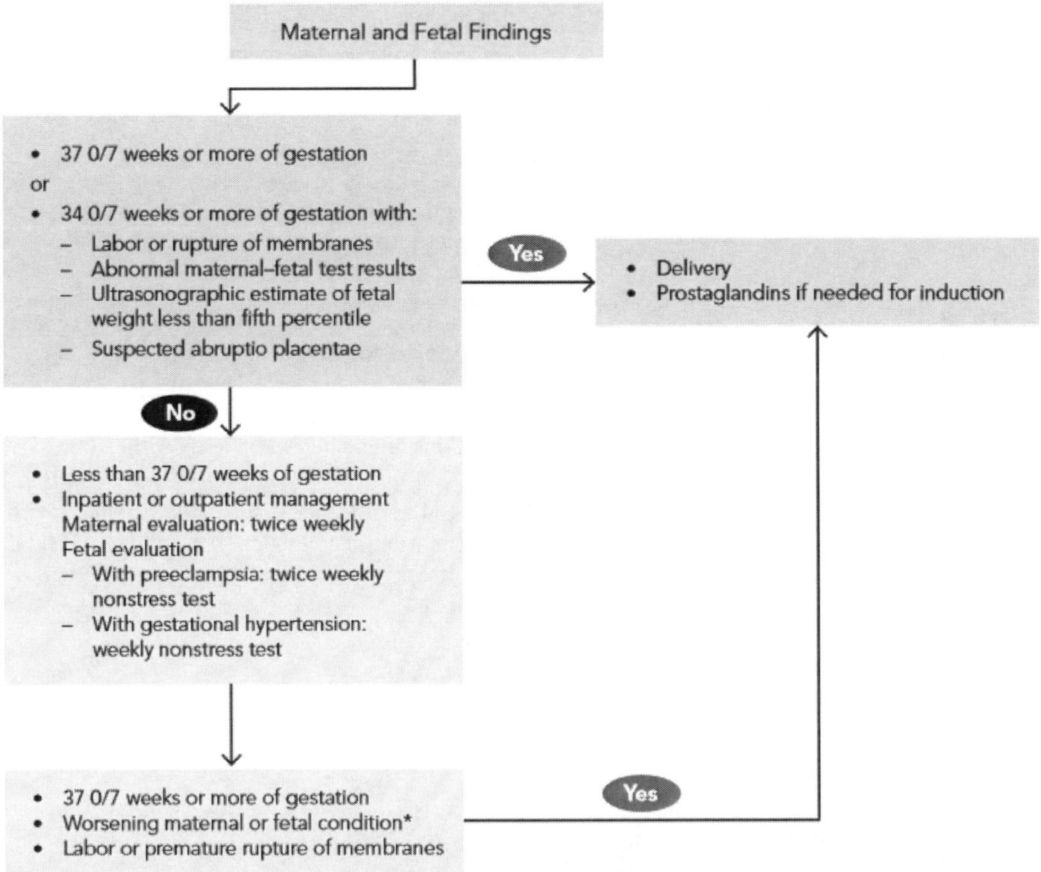

Figure 10. Management of mild gestational hypertension or preeclampsia without severe features (Roberts et al., 2012).

7.5.4. Severe Preeclampsia

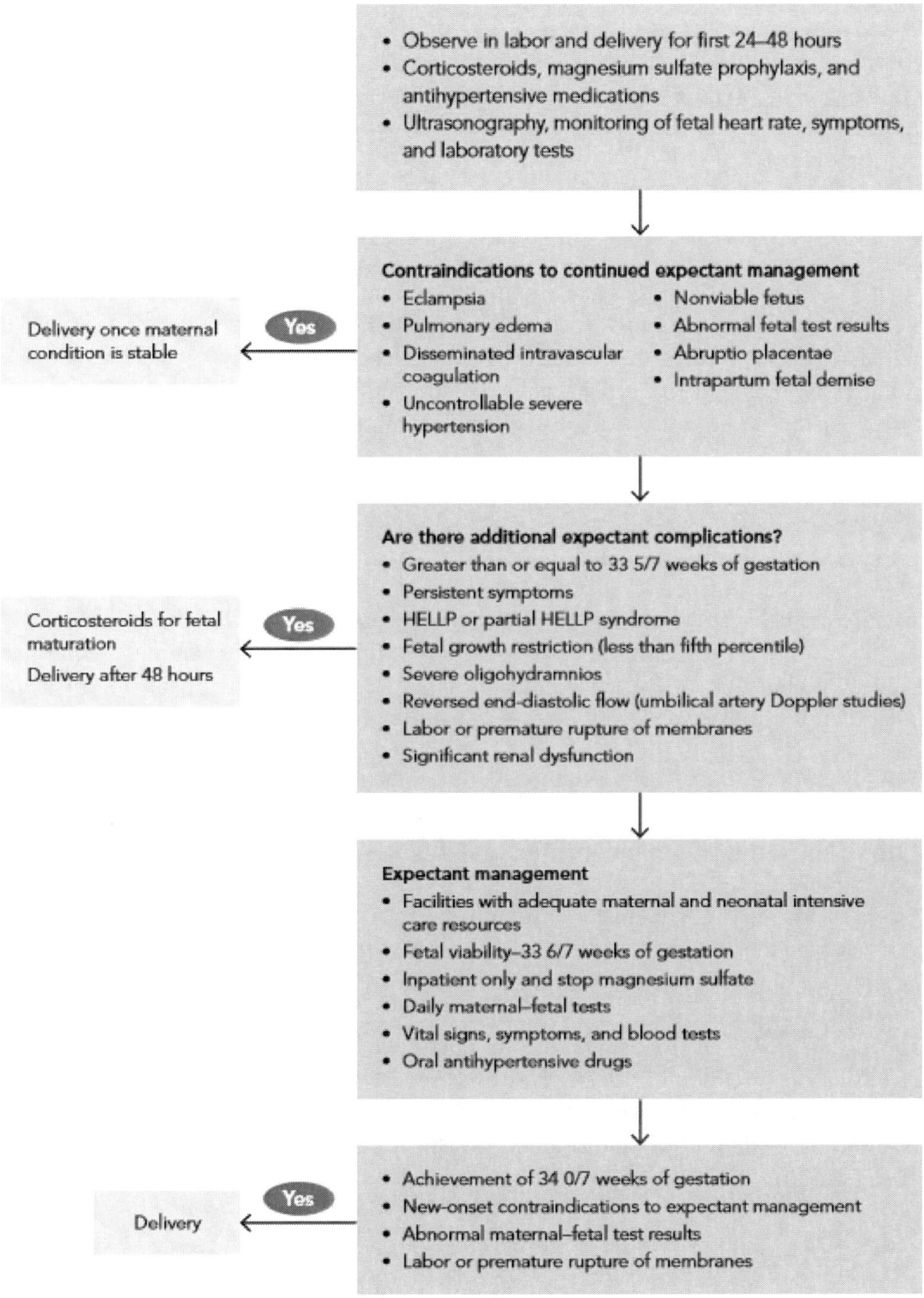

Figure 11. Management of severe preeclampsia at less than 34 weeks of gestation (Roberts et al., 2012).

8. PREVENTION

Many different strategies to prevent preeclampsia have been investigated, but none have been found to be widely effective. It is not surprising that these simple approaches have been unsuccessful, given the complexities in pathogenesis and the likelihood that multiple etiologies cause the syndrome even though the clinical manifestations of elevated blood pressure and proteinuria are common to most cases (August, 2014).

8.1. Antiplatelet Agents

It has been hypothesized that alterations in systemic prostacyclin–thromboxane balance contribute to preeclampsia. Low-dose aspirin, an antiinflammatory agent that blocks the production of thromboxanes, has been studied in dozens of trials for the prevention of preeclampsia, both in high-risk groups and in healthy nulliparous women. For women at high risk of preeclampsia, several small, early trials suggested daily aspirin had a significant protective effect.

8.2. Antioxidant Supplementation with Vitamin C and Vitamin E

Because oxidative stress appears to contribute to the pathogenesis of preeclampsia, it has been suggested that antioxidants may prevent preeclampsia. There were an initial enthusiasm for using a combination of the antioxidants vitamin C and vitamin E, but recent studies confirmed that used vitamin C and vitamin E for the prevention of preeclampsia found no benefit.

8.3. Other Nutritional Interventions and Lifestyle Modifications

Several studies have examined the effectiveness of calcium supplementation to prevent preeclampsia, and the benifits only have been showed in women with nutritional deficiency of calcium (low baseline calcium intake, less tan 600mg/day). Another study nutrient is vitamin D, the deficiency has been suggested as a factor contributing to preeclampsia, but the benefit is unknown. No consensus exists in restricting salt intake or activity for primary prevention of preeclampsia or progression of disease. However, reduced physical activity may be useful for improving uterine blood flow in pregnancies with fetal growth restriction, and may be a useful adjunct to antihypertensive therapy in women with high blood pressure (August, 2014) (Roberts et al., 2012).

References

Akolekar, R., Syngelaki, A., Poon, L., Wright, D. & Nicolaides, K. H. (2013). Competing Risks Model in Early Screening for Preeclampsia by Biophysical and Biochemical Markers. *Fetal Diagnosis and Therapy*,2013, 33, 8–15. DOI: 10.1159/000341264.

Akolekar, R., Syngelaki, A., Sarquis, R., Zvanca, M. & Nicolaides, K. H. (2011). Prediction of early, intermediate and late pre-eclampsia from maternal factors, biophysical and biochemical markers at 11-13 weeks. *Prenatal Diagnosis*, *31*(1), 66-74. Doi: 10.1002/pd.2660.

August, P. (2014). Management of hypertension in pregnant and postpartum women. *UpToDate 2014*. www.uptodate.com.

August, P. (2014). Preeclampsia: Prevention.*UpToDate 2014*. www.uptodate.com.

August, P. & Sibai, B. M. (2014). Preeclampsia: Clinical features and diagnosis. *UpToDate 2014*. www.uptodate.com.

Di Lorenzo, G., Ceccarello, M., Cecotti, V., Ronfani, L., Monasta, L., Vecchi Brumatti, L., et al. (2012). First trimester maternal serum PIGF, free beta-hCG, PAPP-A, PP-13, uterine artery Doppler and maternal history for the prediction of preeclampsia. *Placenta 2012*, *33*, 495–501.

Duckitt, K. & Harrington, D. (2005). Risk factors for pre-eclampsia at antenatal booking: systematic review of controlled studies. *British Medical Journal (Clinical research ed.)*, *330*(7491), 565.

Giguére, Y., Massé, J., Thériault, S., Bujold, E., Laford, J., Rousseau, F. & Forest, J. C. (2014). Screening for pre-eclampsia early in pregnancy: performance of a multivariable model combining clinical characteristics and biochemical markers. *British Journal of Obstetrics and Gynaecology 2014*. DOI: 10.1111/1471-0528.13050.

Hernández, S., Gómez, D., Bellart, J., Domenech, M., Peguero, A., Mazarico, E., Plaza, A., Figueras, F. (2013). Protocolo hipertensión y gestación. *Guías clínicas de medicina materno-fetal. Hospital Clínic.* http://www.medicinafetalbarcelona.org/clinica/images/protocolos/patologia_materna_obstetrica/hipertensi%F3n%20y%20gestaci%F3n.pdf.

Khalil, A. & Nicolaides, K. H. (2013). How to record uterine artery Doppler in the first trimester. *Ultrasound in Obstetrics and Gynecology 2013*, *42*, 478–479. DOI: 10.1002/uog.12366.

Karumanchi, S. A, Lim, K. H. & August, P. (2014). Preeclampsia: Pathogenesis.*UpToDate 2014*. www.uptodate.com.

Lahera, V., Cediel, E., de las Heras, N., Vázquez-Pérez, S., Sanz-Rosa, D., Vázquez-Cruz, B. & Cachofeiro, V. (2003). Alteraciones del endotelio en la hipertensión. *Nefrología2003*. Vol. *XXIII*. Suplemento 4.

Magee, L. A., Pels, A., Helewa, M., Rey, E., Dadelszen, P. von, Hypertension Guideline, C., Audibert, F., et al. (2014). Diagnosis, evaluation, and management of the hypertensive disorders of pregnancy: executive summary. *J Obstet Gynaecol Can*, *36*(5), 416-438.

Magloire, L. & Funai, E. F. (2014). Gestational hypertension. *UpToDate 2014.* www.uptodate.com.

Maynard, S. E. & Karumanchi, S. A. (2011). Angiogenic Factors and Preeclampsia. *Seminars in Nephrology*, *31*(1), 33-46.

Meher, S. & Alfirevic, Z. (2013). Aspirin for pre-eclampsia: Beware of subgroup meta-analysis. *Ultrasound in Obstetrics and Gynecology2013*, *41*, 479–48. DOI: 10.1002/uog.12470

Myatt, L., Clifton, R. G., Roberts, J. M., Spong, C. Y., Hauth, J. C., Varner, M. W., et al. (2012) First-trimester prediction of preeclampsia in nulliparous women at low risk. *Obstet Gynecol 2012*, *119*, 1234–42.

Myers, J., Kenny, L., McCowan, L., Chan, E., Dekker, G., Poston, L., et al. (2013). Angiogenic factors combined with clinical risk factors to predict preterm pre-eclampsia in nulliparous women: a predictive test accuracy study. *British Journal of Obstetrics and Gynaecology 2013*, *120*, 1215–23.

NICE clinical guideline 107 (2011) Hypertension in pregnancy. The management of hypertensive disorders during pregnancy. *National Institute for Health and Clinical Excellence 2011.* guidance.nice.org.uk/cg107.

Nicolaides, K. H. (2011). Turning the pyramid of prenatal care. *Fetal Diagnosis and Therapy*, *29*(3), 183-196. Doi: 10.1159/000324320.

Norwitz, E. R. (2014). Eclampsia. *UpToDate 2014.* www.uptodate.com.

Norwitz, E. R. & Repke, J. T. (2014). Preeclampsia: Management and prognosis. *UpToDate 2014.* www.uptodate.com.

Norwitz, E. R. (2014). Prediction of preeclampsia. *UpToDate 2014.* www.uptodate.com.

Pickering, T. G., Hall, J. E., Appel, L. J., Falkner, BE., Graves, J., Hill, M. N., et al. (2005). Recommendations for blood pressure measurement in humans and experimental animals: Part 1: blood pressure measurement in humans: a statement for professionals from the Subcommittee of Professional and Public Education of the American Heart Association Council on High Blood Pressure Research. Subcommittee of Professional and Public Education of the American Heart Association Council on High Blood Pressure Research. *Hypertension 2005*, 45, 142–61.

Poon, L. C. & Nicolaides, K. H. (2014). Early Prediction of Preeclampsia. *Obstetrics and Gynecology International Volume 2014*, Article ID 297397, 11 pages. doi: 10.1155/2014/297397.

Poon, L. C. Y., Syngelaki, A., Akolekar, R., Lai, J. & Nicolaides, K. H. (2013). Combined screening for preeclampsia and small for gestational age at 11-13 weeks. *Fetal Diagnosis and Therapy*, *33*(1), 16-27. doi: 10.1159/000341712.

Roberts, J. M., Druzin, M., August, P. A., Gaiser, R. R., Bakris, G., Granger, J. P., Barton, J. R., et al. (2012). ACOG Guidelines: Hypertension in pregnancy. *American College of Obstetricians and Gynecologists*. doi: 10.1097/01.AOG.0000437382.03963.88.

Scazzocchio, E., Figueras, F., Crispi, F., Meler, E., Masoller, N., Mula, R., et al. (2013) Performance of a first-trimester screening of preeclampsia in a routine care low-risk setting. *Am J Obstet Gynecol 2013*, 208, 203 e1–10.

Sibai, B. M. (2014). HELLP síndrome. *UpToDate 2014*. www.uptodate.com.

Thadhani, R. I. & Maynard, S. E. (2014). Proteinuria in pregnancy: Evaluation and management. *UpToDate 2014*. www.uptodate.com.

Than, N. G., Balogh, A., Romero, R., Kárpáti, E., Erez, O., Szilágyi, A., Kovalszky, I., Sammar, M., Gizurarson, S., Matkó, J., Závodszky, P., Papp, Z. & Meiri, H. (2014).. Placental Protein 13 (PP13) – A Placental Immunoregulatory Galectin Protecting Pregnancy. *Frontiers in Immunology 2014*, *5*, 348. doi: 10.3389/fimmu.2014.00348.

Vargas-Hernández, V. M., Acosta, G. & Moreno, M. A. (2012). La preeclampsia un problema de salud pública mundial.Rev *Chil Obstet Ginecol 2012*, *77*(6), 471 – 476. Doi: 10.4067/S0717-75262012000600013.

Velauthar, L., Plana, M. N., Kalidindi, M., Zamora, J., Thilaganathan, B., Illanes, S. E., Khan, K. S., et al. (2014). First-trimester uterine artery doppler and adverse pregnancy outcome: A meta-analysis involving 55974 women. *Ultrasound in Obstetrics and Gynecology*. doi: 10.1002/uog.13275.

In: Handbook for High Risk Pregnancy: Clinical Management ISBN: 978-1-63482-299-2
Editors: E. González-Mesa and D. Abehsera

Chapter 5

PERINATAL INFECTIONS: LISTERIA, TOXOPLASMA, CYTOMEGALOVIRUS, HERPES AND HIV

Yolanda Romero Espinar[1,*]***, Ana Nieto Moreno***[1]
and María Jesús Teva García[2]
[1]Obstetrics and Gynecology Department, Quirón University Hospital, Málaga, Spain
[2]Obstetrics and Gynecology Department, High Resolution Obstetric Care Center, Guadix, Granada, Spain

INTRODUCTION

Perinatal infections are transmitted in utero or during the postnatal period that immediately follows, and they play a major role in newborn mortality and morbidity rates. In the 1970s, the term TORCH was created to group the agents that could cause perinatal infections: Cytomegalovirus, rubeolla, toxoplasma, syphilis and herpes.

However, in recent years, the following have been added as causes of these types of infections in fetuses and newborns: hepatitis, varicella-zoster, tuberculosis, HIV, enterovirus, parvovirus B19, Listeria monocytogenes, and in certain geographic regions, Plasmodium, Trypanosoma cruzi and Borrelia burgdorferi (Lyme disease). As a result, the TORCH acronym falls short, and the term perinatal infections is preferred.

These infections may be bacterial, viral or parasitic, and they can be transmitted from the mother to the fetus or newborn in a number of ways:

Intrauterine: This includes transplacentary transmission or vertical transmission through the vagina, which occurs primarily when the membranes rupture prematurely.

During delivery or immediately after birth. Infectious agents that affect newborns may be present in the birth canal. Immediately after birth, certain infections present in mothers can be transmitted to newborns through contact between the two or through breastfeeding.

The process of diagnosing perinatal infections is complex because each agent must be analyzed individually. Maternal IgG are transported through the placenta, so their detection in newborns does not imply infection. The detection of IgM and IgA antibodies is a diagnosis,

* Corresponding author: Email: yolanre83@hotmail.com.

but its sensitivity is not always high. Certain agents must be searched using direct methods, so searching for antibodies is of limited use.

The aim of this chapter is to highlight the most important aspects of perinatal infections caused by toxoplasma, Listeria monocytogenes, herpes simplex virus, cytomegalovirus and HIV.

1. Listeria Monocytogenes

Listeria monocytogenes is a facultatively anaerobic, short, gram-positive coccobacilli that is capable of growing in a wide range of temperatures (-7° to 45°C) and pH levels (4.4 to 9.4), and in high salt concentrations, allowing it to survive longer in adverse environmental conditions.

It appears extensively in the environment, and it has been isolated in dirt, vegetation, forage, fecal matter and water. It is frequently present in raw meats and vegetables, unpasteurized milk, and also in cooked products that have been contaminated after the cooking process.

Infection occurs through transplacentary transmission, vertical transmission or during childbirth.

Listeriosis is a relatively uncommon illness. The estimated prevalence rate in Europe and the U.S. is 13/100,000 live births.

Its incidence in Europe and the U.S. dropped significantly after the early 90s thanks to programs aimed at avoiding the sale of contaminated foods. However, the rise in the consumption of precooked meals has increased the incidence of listeriosis from 0.2 to 0.8 for every 1,000 deliveries as of 2002.

During the first and second trimester, infected pregnant women may present only a mild illness, similar to the flu or diarrhea, and in the third trimester, the infection tends to appear as clinical chorioamnionitis.

Listeriosis is an underestimated illness with serious fetal repercussions. Throughout the world, it has a fetal or neonatal mortality of 40-50%.

If the vertical infection occurs during the first or second trimester (20% of cases), it causes septic abortions and intrauterine fetal death. If it occurs in the third trimester (80% of cases), it causes chorioamnionitis and premature delivery, with a perinatal death rate of 20%. It can be asymptomatic in fetuses/newborns in one-third of cases.

If it is transmitted through the birth canal or post-delivery, the most common clinical manifestation is meningitis.

Serological tests are useless in its diagnosis. Amniocentesis for microbiological study (Gram stain and culture) has a 33% detection rate since it is an intracellular germ that can be easily confused with diplococcus, diphtheroid agents and Haemophilus.

Diagnostic confirmation is only possible through sterile fluid or tissue cultures such as blood, neonatal CSF, amniotic fluid or the placenta.

When the infection occurs during pregnancy, antibiotics administered immediately may prevent infection of the fetus or newborn.

Ampicillin, 2-6 g/day, divided into four, equal, intravenous doses during 14 days. Other alternatives include penicillin and trimethoprim-sulfamethoxazole.

For the initial empirical treatment of serious infections, association with aminoglycosides (gentamicin) is recommended.

Pregnant women must be informed of preventive measures.

Cooking meat thoroughly, washing raw vegetables before eating them, avoiding milk or foods made with unpasteurized milk (such as fresh cheese).

Consuming perishable foods while they are fresh and ingesting pâtés, spreadable meats and canned/packaged smoked fish/seafood products before their expiration date.

2. TOXOPLASMA

Toxoplasma gondii is an intracellular protozoon that frequently infects the general population. The incidence of infection varies in different geographic regions. There are a number of strains of Toxoplasma gondii, and genotype II is the most common in Europe. Genotype I and other atypical genotypes are the most common in South America, and they cause more severe forms of the illness.

The infection is contracted primarily by consuming or handling undercooked or raw meat (especially pork, lamb or wild animals) that contains cysts, or by ingesting vegetables or water contaminated with oocysts shed in the feces of infected cats. Contact with domestic cats is considered low risk.

Maternal infections during the first or second trimester of pregnancy are less common (9-27%) than in the third trimester (up to 60%). However, the consequences are more serious if it is contracted at an early stage as this may result in spontaneous abortion, fetal death or serious congenital toxoplasmosis.

Therefore, the clinical presentation in newborns will vary depending on the stage of pregnancy when it was contracted. Earlier cases may include hydrocephalus, microcephaly, chorioretinitis, brain calcifications and convulsions. Approximately 50-80% of cases present subclinical toxoplasmosis (they are asymptomatic at birth), but there is a high risk of developing long-term retinal and neurological damage.

The diagnosis is done through the clinical profile or using indirect serological methods:

During the first gestational visit, the IgG titers may be determined as a screening method.

If the result is negative, there is a risk of contracting the infection and preventive measures must be taken. In addition, the antibody titer must be repeated during the second or third trimester in order to confirm that seroconversion has not occurred.

If during the first visit the IgG test gives a positive result, the woman may be immunized or, on the contrary, infected. The avidity test is used to differentiate the mother's condition. If the infection occurred recently (less than four months), the avidity will be low (<20%). If the avidity is high (>30-40%), the infection most likely occurred before gestation.

The definitive diagnosis of the acute maternal infection may be confirmed if a negative titer becomes positive or if a low titer increases significantly to a higher one.

The detection of specific IgM is a fairly unreliable marker and its use is not recommended for screening because low IgM levels may persist for many months or years after the primary infection.

The Polymerase Chain Reaction (PCR) test performed on amniotic fluid allows the early prenatal diagnosis of congenital toxoplasmosis, avoiding other procedures that are more invasive, such as cordocentesis.

An ultrasound scan can detect certain serious lesions, but these may appear late.

The most characteristic images are: hydrocephalus and brain calcifications (hyperechoic nodules or intracranial densities). Isolated hyperechoic nodules have an uncertain prognosis. In general, they are not associated with neurological after-effects, but they do increase the risk of chorioretinitis.

There is no evidence of association with restricted fetal growth.

Although a definitive treatment does not exist, clinical recommendations include treating with spiramycin during the first trimester and at the beginning of the second trimester, up until amniocentesis is performed. In the case of a positive PCR test result or when the probability of fetal infection is high (in other words, the mother has contracted the infection at the end of the second trimester or during the third trimester), the recommended treatment consists of pyrimethamine/sulfadiazine, which may be alternated with spiramycin.

Folinic acid is added to the treatment with pyrimethamine in order to reduce bone marrow suppression, and hematotoxicity must be carefully monitored.

In most countries, the fetus's treatment is continued throughout the infant's first year of life.

Since a toxoplasma vaccine does not exist, prevention is primarily based on educating pregnant women:

Avoiding the consumption of raw or undercooked meat, washing all raw vegetables, using gloves when working with dirt, avoiding contact with cats and their feces, avoiding the consumption of untreated or unfiltered drinking water.

3. Cytomegalovirus

Cytomegalovirus (CMV) is a double-stranded DNA virus that belongs to the herpes virus family.

CMV is the most common congenital viral infection, and it appears in approximately 1% of newborns. In general, the prevalence of immunity against CMV is higher in developing countries and in women of lower socio-economic levels. Therefore, the incidence and seriousness of congenital CMV infections varies throughout the world.

CMV is transmitted through human contact via the infected individual's saliva, blood, urine, semen, cervical/vaginal secretions or breast milk. It is able to survive in fomites, including diapers, toys and hands.

Women at a higher risk of a primary (initial) infection during pregnancy are those who are in contact with preschool children because after the primary infection, children excrete the virus in their urine and saliva for an average of 18 months (a much longer period than adults).

Newborns can be infected through transplacentary transmission, during birth or post-delivery through breast milk or contact with secretions.

The risk of vertical transmission is higher during a primary infection and as gestation progresses. However, the fetus is affected more severely, especially when the maternal infection occurs during the first trimester.

Neonatal infections transmitted in the birth canal or through breastfeeding have no effect on subsequent neurological development, but there have been cases of sepsis in premature infants < 32 weeks.

The primary CMV infection in pregnant women can be asymptomatic or cause non-specific symptoms that disappear spontaneously. The virus then becomes latent but reactivates periodically during mild immunodeficient episodes.

90% of newborns that have been infected congenitally are asymptomatic at birth, and of these, 8-15% will develop complications such as hepatomegaly, splenomegaly, microcephaly, jaundice and petechia. Between 5% and 15% can develop (even in the long term) alterations such as sensorineural hypoacusis, motor alterations, mental retardation, chorioretinitis and dental alterations. Approximately 5% of infants born with the congenital infection have the general illness, characterized by multiple organs that are affected (primarily the reticuloendothelial system and the central nervous system).

Diagnosis through serologies is non-specific. The ultrasound examination of intracranial calcifications, cerebral ventriculomegaly or hydrops has a low sensitivity and specificity for fetal illnesses.

The best way to diagnose a fetal infection is through fetal amniocentesis. The detection of CMV DNA through PCR after 22 weeks of gestation allows diagnosing the fetal infection. Any attempts to diagnose CMV prior to 22 weeks are much less reliable.

There is controversy regarding the treatment's effectiveness and safety.

However, certain preliminary evidence confirms that the CMV hyperimmune globulin could prevent mother-to-child transmission or the fetal illness.

Measures for prevention and control focus on maximum hygiene for women with children under the age of three.

4. Herpes Simplex

The herpes simplex virus appears throughout the world. There are two sub-types: HSV-1 and HSV-2.

The majority of genital herpes cases are caused by HSV-2 and they are almost always the result of sexual transmission.

HSV-1 is more common. It causes an oral infection that is contracted during childhood and it may also be asymptomatic. However, the sexual transmission of HSV-1 is becoming increasingly common, especially through oral-genital contact.

Neonatal HSV infections have a low incidence rate of 3-13/100,000 live births.

Most cases are related to HSV-2, and 15% to 20% could be related to HSV1. Most neonatal herpes simplex cases occur as a result of contact with the herpes simplex virus during vaginal delivery. Neonatal herpes resulting from transplacentary or vertical transmission is much less common, as is the case of a postnatal infection of HSV-1 through close contact with people who have oral herpes.

Women who contract genital herpes shortly before childbirth have a high risk of transmitting it to their newborn (30-50%). If genital herpes is contracted during the first half of gestation or if the mother has recurrent genital herpes lesions, the risk of transmitting it to the newborn is low (<1%).

Although the neonatal infection of herpes simplex is rare, it may appear as a syndrome of the neonatal herpes virus and/or severe encephalitis, which are often lethal or have severe after-effects.

HSV may be diagnosed through ultrasound markers: microcephaly, hydranencephaly, intracranial calcifications, microphthalmia, cutaneous lesions (thickened skin, cutaneous hyperechogenicity), IUGR and fetal hydrops.

Indirect serologies provide limited results, so isolating the virus through culture is the definitive diagnostic method for detecting HSV, especially in the skin and mucous membranes. Direct immunofluorescence staining with monoclonal antibodies of the cells scraped from vesicular lesions provides a quick alternative diagnosis at a low cost.

Polymerase Chain Reaction (PCR) tests for herpes simplex DNA are more sensitive than culturing the virus, and they are the preferred method for detecting HSV in amniotic fluid.

The main objective of treating genital herpes during gestation is to prevent vertical transmission at birth. Performing a cesarean section if herpes lesions are present when labor begins and reducing asymptomatic viral excretions by administering antiviral medications (aciclovir and valaciclovir) are the best prophylactic measures available.

According to the latest revision, the use of systematic antiviral agents to reduce the high morbidity and mortality rates of the neonatal herpes virus helped improve the mortality rates of newborns with a central nervous system disease or an infection spread by HSV. There is insufficient evidence from trials to support a preference between the use of aciclovir or valaciclovir, or a higher dosage and a longer duration of the aciclovir treatment for this condition.

5. HIV

The human immunodeficiency virus (HIV) is a retrovirus that infects the immune system's T lymphocytes, causing a progressive reduction in their number and with time, the Acquired Immune Deficiency Syndrome.

HIV is a pandemic disease that affects more than 2.5 million children throughout the world.

Vertical transmission is the most common way through which children contract HIV around the world. Vertical transmission may occur at three different points in time during pregnancy and the post-delivery period: in utero, (25-40% of cases), intrapartum (60-70% of cases) and through breastfeeding, which increases the risk in 16% of established infection cases and in 29% of primary infection cases.

Advances in treatment and preventive measures have reduced the prevalence of vertical transmission to less than 2% in developed nations, but it remains high in developing countries, especially in Sub-Saharan Africa.

In developed nations, the prevalence of HIV in mothers of newborns is estimated to be between 1.6 and 1.9.

The increased prevalence of pregnant women who are HIV positive and expose their children to infection is due to two factors:

A constant increase of HIV infections in women.

An improved life expectancy for infected women as a result of treatment.

The disease's clinical profile goes unnoticed during the first weeks after an individual is infected with HIV because symptoms include fever, general discomfort, lymphadenopathy, and rashes in 40% to 90% of cases, and these symptoms may be easily confused with the flu.

After the acute phase, infected individuals may not show any clinical signs or symptoms during many months or years, and the disease may subsequently appear through opportunistic infections and certain cancers that arise as the immune system is progressively weakened by the HIV infection.

Pregnant women may face obstetric complications, primarily prematurity, preeclampsia, IUGR or fetal death.

They must also be informed of possible maternal or fetal toxicity as a result of treatment.

The diagnosis must be based on serologies. The antibody against HIV is detectable in more than 95% of patients within three months after infection.

This test should be performed in the first gestational visit and then repeated during the third trimester in order to rule out seroconversion. It should be performed each trimester if risk factors are present.

Reactive detection tests should be confirmed by an additional confirmation test--the Western blot analysis.

The rapid or instant ELISA test provides results in 30 minutes and it is used on patients who begin labor without prior serologies. If the test is positive, prophylaxis should commence with antiretrovirals without waiting for the results of the confirmation test.

If the mother has HIV, her analyses each trimester should include:

CD4+ count (degree of immunodeficiency).

RNA plasma level (viral load) (risk of the disease's progression).

In terms of the neonatal diagnosis, it is important to take into consideration that the antibody against maternal HIV passes through the placenta. During the 6-18 month period after birth, it is likely for HIV antibody test results to be positive for the serum of infected and non-infected newborns. Therefore, the preferred test is HIV DNA Polymerase Chain Reaction (PCR), which detects this DNA in the mononuclear cells of peripheral blood.

Antiretroviral treatment (HAART) for women with HIV reduces the risk of vertical transmission of HIV.

It is necessary to know the most effective treatment, the medication's repercussion on the vertical transmission of HIV, and the potential complications of the treatment for the mother and the fetus.

Women diagnosed with HIV during pregnancy who are eligible for treatment with antiretroviral medications should begin treatment as soon as possible. Treatment may begin after the first trimester if the necessary criteria are not met, but if a woman is seriously ill, the benefits are greater than any potential risks to the fetus.

HAART is the ideal treatment during pregnancy.

Zidovudine must be included in HAART as long as there is no resistance to it or in the case of patients with severe anemia. However, zidovudine monotherapy after 20-28 weeks is less effective in preventing vertical transmission. Therefore, it is recommended to combine other medications after 20-28 weeks or when the viral load is higher than 1,000 cop/ml.

Standard treatment guidelines include the use of two nucleotide analog reverse-transcriptase inhibitors + one protease inhibitor.

In the case of pregnant women with CD4 counts higher than 250/ mm3, it is not recommended to begin treatment with nevirapine due to its potential hepatotoxicity. In the case of patients who have already received nevirapine, treatment should not be stopped.

Efavirenz is classified as Food and Drug Administration (FDA) Pregnancy Category D, so it is not recommended during the first trimester due to its teratogenic effect.

During labor and in the absence of prior treatments, it is advised to administer intrapartum intravenous zidovudine three hours before a cesarean section, followed by a six-week treatment for the newborn.

It is recommended to perform a post-partum analysis of the mother with a CD4+ count and HIV RNA copy number, and assess the appropriate treatment. If treatment is given during delivery, the same guidelines should be followed, but with the addition of intrapartum zidovudine.

The recommended delivery method is an elective cesarean section scheduled at 38 weeks because this significantly reduces perinatal HIV transmission. However, there is no evidence showing that an elective cesarean section reduces vertical transmission of HIV after the mother's membranes rupture or once labor begins.

The risk of perinatal HIV transmission can be significantly lowered through: Universal prenatal HIV screening, access to antiretroviral treatment, elective cesarean section scheduled at 38 weeks, lactation suppression, and multiple micronutrient supplementation.

REFERENCES

Jones, CA; Walker, KS; Badawi, N. Antiviral agents for treatment of herpes simplex virus infection in neonates. *Cochran Database of Systematic Reviews.*, 2009, 3, CD 004206. Doi: 10.1002/14651858. CD 004206. Pub2.

McCarthy, FP; Giles, ML; Rowlands, S; Purcell, KJ; Jones, CA. Antenatal interventions for preventing the transmission of cytomegalovirus (CMV) from the mother to fetus during pregnancy and adverse outcomes in the congenitally infected infant. *Cochrane Database of Systematic Reviews.*, 2001, 3, CD 008271. Doi:10.1002/14651858. CD 008371. Pub2.

Peyron, F; Wallon, M; Liou, C; Garner, P. Treatments for toxoplasmosis in pregnancy. *Cochrane Database of Systematic Reviews.*, 1999, 3, CD001684. Doi: 10.1002/14651858.CD001684.

Polo Rodríguez, R; Muñoz, Galligo, E; Iribarren, JA. Consensus statement on monitoring of HIV: pregnancy, birth, and prevention of mother-to-child transmission. *Enferm Infecc Microbiol Clin.*, 2014, 32, 310-3.

Sturt, AS; Dokubo, EK; Sint, TT. Antiretroviral therapy (ART) for treating HIV infection in ART-eligible pregnant women. *Cochrane Database of Systematic Review.* 2010, *3*, CD008440. Doi: 10.1002/14651858.CD008440.

Ramaswamy, V; Cresence, VM; Rejitha, JS; Lekshmi, MU; Dharsana, KS; Prasad, SP. Listeria-review of epidemiology and pathogenesis. *J Microbiol Immunol Infect.*, 2007; 40: 4-13.

Swaminathan, B; Gerner-Smidt, P. Epidemiology of human listeriosis. *Microbes Infect.*, 2007, 9, 1236-43.

Swanson, EC; Schleiss, MR. Congenital cytomegalovirus infection: New prospects for prevention and therapy. *Pediatr Clin North Am.*, 2013, 60, 335-49.

In: Handbook for High Risk Pregnancy: Clinical Management ISBN: 978-1-63482-299-2
Editors: E. González-Mesa and D. Abehsera

Chapter 6

UROLOGIC DISORDERS DURING PREGNANCY

Marta de la Peña Rodríguez de Medina*[*], *Laura López Casañas* and *Andrés Carlos López Díaz
Obstetrics and Gynecology Department, University Quirón Hospital, Málaga, Spain

INTRODUCTION

Pregnancy affects both the kidney and the remainder of the urinary tract.

1. Increased renal size: Both kidneys increase in size by 1 to 1.5 cm during pregnancy (Bailey et al., 1971). Kidney volume increases by up to 30 percent, primarily due to an increase in renal vascular and interstitial volume. There are no histological changes or changes in number of nephrons, but the glomerular filtration rate is also increased. The renal pelvises and caliceal systems may be dilated as a result of progesterone effects and mechanical compression of the ureters at the pelvic brim.
2. Ureters: Dilatation of the ureters and renal pelvis is more prominent on the right than the left and is seen in up to 80 percent of pregnant women (Rasmussen et al., 1988). These changes can be visualized on ultrasound examination by the second trimester, and may not resolve until 6 to 12 weeks postpartum.
   The dilated collecting system can hold 200 to 300 mL of urine. The resulting urinary stasis can serve as a reservoir for bacteria, which may contribute to the increased risk of pyelonephritis in pregnancy.
   Hydroureter and hydronephrosis in pregnancy have been attributed to hormonal effects, external compression, and intrinsic changes in the ureteral wall (Beydoun et al., 1985). The following factors may contribute:
   - High concentrations of progesterone reduce ureteral tone, peristalsis, and contraction pressure.
   - More prominent involvement of the right ureter may be due to dextrorotation of the uterus by the sigmoid colon, kinking of the ureter as it crosses the right iliac artery, and/or proximity to the right ovarian vein.

[*] Corresponding author: Email: marta.dlp.rdm@gmail.com.

- The vessels in the suspensory ligament of the ovary enlarge and may compress the ureter at the brim of the bony pelvis.
- Uterine enlargement may cause the ureters to become elongated, tortuous, and displaced laterally as pregnancy advances. In rare cases, compression of the ureter causes pain and true urinary obstruction, which resolves with placing the mother on her side, insertion of stents, and/or delivery (Irving et al., 2002).
- Hypertrophy of Waldeyer's sheath (the connective tissue that surrounds the ureters within the true pelvis) may prevent hormone-induced dilatation below the pelvic brim (Dure-Smith et al., 1970).

3. Bladder: The bladder mucosa is edematous and hyperemic in pregnancy. Although progesterone-induced bladder wall relaxation may lead to increased capacity, the enlarging uterus displaces the bladder superiorly and anteriorly, and flattens it, which can decrease capacity.
4. Renal hemodynamic: Normal pregnancy is characterized by widespread vasodilatations, with increased arterial compliance and decreased systemic vascular resistance. These global hemodynamic changes are accompanied by increases in renal perfusion and glomerular filtration rate. In late gestation, assumption of the left lateral position is associated with increases in glomerular filtration rate and sodium excretion (Almeida et al., 2009).

NEPHROLITHIASIS DURING PREGNANCY

The development of a symptomatic stone during pregnancy is a rare event, occurring in about one in every 1500 to 3000 pregnancies (Stothers et al., 1992; Butler el al, 2000). This rate is similar to non-pregnant women of child-bearing age (Curhan et al., 2004).

Affected patients usually present in the second or third trimester with acute flank pain (90 percent), which often radiates to the groin or lower abdomen. Hematuria is present in 75 to 95 percent. One third of women have gross hematuria, and approximately 40 percent will have pyuria (Stothers et al., 1992; Butler el al, 2000).

Most of these women do not have a prior history of stone disease (Butler el al, 2000). However, it is not clear if such women have an underlying tendency to stone formation or if factors related to pregnancy are responsible. Normal pregnancy is associated with a mild increase in urine calcium excretion, lesser increases in urine citrate and magnesium excretion, and a rise in urine pH but not urine volume (Maikranz et al., 1989). Additional factors that contribute to stone formation during pregnancy include urinary stasis, secondary to increased progesterone levels and diminished fluid intake, as a result of decreasing bladder capacity from the gravid uterus. Most stones appear to be predominantly composed of calcium phosphate (Ross et al., 2008).

Renal and pelvic ultrasound scan should be performed when an obstructing calculus is suspected (Butler el al, 2000). This is useful for detecting secondary signs of obstruction, such as hydronephrosis or hydroureter. Rarely, pelvic ultrasound may identify a stone obstructing the distal uréter.

Most (75 to 85 percent) stones pass spontaneously, due in part to the normally dilated urinary tract in pregnant women (Stothers et al., 1992; Butler el al, 2000).

Cystoscopy with insertion of a ureteral stent or ureteroscopy to remove or fragment the stone may be required in the patient who is septic, has persistent severe pain, or has obstruction in a solitary functioning kidney (Scarpa et al., 1996; McAleer et al., 2004). Ureteral stenting or placement of a nephrostomy tube to relieve obstruction or pain is a valid option for managing pregnant patients. However, pregnancy significantly increases the risk of stent encrustation, necessitating the need for frequent ureteral stent change every four to six weeks until delivery of the baby (Parulkar et al., 1998).

URINARY TRACT INFECTIONS AND ASYMPTOMATIC BACTERIURIA IN PREGNANCY

Asymptomatic Bacteriuria

The term asymptomatic bacteriuria refers to the presence of a positive urine culture in pregnant women in the absence of clinical symptoms.

Its prevalence is 2-7% being more common in multiparous women with low socioeconomic status, previous urinary tract infection, diabetes and other diseases (Stenqvist et al., 1987). The frequency of asymptomatic bacteriuria during pregnancy did not differ from that of a non-pregnant woman of the same age. Although pregnancy does not increase its appearance, it does aggravate their consequences and favors the appearance of symptomatic forms, complicating up to 35% of patients with acute pyelonephritis (Smaill et al., 2007).

Moreover asymptomatic bacteriuria has been associated with multiple complications during pregnancy, such as low birth weight of the newborn, preterm delivery, maternal hypertension and anemia (Delzell JE Jr et al., 2000). There are also multiple studies showing that treatment reduces the incidence of these complications (Whalley et al., 1965; Rouse et al., 1995; Mittendorf et al., 1992).

Asymptomatic bacteriuria is detectable during the first weeks of pregnancy. The American College of Obstetricians and Gynecologists recommends screening all pregnant women for the detection of asymptomatic bacteriuria during the first trimester of pregnancy. The goal of screening is to perform treatment and control these pregnant women to avoid complications (Nicolle et al., 2005).

If the urine culture is negative, a new screening is not recommended in low-risk women; although it is desirable to repeat in pregnant women at high risk of infection (recurrent infections, urinary tract anomalies, preterm labor) (Gratacos et al., 1994).

The diagnosis of asymptomatic bacteriuria should be based on the culture sample of a urine specimen collected in a manner that minimizes contamination, with> 100,000 CFU / mL of a single uropathogenic germ in a patient without urinary symptoms. If counts between 10,000 and 100,000 CFU / ml or polymicrobial cultures samples should be repeated. The samples should be obtained with extreme caution to avoid contamination and also when taking then to the laboratory. The presence of more than one kind of bacteria generally indicates contamination. (Nicolle et al., 2005; McNair et al., 2000).

Antibiotic treatment will be based on the antibiogram although Escherichia Coli is present in the majority of asymptomatic bacteriuria, which can be treated with any of these regimens. None has proven to be superior to others (Guinto et al., 2010):

- Amoxicillin 500 mg to be taken every 8 hours for three to seven days
- Amoxicillin-clavulanate 500 mg to be taken every 8 hours for three to seven days
- Fosfomycin 3 g single oral dose
- Cephalexin 500 mg to be taken every 12 hours for three to seven days
- Cefuroxime 250 mg to be taken every 12 hours for three to seven days
- Nitrofurantoin 100 mg to be taken every 6 hours for three to seven days

A follow-up culture sample should be done one week after following the treatment to ensure that bacteriuria is eliminated (Patterson et al., 1997).

In 20% to 30% of patients a short-course antibiotic therapy will fail. In these cases, a repeat 7 to 10 day antibiotic course with a culture-specific antimicrobial sample is appropriate (Andriole et al., 1975).

As there is a high risk of recurrence in pregnant women. Conducting periodic urine cultures until delivery is recommended after asymptomatic bacteriuria is detected. Currently, there are no adequate clinical studies that provide sufficient evidence to indicate the frequency in testing pregnant women with asymptomatic bacteriuria.

Acute Cystitis

Cystitis is a symptomatic bladder infection that causes urgency, frequency, dysuria and suprapubic pain in the absence of symptoms of systemic involvement (fever) and lumbar pain. Acute cystitis occurs in approximately 1 to 2 percent of pregnant women and the incidence does not decrease even treating asymptomatic bacteriuria (Gilstrap et al., 2001).

No correlation has been established between acute cystitis and increased risk of low birth weight, preterm delivery or pyelonephritis, perhaps because pregnant women with symptomatic urinary tract infection usually receive treatment (Millar et al., 1997).

Diagnosis is based on clinical described, the absence of symptoms of upper urinary tract and a positive urine culture with> 1,000 CFU / ml. To confirm the diagnosis it is not considered necessary to obtain a positive urine culture with> 100,000 CFU / ml; it is enough with > 1,000 CFU / ml if the clinical symptoms are suggestive of urinary tract infection (Stamm et al., 1982).

Pregnant women with acute cystitis should be treated with a three to seven day course of antibiotics. A systematic review from Cochrane Database analyzed the most effective agents for the treatment of symptomatic urinary tract infections (cystitis and pyelonephritis) during pregnancy in terms of treatment rates, recurrent infection, incidence of preterm delivery and the need to change the course of antibiotics. All of the antibiotics studied were very effective and complications were rare. There was not enough evidence to recommend a particular treatment scheme (Vazquez et al., 2000).

A follow-up culture sample for treating cystitis should be obtained a week after completion of antibiotic therapy. It is also useful to repeat urine cultures a month after the completion of the pregnancy to evaluate for persistent or recurrent bacteriuria.

ACUTE PIELONEFRITIS

It is an infection of the renal parenchyma that usually occurs in the second or third trimester of pregnancy because stasis and hydronephrosis are more evident (Gilstrap et al., 2001). The incidence of acute pielonefritis is 1-2% and is almost always secondary to an undiagnosed or improperly treated asymptomatic bacteriuria. In fact, 20-40% of patients with untreated asymptomatic bacteriuria develop pyelonephritis (Schaeffer et al., 2002).

The predisposition for pyelonephritis during pregnancy is primarily due to pregnancy-related anatomic changes in the urinary tract, such as pressure on the bladder from the enlarging uterus and an increase in the size of the ureters due to smooth muscle relaxation. In addition, the immunosuppression of pregnancy may also contribute (Petersson et al., 1994).

The germ that is found in most cases (70%) is E-Coli. Other germs can also be present as Klebsiella, Enterobacter, Proteus and Streptococcus Group B.

Diagnosis is mainly clinical. The usual symptoms are lumbar pain, fever, chills, nausea, vomiting. There are usually no symptoms of cystitis.

Many studies have described a relationship between maternal urinary tract infection, particularly asymptomatic bacteriuria, and adverse pregnancy outcomes (eg, preterm birth, low birthweight). It has been suggested that acute pyelonephritis has a similar association, but the strength of this association is not known because of confounding variables such as socioeconomic status and previous preterm delivery (Millar et al., 2003).

There are some complications associated with pyelonephritis like anemia, hypertension, renal failure, acute respiratory distress and sepsis (Gilstrap et al., 2001).

Treatment is initially parenteral until the patient remains afebrile 48-72 h (Schaeffer et al., 2002). In the empirical treatment third-generation cephalosporins are preferred like ceftriaxone at a dose of 1 g / 24 h intravenously or intramuscularly. In cases of allergy to beta-lactam use Gentamicin 80 mg / 8 h.

When the patient is afebrile it is posible to begin with oral therapy, which will continue to complete 14 days of treatment. If antibiogram is available, it is recommended to use narrower spectrum antibiotic. If not available, empirical treatment with cefuroxime 250 mg / 12 h per oral to meet 14 days of treatment (American College of Obstetricians and Gynecologists, 1998). It is important to repeat a urine culture 1-2 weeks after treatment and then monthly until delivery.

The recurrent pyelonephritis during pregnancy occurs in 6-8% of patients (Wing et al., 1998). In these cases, antibiotic prophylaxis should be used. The recommended drugs are nitrofurantoin 50 mg / 24 hours (given at night) or Cephalexin 250 mg / 24 h (given at night) (American College of Obstetricians and Gynecologists, 1998).

KIDNEY TRANSPLANTATION AND PREGNANCY

Chronic renal failure is often associated with sexual dysfunction and infertility. After kidney transplantation sex life and fertility are improved (Pezeshki et al., 2004)

However, the rates of both pregnancy and successful pregnancy (ie, resulting in a live birth) remain far lower than in the general population (Gill et al., 2009, Levidiotis et al., 2009). During the first three post transplant years, the unadjusted pregnancy rate was 33 per 1000 women, compared with more than 100 per 1000 women in the general population (Gill et al., 2009).

Pregnancy Planning

Ideally, pregnancy should be planned at a time of good general and organ transplant health, the second year after transplantation is the ideal period for conception (Bar et al., 2000). In pregnancy occurring some years after transplantation, there is a risk that some chronic rejection and/or some deterioration of renal function may have developed.

Pregnancy should be planned when renal function and immunosuppressive therapy are stable and there are no signs of rejection, hypertension, proteinuria, hydronephrosis or chronic infection (Stratta et al., 2003).

The American Society of Transplantation Consensus Opinion states that the patient can safely proceed with pregnancy providing the following conditions are met (McKay et al., 2005):

- Normal renal function with creatinine <1.5 mg / dL with <500 mg/24 hour protein excretion
- No fetotoxic infections such as CMV
- The patient is not treated with fetotoxic or teratogenic medication
- The immunosuppressive regimen is stable at maintenance levels

Early detection of pregnancy is important so that monitoring and adjustment of immunosuppressive therapy can begin as soon as possible.

Risks to Patient and Organ Transplant

Even if the transplanted woman presents good general health, pregnancy presents a risk for the patient and the organ transplant. The greatest risks are rejection due to changes in the metabolism of immunosuppressive medication and organ transplant failure due to increased filtration that occurs during pregnancy.

There are various factors that may affect renal transplantation during pregnancy such as high blood pressure, hemodynamic alterations, impaired renal function, urinary infection or rejection (clinical guideline on renal transplant of the European Association of Urology)

Care during Pregnancy

Pregnancies in transplanted women are often unproblematic, but these patients should always be considered high risk and require shared care by an obstetrician, nephrologist, and an urologist (grade B recommendation in clinical renal transplant guide of the European Association of urology). Attendance during pregnancy should focus primarily on controlling the risk factors that may affect the renal transplant:

- Control of proteinuria
- Control of hypertension (preeclampsia may affect 30% of patients)
- Control of renal function
- Early rejection
- Detection of urinary tract infections by testing monthly urine samples and always treating bacteriuria, whether the transplanted woman is symptomatic or asymptomatic.

Immunosuppressive Treatment

The standard immunosuppressive treatment used during pregnancy and recommended by the European Society of Urology is cyclosporine with or without azathioprine and prednisone (Fischer et al., 2005; Armenti et al., 1998). These drugs cross the placental barrier, but apparently do not increase the risk of teratogenicity.

Cyclosporine does not seem to be a major teratogen as suggested by the results of a meta-analysis of 15 studies (Bar et al., 2001).

Recent research suggests that the new drug *Tacrolimus* (Kainz et al., 2000; Jain et al., 1997) used in kidney, heart and liver transplantation might also be safe.

Mycophenolate mofetil: is contraindicated in pregnancy because this medication is listed as a category-D drug for use in pregnancy. Increased risk in first and second trimester of fetal and congenital malformations such as cleft lip, cleft palate and cardiac abnormalities, esophageal and renal losses. MMF should be discontinued at least six weeks prior to attempted conception (Sifontis et al., 2006).

Sirolimus: is contraindicated in pregnancy because it has been shown to be embryotoxic and foetotoxic in animal studies. Its use should also be discontinued at least 12 weeks prior to attempted conception (European Best Practices Guidelines (Part 2), 2002).

Pregnancy Outcome

Transplanted patients are more likely to suffer complications during pregnancy (Deshpande et al., 2011; Bramham et al., 2013; Davison et al., 1997; Sgro et al., 2002):

- The rate of fetal loss is greater than in the general population. In patients transplanted for 55% of pregnancies result in birth compared with about 70% in the general population.
- Preeclampsia: According to different studies, 24-27% of transplanted patients were affected by preeclampsia during pregnancy, compared to 4% in the general population.

- Gestational Diabetes: Some studies document an 8% risk of gestational diabetes with women who have had a kidney transplant versus other groups which found no difference with the general population.
- Premature birth: There is a high incidence of prematurity due to kidney transplantation these are: uncontrolled hypertension, fetal distress or rupture of membranes weakened by the use of steroids. There are several studies documenting that between 46-52% of transplanted patients completed pregnancy before 37 weeks, compared with 8-13% in the general population
- Approximately 20-24% of newborns have low birth weight (mean birth weight 2.5 ± 0.67 kg versus normal weight of 3.5 ± 0.53 kg)
- Congenital anomalies are not higher than in the general population.

Mode of Delivery

In general, vaginal delivery is recommended, as long as there are no circumstances that contraindicate this. The pelvic transplant will not obstruct the birth canal in most women. The use of ultrasound scan will help the physicians locate the transplanted kidney and ureter being able to determine if the patient will be a candidate for a vaginal birth delivery or lower segment cesarean section.

Postpartum

Breastfeeding is not recommended because of the baby's risk of ingesting immunosuppressive agents. A close follow-up of the mother in the first three post-partum months is suggested, including weekly renal function tests. It is also recommended to delay vaccinations until the infant is six months old.

References

Almeida, F. A., Pavan, M. V. & Rodrigues, C. I. (2009). The haemodynamic, renal excretory and hormonal changes induced by resting in the left lateral position in normal pregnant women during late gestation. *British Journal of Obstetrics and Gynaecology*, *116*, 1749.

American College of Obstetricians and Gynecologists. (1998). Antimicrobial therapy for obstetric patients. ACOG educational bulletin 245. Washington, DC.

Andriole, V. T. (1975). Urinary tract infections in pregnancy. *Urologic Clinics of North America*, *2*(3), 485–98.

Armenti, V. T., Moritz, M. J. & Davison, J. M. (1998). Drug safety issues in pregnancy following transplantation and immunosuppression: effects and outcomes. *Drug Saf*, 19(3), 219-32.

Bailey, R. R. & Rolleston, G. L. (1971). Kidney length and ureteric dilatation in the puerperium. *The Journal of obstetrics and gynaecology of the British Commonwealth*, *78*, 55.

Bar, J., Ben-Rafael, Z., Pados, A., Orvieto, R., Boner, G. & Hod, M. (2000). Prediction of pregnancy outcome in subgroups of women with renal disease. *Clin Nephrol*, *53*(6), 437-44.

Bar, Oz B., Hackman, R., Einarson, T. & Koren, G. (2001). Pregnancy outcome after cyclosporine therapy during pregnancy: a meta-analysis. *Transplantation*, *71*, 1051.

Beydoun, S, N. (1985). Morphologic changes in the renal tract in pregnancy. *Clinical Obstetric and Gynecology*, *28*, 249.

Bramham, K., Nelson-Piercy, C., Gao, H., et al. (2013). Pregnancy in renal transplant recipients: a UK national cohort study. *Clin J Am Soc Nephrol*, *8*, 290.

Butler, E. L., Cox, S. M., Eberts, E. G. & Cunningham, F. G. (2000). Symptomatic nephrolithiasis complicating pregnancy. *Obstetrics and Gynecology*, *96*, 753.

Curhan, G. C., Willett, W. C., Knight, E. L. & Stampfer, M. J. (2004). Dietary factors and the risk of incident kidney stones in younger women: Nurses' Health Study II. *Archives of Internal Medicine*, *164*, 885.

Davison, J. M. & Milne, J. E. (1997). Pregnancy and renal transplantation. *Br J Urol*, *80*(Suppl 1), 29

Delzell, J. E. Jr. & Lefevre, M. L. (2000). Urinary tract infections during pregnancy. *American Family Physician*, *61*, 713.

Deshpande, N. A., James, N. T. & Kucirka, L. M., et al. (2011). Pregnancy outcomes in kidney transplant recipients: a systematic review and meta-analysis. *Am J Transplant*, *11*, 2388.

Dure-Smith, P. (1970). Pregnancy dilatation of the urinary tract. The iliac sign and its significance. *Radiology*, *96*, 545.

European Best Practices Guidelines (Part 2). (2002). *Nephrol Dial Transplant*, *17* (Suppl 4), 50.

Fischer, T., Neumayer, H. H., Fischer, R., Barenbrock, M., Schobel, H. P., Lattrell, B. C., Jacobs, V. R., Paepke, S., von Steinburg, S. P., Schmalfeldt, B., Schneider, K. T. & Budde, K. (2005). Effect of pregnancy on long-term kidney function in renal transplant recipients treated with cyclosporine and with azathioprine. *Am J Transplant*, *5*(11), 2732-9.

Gill, J. S., Zalunardo, N., Rose, C. & Tonelli, M. (2009). The pregnancy rate and live birth rate in kidney transplant recipients. *Am J Transplant*, *9*, 1541.

Gilstrap, L. C. 3rd & Ramin, S. M. (2001). Urinary tract infections during pregnancy. *Obstetric and Gynecology Clinics of North America*, *28*, 581.

Gratacos, E., Torres, P. J., Vila, J., et al. (1994). Screening and treatment of asymptomatic bacteriuria in pregnancy prevent pyelonephritis. *The journal of infectious diseases*, *169*(6), 1390–2.

Guinto, V., De Guia, B., Festin, M. & Dowswell, T. (2010). Diferentes regímenes de antibióticos para el tratamiento de la bacteriuria asintomática en el embarazo. Cochrane Database of Systetic Reviews.

Irving, S. O. & Burgess, N. A. (2002). Managing severe loin pain in pregnancy. *British Journal of Obstetrics and Gynaecology*, *109*, 1025.

Jain, A., Venkataramanan, R., Fung, J. J., Gartner, J. C., Lever, J., Balan, V., Warty, V. & Starzl, T. E. (1997). Pregnancy after liver transplantation under tacrolimus. *Transplantation*, *64*(4), 559-65.

Kainz, A., Harabacz, I., Cowlrick, I. S., Gadgil, S. D. & Hagiwara, D. (2000). Review of the course and outcome of 100 pregnancies in 84 women treated with tacrolimus. *Transplantation*, *70*(12), 1718

Levidiotis, V., Chang, S. & McDonald, S. (2009). Pregnancy and maternal outcomes among kidney transplant recipients. *J Am Soc Nephrol*, *20*, 2433.

Maikranz, P., Holley, J. L., Parks, J. H., et al. (1989). Gestational hypercalciuria causes pathological urine calcium oxalate supersaturations. *Kidney International Supplements*, *36*, 108.

McAleer, S. J. & Loughlin, K. R. (2004). Nephrolithiasis and pregnancy. *Current Opinion in Urology*, *14*, 123.

McKay, D. B., Josephson, M. A., Armenti, V. T., et al. (2005). Reproduction and transplantation: report on the AST Consensus Conference on Reproductive Issues and Transplantation. *Am J Transplant*, *5*, 1592.

McNair, RD., MacDonald, SR., Dooley, SL., et al. (2000). Evaluation of the centrifuged and Gram-stained smear, urinalysis, and reagent strip testing to detect asymptomatic bacteriuria in obstetric patients. American Journal of *Obstetrics and Gynecology*, *182*(5), 1076–9.

Millar, L. K. & Cox, S. M. (1997). Urinary tract infections complicating pregnancy. *Infectious Disease Clinics of North America*, *11*, 13.

Millar, L. K., DeBuque, L. & Wing, D. A. (2003). Uterine contraction frequency during treatment of pyelonephritis in pregnancy and subsequent risk of preterm birth. *Journal of Perinatal Medicine*, *31*, 41.

Mittendorf, R., Williams, M. A. & Kass, E. H. (1992). Prevention of preterm delivery and low birth weight associated with asymptomatic bacteriuria. *Clinical infectious diseases: an official publication of the Infectious Diseases Society of America*, *14*, 927.

Nicolle, L. E., Bradley, S., Colgan, R., et al. (2005). Infectious Diseases Society of America guidelines for the diagnosis and treatment of asymptomatic bacteriuria in adults. *Clinical infectious diseases: an official publication of the Infectious Diseases Society of America*, *40*, 643.

Parulkar, B. G., Hopkins, T. B., Wollin, M. R., et al. (1998). Renal colic during pregnancy: a case for conservative treatment. *The Journal of Urology*, *159*, 365.

Patterson, T. F. & Andriole, V. T. (1997). Detection, significance, and therapy of bacteriuria in pregnancy. Update in the managed health care era. *Infectious Disease Clinics of North America*, *11*, 593.

Petersson, C., Hedges, S., Stenqvist, K., et al. (1994). Suppressed antibody and interleukin-6 responses to acute pyelonephritis in pregnancy. *Kidney International*, *45*, 571.

Pezeshki, M., Taherian, AA., Gharavy, M. & Ledger, W. L. (2004). Menstrual characteristics and pregnancy in women after renal transplantation. *Int J Gynaecol Obstet*, *85*, 119-25.

Rasmussen, P. E. & Nielsen, F. R. (1988). Hydronephrosis during pregnancy: a literature survey. *European Journal of Obstetrics and Gynecology and Reproductive Biology*, *27*, 249.

Ross, A. E., Handa, S., Lingeman, J. E. & Matlaga, B. R. (2008). Kidney stones during pregnancy: an investigation into stone composition. *Urological Research*, *36*, 99.

Rouse, D. J., Andrews, W. W., Goldenberg, R. L. & Owen, J. (1995). Screening and treatment of asymptomatic bacteriuria of pregnancy to prevent pyelonephritis: a cost-effectiveness and cost-benefit analysis. *Obstetrics and gynecology*, *86*, 119.

Scarpa, R. M., De Lisa, A. & Usai, E. (1996). Diagnosis and treatment of ureteral calculi during pregnancy with rigid ureteroscopes. *The Journal of Urology*, *155*, 875.

Schaeffer, A. J. Infections of the urinary tract. (2002). In: Walsh PC, Retik AB, Vaughan ED Jr, et al., editors. Campbell's Urology. 8th edition. Philadelphia: WB Saunders, 516–602.

Sgro, M. D., Barozzino, T., Mirghani, H. M., Sermer, M., Moscato, L., Akoury, H., Koren, G. & Chitayat D. A. (2002). Pregnancy outcome post renal transplantation. *Teratology*, *65*(1), 5-9.

Sifontis, N. M., Coscia, L. A., Constantinescu, S., et al. (2006). Pregnancy outcomes in solid organ transplant recipients with exposure to mycophenolate mofetil or sirolimus. *Transplantation*, *82*, 1698.

Smaill, F. & Vazquez, J. C. (2007). Antibiotics for asymptomatic bacteriuria in pregnancy. Cochrane Database of Systetic Reviews.

Stamm, W. E., Counts, G. W., Running, K. R., et al. (1982). Diagnosis of coliform infection in acutely dysuric women. *The New England of Journal of Medicine*, *307*, 463.

Stenqvist, K., Sandberg, T., Lidin-Janson, G., et al. (1987). Virulence factors of Escherichia coli in urinary isolates from pregnant women. *The journal of infectious diseases*, *156*, 870.

Stothers, L. & Lee, L. M. (1992). Renal colic in pregnancy. *The Journal of Urology*, *148*, 1383.

Stratta, P., Canavese, C., Giacchino, F., Mesiano, P., Quaglia, M. & Rossetti, M. (2003). Pregnancy in kidney transplantation: satisfactory outcomes and harsh realities. *J Nephrol*, *16*(6), 792-806.

Vazquez, J. C. & Villar, J. (2000). Treatments for symptomatic urinary tract infections during pregnancy. Cochrane Database Syst Rev.

Whalley, P. J., Martin, F. G. & Peters, P. C. (1965). Significance of asymptomatic bacteriuria detected during pregnancy. *The Journal of the American Medical Association*, *193*, 879.

Wing, D. A., Hendershott, C. M., Debuque, L. & Millar, L. K. (1998). A randomized trial of three antibiotic regimens for the treatment of pyelonephritis in pregnancy. *Obstetrics and gynecology*, *92*, 249.

In: Handbook for High Risk Pregnancy: Clinical Management ISBN: 978-1-63482-299-2
Editors: E. González-Mesa and D. Abehsera

Chapter 7

THROMBOPHILIA AND PREGNANCY

Carolina Monedero Mora, MD [*]
Obstetrics and Gynecology Department,
Quiron University Hospital Málaga, Spain

1. INTRODUCTION

The risk of venous thromboembolic events is high during pregnancy. Fifty percent of the patients with thrombosis during pregnancy will be found to have an underlying thrombofilia.

Pulmonary thromboembolism (PTE) remains a major cause of direct maternal mortality, with many deaths associated with a failure to obtain objective diagnoses (often because of unfounded concerns such as radiation exposure for the fetus) and lack of adequate treatment. (Lewis, 2004). Effective primary prevention and acute management of venous thromboembolism in pregnancy are important to reduce maternal mortality and morbidity. (Greer and Nelson-Piercy, 2005).

Venous thromboembolism complicates approximately 1 in 1600 births and is a leading cause of maternal morbidity in the United States. There is a strong association between inherited thrombophilias and venous thromboembolism, which makes detection of these mutations a logical target for prevention strategies (ACOG, 2010).

2. THROMBOGENICITY OF THE PERIPARTUM PERIOD

Pregnancy requires the avoidance of hemorrhage during implantation, endovascular cytotrophoblast remodelling of maternal spiral arteries, and during the third stage of labour, yet also requires the maintenance of a fluid uteroplacental circulation. Maintaining hemostatic balance during pregnancy requires alterations in both local uterine and systemic clotting, as well as anticoagulant and fibrinolytic proteins (ACOG, 2010). Von Villebrand factor, factor VII, factor VIII, factor X and fibrinogen are elevated as a result of hormonal changes.

[*] Correspondence: cmonederomora@gmail.com.

The activity of protein S is decreased due to changes in the total protein S antigen level and the resistance to activated protein C increases in the second and third trimesters. There is an increase of inhibitors of the fibrinolytic pathway such as activatable fibrinolytic inhibitor and plasminogen activator inhibitor 1 and 2. The physical changes of pregnancy result in an increased thrombotic state (Battinelli, Marshall and Connors, 2013).

3. THROMBOPHILIAS

3.1. Inherited Thrombophilias

3.1.1. V Leiden Mutation

Contributes to activated protein C resistance through disrupting factor Va inactivation. (Battinelli, Marshall and Connors, 2013) The prevalence of the factor V Leiden mutation in European populations is approximately 5% (ACOG, 2010). The risk of homozygous factor V Leiden for thrombosis in pregnancy is associated with an odds ratio of 43.4; Heterozygosity, with 8.3 odds ratio.

3.1.2. Prothrombin Gene Mutation

Contributes to increase the level of plasma prothrombin (Battinelli, Marshall and Connors, 2013). The prevalence is present in approximately 3% of European population.

The combination of factor V Leiden and prothrombin G20210 mutations has synergistic hypercoagulable effects (ACOG, 2010). The risk of homozygous prothrombin mutation for thrombosis in pregnancy is associated with an odds ratio of 24.4; Heterozygosity, with 6.8 odds ratio.

3.1.3. Protein C Deficiency

The risk for thrombosis in pregnancy is associated with an odds ratio of 4.8. (Battinelli, Marshall and Connors, 2013). There are more than 160 different mutations that produce a highly variable phenotype. The prevalence of this deficiency is 0.2-0,3% when is determined by a functional assay with a cut off of 50%-60%.(ACOG, 2010)

3.1.4. Protein S Deficiency

The risk for thrombosis in pregnancy is associated with an odds ratio of 3.2 (Battinelli, Marshall and Connors, 2013). Protein S deficiency generally has two causes, a silenced gene, or a mutation, which results in reduced free protein S antigen levels and activity. As with protein C deficiency, homocygous protein S deficiency results in neonatal purpura fulminans. (ACOG, 2010)

3.1.5. Antithrombin Deficiency

The risk for thrombosis in pregnancy is associated with an odds ratio of 4.7 (Battinelli, Marshall and Connors, 2013). There are more than 250 associated mutations that can decrease gene transcription, leading to reductions in both antigen and activity, or alter structure and function leading to normal antigen levels but decreased activity (ACOG, 2010).

3.1.6. Mutations in MTHFR

The homocygosis mutations in the MTHFR gene are not significantly associated with increased risk of thrombosis during pregnancy, with an odds ratio of 0.7 (Battinelli, Marshall and Connors, 2013). Homocygosity for the MTHFR C677T is present in 10-16% of all Europeans. There is insufficient evidence to support assessment of MTHFR polymorphism or measurement of fasting homocysteine levels in the evaluation of a thrombophilic etiology for venous thromboembolism and, therefore, it is not recommended. (ACOG, 2010)

3.2. Acquired Thrombophilias

Antiphospholipid antibody syndrome: has been associated with an odds ratio of 15.8 (Battinelli, Marshall and Connors, 2013).

Criteria diagnosis: One or more episodes of thrombosis and/or recurrent early miscarriages occurring in the first 10 weeks of gestation, 1 or more fetal losses occurring after 10 weeks or preterm delivery at <34 weeks for preeclampsia or placental insufficiency. Laboratory criteria: lupus anticoagulant present in the plasma on 2 separate occasions at least 12 weeks apart and/or anticardiolipin antibody of either the IgG or IgM isotype present in plasma at medium to high titers, or the present of anti-beta2-glycoprotein of IgG or IgM must be present on 2 or more occasions again at least 12 weeks apart.

4. Laboratory Tests (ACOG, 2010)

4.1. Factor V Leiden: activated protein C resistance assay. If abnormal, DNA analysis.
4.2. Prothrombin gene mutation G20210A: DNA analysis.
4.3. Protein C deficiency: Protein C activity (<60%).
4.4. Protein S deficiency: Functional assay (<55%)
4.5. Antithrombin deficiency: Antithrombin activity (<60%)

They should be performed after 6 weeks from the thrombotic event and while the patient is not pregnant and not taking anticoagulation or hormonal therapy. Screenig with fasting homocysteine levels or MTHFR mutation analyses are not recommended.

5. Disorders Associated with Thrombophilias

5.1. Repeated Implantation Failure (RIF)

Is determined when transferred embryos fail to implant following several in vitro fertilization treatment cycles. The definition of RIF is a failure of implantation in at least three consecutive IVF attemps, in which 1-2 embryos of high grade quality are transferred in each cycle. Any abnormality attributed to the embryo, the endometrium or the immune system will result in implantation failure. RIF and Thrombophilia: although the thrombophilic state, either inherited or acquired, has been mainly associated with repeated pregnancy loss, several investigators have reported an association between RIF and a tendency of hypercoagulable conditions (Azem F et al., 2004) (Grandone et al., 2001). Still the association between the hypercoagulable state and RIF is still debatable, since other investigators did not find a higher prevalence of thrombophilia in patients with RIF compared to controls. Nevertheless, when summarizing all studies focusing on gene polymorphism and the thrombophilia trait, it seems that prothrombotic disorders are more prevalent in RIF patients than in controls. It is recommended that patients diagnosed with RIF be investigated for acquired as well as hereditary thrombophilia disorders, and be treated accordingly.

In recurrent miscarriages, patients are advised to undergo blood test for thrombophilia as well as for connective tissue diseases that involve antiphospholipide antibodies. However, thrombophilia and antiphospholipids antibodies may also be associated with risk of RIF. Patients with no history of thrombotic events, personally or among close relatives, and who already experienced several uneventful IVF treatments, may be considered suitable to start low molecular weight heparin on the day of de embryo transfer. Patients with antiphospholipic antibodies syndrome or with a history of a disease that can be attributed to a hypercoagulability trait should start anticoagulation concomitant with gonadotropin administration. Treatment with low molecular weight heparin should be stopped 24 h before egg retrieval and reinitiated the day following ovum pick-up. Empirical treatment with low molecular weight heparin, aspirin or corticosteroids was not found to be effective, and is not advocated for women with RIF who were negative for thrombophilic tests (Simon and Laufer, 2012)

5.2. Pregnancy Loss and Inherited Thrombosis

Recurrent pregnancy loss is a common health problem, with three or more losses affecting 1-2% and two or more losses affecting up to 5% of women at the reproductive age (Alireza Parand et al., 2013).

The presence of the Factor V Leiden or Prothrombin gene mutation was associated with increased risk of pregnancy loss in the first or second trimester as well as with recurrent pregnancy losses. The role of the other thrombophilias is less clear (Battinelli, Marshall and Connors, 2013) (Alireza Parand et al., 2013). Whereas meta-analyses and a retrospective cohort study have revealed an association between inherited thrombophilias and first-trimester pregnancy loss, prospective cohort studies have found no association between inherited thrombophilias and fetal loss (ACOG, 2010).

5.3. Preeclampsia

The cases associated with thombophilia appear to have a severe phenotype with an increased risk of HELLP (Battinelli, Marshall and Connors, 2013). There is insufficient evidence to conclude that inherited thrombophilias are associated with an increased occurrence of preeclampsia (ACOG, 2010).

5.4. Intrauterine Growth Delay

Its etiology is unknown in most cases. It has been suggested to be associated with abnormal placental vascular and disturbance of homeostasis leading to inadequate maternal-fetal circulation. Intrauterine growth restriction is a frequent cause of perinatal morbidity and mortality. Some studies showed association between inherited thrombophilia and complications, such as intrauterine fetal death, preeclampsia and placental abruption but association between intrauterine growth restriction is controversial. Correlation of hereditary thrombophilia and intrauterine growth restriction has been suggested in many studies, but there is no accepted guideline for screening pregnant women (Fatemed, MD and Farzad-smahajer MD, 2013). There are many studies not definitive because of the small sample size of the component studies included. There are no definitive conclusions.

5.5. Placental Abruption

A consistent association has not been established. ACOG guidelines do not recommend screening women with a history of recurrent or nonrecurrent early fetal losses or adverse pregnancy outcomes due to lack of evidence from clinical data.

6. Diagnostic Algorithm in Suspected Deep Vein Thrombosis During Pregnancy

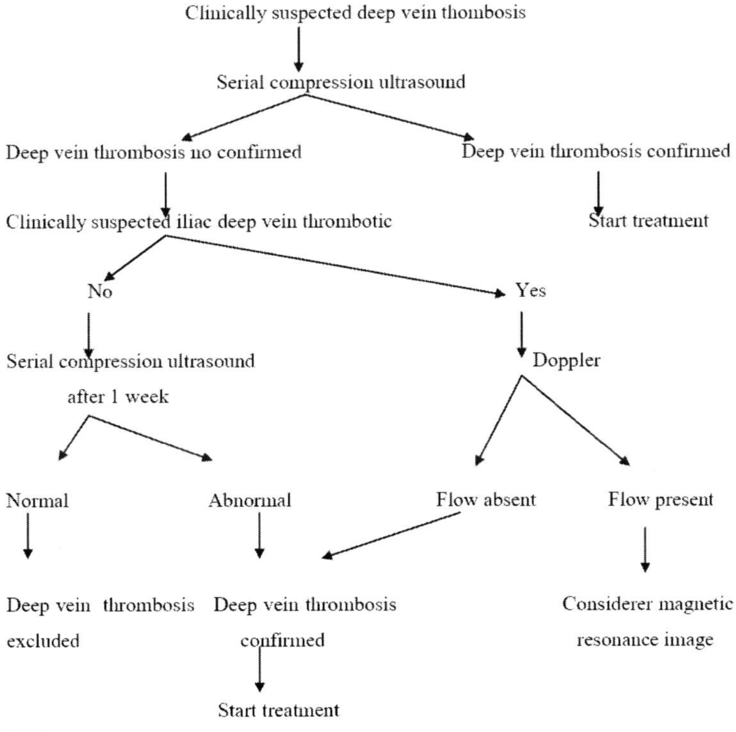

(Paramo et al., 2014).

7. Diagnostic Algorithm in Suspected Pulmonary Embolism during Pregnancy

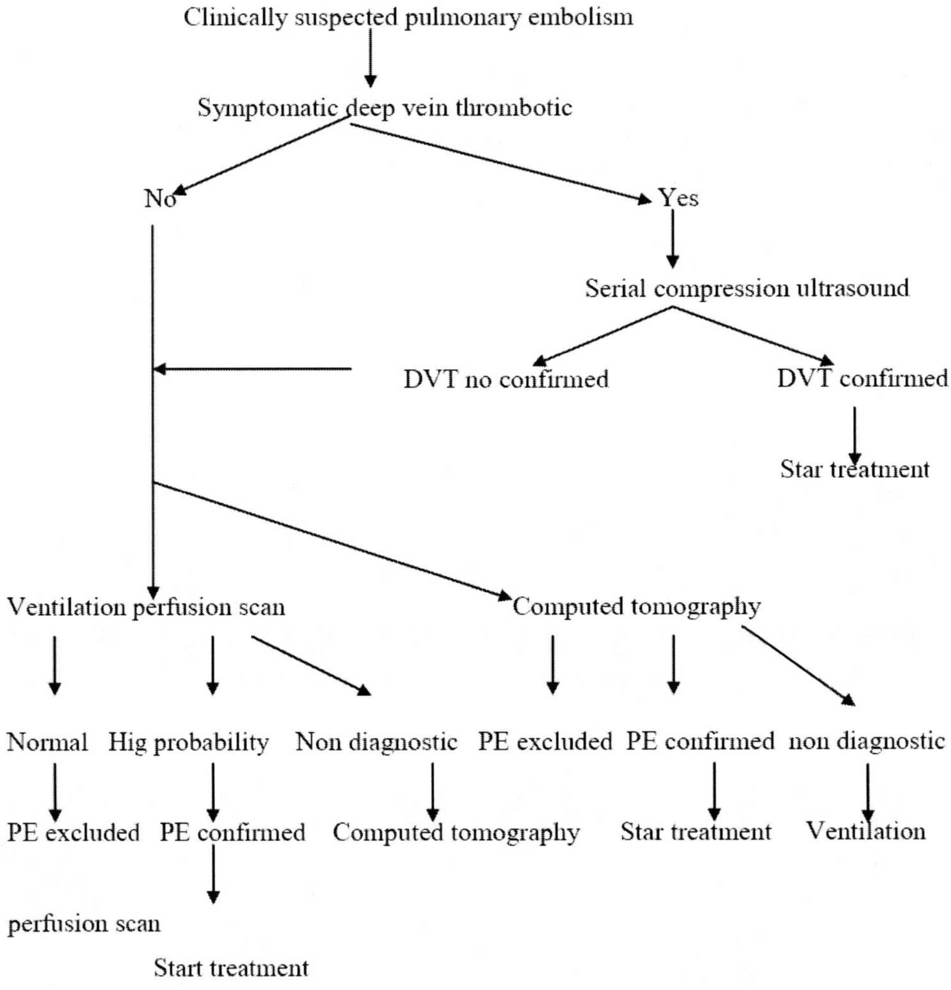

(Paramo et al., 2014).

If there is a delay in obtaining objective testing, anticoagulant therapy should be commenced until testing is available unless there are strong contraindications to its use. Some practitioners use D-dimer measurements after the initial negative ultrasound scan and when there is an elevated D-dimer, a repeat ultrasound is performed. However, D- dimmer levels increase in normal pregnancy, increasing as gestational advances. D-dimer levels also increase with complications such as preeclampsia and abruption, which are themselves associated with an increase in risk for venous thromboembolism. D-dimer have not been evaluated in prospected management studies (Greer, 2012).

8. Candidates for Thrombophilia Evaluation (ACOG, 2010)

Screening may be considered in this clinical settings:

- A personal history of venous thromboembolism that was associated with a nonrecurrent risk factor (e.g., fractures, surgery, and prolonged immobilization).
- A first-degree relative (e.g., parent or sibling) with a history of high-risk thrombophilia or venous thromboembolism before age 50 years in the absence of other risk factors in as much as affected women should receive prophylaxis.
- Screening for antiphospholipid antibodies may be appropriate in patients experiencing fetal loss.

9. Anticoagulation during Pregnancy

Vitamin K antagonists cross the placenta. They are associated with embryopathy with first trimester exposure and with an increased risk of pregnancy loss. Coumarin can be used postpartum if required, because there is no significant excretion in breast milk.

There are no significant data supporting the use of new oral direct thrombin inhibitors (dabigatran) or the new anti-Xa inhibitors (rivaroxaban, apixaban). (Bates and Greer, 2012) Low molecular weight heparin has half-life better bioavailability, it is easy of use and has decreased incidence of bone loss in comparison to unfractioned heparin. Is more effective, has a lower risk of bledding, and is associated with lower mortality than unfractionated heparin for the initial treatment of deep venous thrombosis in nonpregnant patients.

Is equivalent the efficacy of low molecular weight heparin and unfractionated heparin in the initial treatment of pulmonary thromboembolic. (Quinlan, McQuillan and Eikelboom, 2004).

Compared with unfractionated heparin, low molecular weight heparin is associated with a substantially lower risk of heparin induced thrombocytopenia, hemorrhage, and osteoporosis. (Greer, 2012).

Allergic skin reactions are significantly more common with the use of dalteparin than with enoxaparin. In a study with 2777 pregnancies with low molecular weight heparin use, no cases of heparin induced thrombopenia associated with thrombosis were reported. The risk of osteoporosis was 0.04% with the use of low molecular weight heparin (Greer and Nelson-Piercy, 2005).

Greer IA and Nelson-Piercy in 2005 demonstrated that the risk of venous thromboembolism is 1.15% when treatment doses of low molecular weight heparin is use to treat venous thromboembolism in pregnancy. This, compares favourably with recurrence rates of 5% to 8% reported in trials carried out in nonpregnant patients treated with low molecular weight heparin or unfractionate heparin followed by coumarin theraphy who are followed up for 3 to 6 months, and it confirms that low molecular weight heparins are effective in the treatment of acute venous thromboembolism in pregnancy. They demonstrate that low molecular weight heparins provide effective thromboprophylacsis in pregnancy. The optimal prophylactic dose of heparin or low molecular weight heparin has not been determined for pregnant women.

Anticoagulation with low molecular weight heparin is usually initiated during the antepartum period.

Anticoagulation should be continued for at least 3-6 month from development of venous thromboembolic events but if venous thromboembolic events is found early in gestation, anticoagulation should be continued throught delivery and for at least 4-6 weeks postpartum.

In the postpartum period, either continuation of low molecular weight heparin or bridging to warfarine are acceptable options (Battinelli, Marshall and Connors, 2013).

9.1 Anticoagulation Regimen Definitions with Low Molecular Weight Heparine of the American College of Obstetricians and Gynecologists (ACOG)

9.1.1Prophylactic Low Molecular Weight Heparin

Enoxaparin, 40mgr subcutaneously once daily; dalteparin 5000 units subcutaneously once daily; tinzaparin 4500 units subcutaneously once daily (although at extremes of body weight modification of dose may be required)

9.1.2. Intermediate-Dose Low Molecular Weight Heparin

Enoxaparin, 40mgr subcutaneously every 12 hours; dalteparin 5000 units subcutaneously every 12 hours.

9.1.3. Adjusted-Dose Low Molecular Weight Heparin

Weight adjusted, full treatment doses of low molecular weight heparin low molecular weight heparin, given once or twice daily (e.g., enoxaparin, 1 mgr/Kg every 12 hours, dalteparin 200 units/Kg or tinzaparin 175 units/Kg once daily or dalteparin 100 units/Kg every 12 hours).

May target an antiXa level in the therapeutic range (0.6-1 units/mL for twice-daily regimen and slightly higher for a once daily regimen)

9.2. Prophylactic Anticoagulation

In women with history pregnancy loss but without known thombophilias: the use of anticoagulation has not shown significant benefit. Clearly more studies are needed.

9.2.1. Recommendations of the American College of Chest Physicians (ACCP)

9.2.1.1. Antiphospholipid Antibody Syndrome with Previous History of Pregnancy Loss

Should receive low molecular weight heparin and low dose aspirin.

9.2.1.2. Homozygosity for Factor V Leiden or Prothrombin Gene Mutation and a Positive Family History of Venous Thromboembolic Events

Antepartum and postpartum prophylaxis with prophylactic or intermediate dose low molecular weight heparine.

9.2.1.3. Homozygosity for Factor V Leiden or Prothrombin Gene Mutation and No Family History of Venous Thromboembolic Events

Only postpartum prophylaxis for 6 weeks.

9.2.1.4. All Other Known Thrombophilias

Is recommended to undergo close monitoring only.

9.2.1.5. Women With Prior Personal History Of Venous Thromboembolic Events

Postpartum prophylaxis with prophylactic or intermediate dose low molecular weight heparin is suggested.

Clinical decisions should be based on evaluation of each case. (Bates et al., 2012)

9.2.2. Recommendations of the American College of Obstetricians and Gynecologists (ACOG)

Any increased risk of venous thromboembolism in pregnancy appears to be greatest before 20 weeks of gestation, so if antepartum prophylaxis is used, it should be iniciated in the first trimester. Postpartum treatmen levels should be greater tha or equal to antepartum treatment. Low risk thrombophilias are: factor V Leiden heterozygous, prothrombin G20210A heterozygous, protein C or S deficiency.

High risk thrombophilias are: factor V Leiden homozygous, prothrombin G20210A homozygous, double heterozygous for factor V Leiden and prothrombin G20210A mutation, antithrombin deficiency.

9.2.2.1. Low Risk Thrombophilias without Previous Venous Thromboembolism

Surveillance antepartum; surveillance or postpartum anticoagulation with additional risks factors.

9.2.2.2. Low Risk Thrombophilias with a Single Previous Episode of Venous Thromboembolism:

Surveillance or prophylactic or intermediate dose antepartum; postpartum anticoagulation or intermediate dose.

9.2.2.3. High Risk Thrombophilias without Previous Venous Thromboembolism

Prophylactic prepartum; postpartum anticoagulation.

9.2.2.4. High Risk Thrombophilias with a Single Previous Episode of Venous Thromboembolism

Prophylactic or intermediate dose or adjusted dose prepartum; postpartum anticoagulation or intermediate dose for 6 weeks.

9.2.2.5. No Thrombophilia with a Single Previous Episode of Venous Thromboembolism Associated with Transient Risk Factor That is No Longer Present. Excludes Pregnancy, or Estrogen-Related Risk Factor

Surveillance prepartum; postpartum anticoagulation.

9.2.2.6. No Thrombophilia with a Single Previous Episode of Venous Thromboembolism Associated with Transient Risk Factor That Was Pregnancy or Estrogen-Related

Surveillance or prophylactic or intermediate dose antepartum; postpartum anticoagulation or intermediate dose.

9.2.2.7. No Thrombophilia with a Single Previous Episode of Venous Thromboembolism Idiopathic

Surveillance or prophylactic or intermediate dose antepartum; postpartum anticoagulation or intermediate dose.

9.2.2.8. Two or More Episodes of Venous Thromboembolism

Prophylactic or intermediate dose or adjusted dose prepartum; postpartum anticoagulation or intermediate dose for 6 weeks.

9.2.2.9. Two or More Episodes of Venous Thromboembolism Receiving Long Term Anticoagulation

Adjusted dose prepartum; resumption of long term anticoagulation.

9.3. Acute Venous Thromboembolism

In pregnant women, a twice-daily regimen is often recommended. With tinzaparina, once daily dosing may be satisfactory (tinzaparin 175 units/Kg) and may be appropriate in the treatment of venous thromboembolism. Twice-daily dose with enoxaparin (1mgr/Kg twice daily) or dalteparin (100 units/Kg twice daily) in the initial treatment of acute venous thromboembolism until the situation is stable. At that time, once-daily regimen of 1.5mg/Kg of enoxaparin or 1000-18000 units or dalteparin once daily depending on body weight (Greer, 2012).

9.4. Deep Venous Thrombosis

Leg elevation and graduated elastic compression to reduce edema (Greer, 2012). The current American College of Chest Physicians recommendations is to prefer anticoagulation over systemic thrombolysis, reserving consideration of the latter only for patients with all of the following criteria: ilio-femoral deep venous thrombosis, symptoms for <14 days, good functional status, life expectancy of >1 year, and low risk of bleeding (Kearon, Akl and Comerota, 2012).

9.5. Life-Threatening Pulmonary Thromboembolism

It is a serious obstetric and medical emergency. This may be defined as a pulmonary embolus associated with hemodynamic compromise.

IT requires rapid assessment by a multidisciplinary resuscitation team of experienced clinicians. The options include: IV unfractionated heparin, thrombolytic theraphy, catheter-assisted thrombus removal and surgical embolectomy. Oxygen should be administered and circulatory support provided with IV fluids and inotropic agents as required. Intravenous unfractionated heparin is the traditional method of heparin administration in massive pulmonary thromboembolism because of its rapid effects and the extensive experience of its use in this situation (Greer, 2012).

There is growing evidence on the use of thrombolytic agents in pregnancy. Streptokinase, and probably other thrombolytic agents as well, do not cross the placenta. No maternal deaths associated with thrombolytic theraphy have been reported, and the maternal bleeding complication rate is approximately 6% (Bates and Greer, 2012). If the patient is not suitable for thrombolysis or is moribund, cardiothoracic surgeons should be consulted urgently for consideration of emergency thoracotomy (Greer, 2012).

9.6. Inferior Vena Cava Filters

Temporary inferior vena cava filters can be considered in the perinatal period for large iliac deep venous thromboembolism, but their value is uncertain. In women with a filter in place who become pregnant, anticoagulation should be continued or restarted with low molecular weight heparin as soon as pregnancy is diagnosed.

10. Monitoring of Low Molecular Weight Heparin Theraphy

Anti X-a monitoring is not useful in predicting either recurrent thrombosis or bleeding risk, at least in part because of variability in the assay (Greer and Hunt, 2005). There may be a case for monitoring levels for women at extremes of body weight (<50 Kg and >90 Kg) or those with other complicating factors such as renal disease, severe thrombophilia and recurrent venous thromboembolism.

If low molecular weight heparin therapy requires monitoring, the aim is to achieve a peak anti-Xa activity of 0.5-1.2 mc/mL 3 hours postinjection for women with venous thromboembolism. Routine platelet count monitoring for evidence of heparin induced thrombopenia is not required in pregnant patients who have received only low molecular weight heparin (Greer, 2012).

11. Duration of Maintenance Treatment of Venous Thromboembolism

For pregnant women with acute venous thromboembolism, it is recommended that anticoagulants should be continued for at least 6 weeks postpartum and for minimum total duration of therapy of 3 months.

12. Delivery and Anticoagulant Treatment

Low molecular weight heparin should be reduced to a once-daily thromboprophylactic dose on the day before induction of labor or caesarean section. The treatment dose recommended approximately 12 hours later. There is an increased risk of wound hematoma after caesarean section with both unfractionated heparin and low molecular weight heparin of approximately 2%. When a woman presents in labor on therapeutic low molecular weight heparin, neuraxial anesthetic techniques should usually be avoided for at least 24 hours after the last dose of low molecular weight heparin. If thrombosis occurs close to term with a consequently high risk of spontaneous labor we can use unfractioned heparin because it can be relatively easily reversed using protamine sulphate and has a short duration of action (Greer, 2012).

Recommendations of the American College of Obstetricians and Gynecologists (ACOG) are this: In patients which are receiving low molecular weight heparin, a consideration should be given to substituting a comparable dose of unfractioned heparin at 36 weeks of gestation to permit induction of neuroaxial anesthesia during labor and delivery. Alternatively, subcutaneous low molecular weight heparin or unfractionated heparin can be discontinued 24-36 hours before an induction of labor or scheduled caesarean delivery to avoid the anticoagulant effect during delivery. 12 hours after a prophylactic dose or 24 hours after a therapeutic dose of low molecular weight heparin, spinal anesthesia should not be withheld because the risk of procedure related bleeding is limited.

13. Postnatal Anticoagulation

Both heparin and coumarin are satisfactory for use postpartum (both heparin and coumarin are satisfactory for use for breastfeeding mothers) (Greer, 2012).

13.1. Postpartum Contraceptives Options for Women with Thrombophilias

Intrauterine devices, including those containing progestin, progestin only pills or implants and barrier methods should be considered. However, screening all women for thrombophilias before iniciating combination contraception is not recommended (ACOG, 2006).

REFERENCES

ACOG. Use of hormonal contraception in women with coexisting medical conditions. ACOG Practice Bulletin No 73. American College of Obstetricians and Gyecologist. *Obstet. Gynecol.* 2008; 107: 1453-72.

Azem F, Many A, Ben Ami I, Yovel I, Amit A, Lessing JB, et al. (2004). Increased rates of thrombophilia in women with repeat IVF failures. *Hum. Reprod.* 19: 368-370.

Bates SM, Greer IA, Middeldorp S, Veenstra DL, Prabulos AM, Vandvik PO. (2012). VTE, thrombophilia, antithrombotic theraphy and pregnancy. *Chest.* 141(2suppl)e691S-e736S.

Battinelli EM, Marshall A, Connors JM. (2013). The role of thrombophilias in pregnancy. *Thrombosis.* 2013:516420. doi: 10.1155/2013/516420.

Benet SA, Bagot CN, Arya R. (2012). Pregnancy loss and thrombophilia: the elusive link. Br *J. Haem. TOL.*17(5):529-542.

Doi:10.5812/ircmj.13708 Quinlan DJ, Mc Quillan A, Eikelboom JW. (2004). Low- molecular weight heparin compared with intravenous unfractionated heparine for treatment of pulmonary embolism : a meta-analysis of randomizede, controlled trials. *Ann. Intern. Med.* 140:175-83.

Fatemeh Mirzaei MD, Zohreh Farzad-Mahajeri MD. (2013). Association of hereditary thrombophilia with intrauterine growth restriction. *Iran J. Reprod. Med.* 11:275-278.

Grandone E, Colaizzo D, Lo Bue A, Checola MG, Cittadini E, Margaglione M. (2001). Inherited thrombophilia and in Vitro fertilization implantation failure. *Fertil. Steril.* 76: 201-202.

Greer I A, Nelson-Piercy C. (2005). Low-molecular-weight heparins for thromboprophylaxis and treatment of venous thromboembolism in pregnancy: a systematic review of safety and efficacy. *Blood.* 106: 401-407.

Greer IA, Hunt BJ. (2005). Low molecular weight heparin in pregnancy: current issues. *Br. J. Haematol.* 128:593-601.

Greer IA. (2012). Thrombosis in pregnancy: updates in diagnosis and management. Hematology Am. Soc. Hematol. Educ. Program. 2012:203-207 doi: 10.1182/ asheducation-2012.1.203

Inherited thrombophilias in Pregnancy. ACOG Practice Bulletin No 113. American College of Obstetricians and Gyecologist. *Obstet. Gynecol* 2010; 116: 212-222.

Jamal A, Hantoshzadeh S, Hekmat H, Abbasi S. (2010). The association of trombophilia with fetal growth restriction. *Arch. Iran Med.* 13: 482-485.

Kearon C, Akl EA, Comerota AJ et al. (2012). Antithrombotic theraphy for VTE disease: antithrombotic theraphy and prevention of trombosis. American College of Chest Physicians evidence based clinical practice guidelines. 9th Ed. Chest. 141(2suppl):e419S-e494S.

Kupferminc MJ, Many A, Bar-Arm A, Lessing JBm Ascher-Iandsberg JA. (2002). Mid-trimester severe intrauterine growth restriction is associated with a high prevalence of thrombophilia. *BJOG.* 109:1373-1376.

Ogueh O, Chen MF, Spuril G, Benjamin A.(2001). A outcome of pregnancy in women with hereditary thrombophilia. *Int. J. Gynecol. Obstet.* 74: 247-253.

Paramo JA, Bounameaux H, Levi M, Yh Lip G, Marco P, Reverter JC, Tosetto A. (2014). Diagnostic algorithm in suspected deep vein thrombosis during pregnancy. Scores and algorithms in haemostasis and thrombosis. Grupo Acción Médica. Madrid. pp22-24.

Parand A, Zolghadri J, Mozhgan N, Afrasiabi A, Hagh-panah S, Karimi M. (2013). Inherited thrombophilia and recurrent pregnancy loss. *Iran J. Reprod. Med.* 15(12):e13708.

Simon A, Neri L.(2012). Assesment and treatment of repeated implantation failure (RIF). J Assit Reprod Genet. 29: 1227-1239. Doi: 10.1007/s10815-012-9861-4 Tincani A, Cavazzana I, Ziglioli T, Lojacono A, De Angelis V, Meroni P. (2012). Complement activation and pregnancy failure. *Clin. Rev. Allergy inmunol.* 39(3) :153-159.

In: Handbook for High Risk Pregnancy: Clinical Management ISBN: 978-1-63482-299-2
Editors: E. González-Mesa and D. Abehsera

Chapter 8

AUTOIMMUNE DISORDERS

***Laura López Casañas*[1], *Andrés Carlos López Díaz*[1] *and Mª Dolores Gómez García*[2]**
[1]Hospital Quirón Málaga, Spain
[2]University Hospital of Bristol, UK

1. INTRODUCTION

Most systemic autoimmune diseases preferentially affect women, usually in the period covering the childbearing age. It is therefore not uncommon coexistence of pregnancy and systemic autoimmune disease with all the (diagnostic, therapeutic and prognostic) implications that entails both, pregnancy and underlying disease.

The prognosis of these diseases has improved in recent decades, from being almost impossible for these women to have offspring, becoming it similar to that of the general population; although close monitoring of these patients is required due the maternal-fetal morbidity and mortality.

Systemic lupus erythematosus (SLE) is the most representative autoimmune disease in which the connection with pregnancy and disease is known. Almost 90% of these patients are women and almost 70% of them are of childbearing age. Moreover we know the favorable role of hormones in the development and activity of disease (Cervera et al.).

2. SYSTEMIC LUPUS ERYTHEMATOUS (SLE) AND PREGNANCY

Systemic lupus erythematosus is a chronic inflammatory disease resulting from an autoimmune dysfunction. It can affect any part of the human body. The etiology is unknown and often occurs in women of childbearing age, with a ratio of female / male 10/1.

The prevalence is estimated at 20 to 150 cases per 100,000 inhabitants and incidence of 1-25 cases per 100,000 persons / year (Teixidó et al.).

It is characterized by a clinical course with periods of activity and remission. Clinical manifestations are highly variable, from fever, fatigue, malaise or can affect even skin, mucous membranes, joints, kidneys, brain, lungs, heart, blood or gastrointestinal tract (Cervera et al.).

As mentioned above, the pregnancy often exacerbates the disease by up to 60% of cases, especially in patients with active disease at the time of conception. We also know that patients with lupus have higher fetal maternal morbidity, with 19% of miscarriages (55% of stillbirths in the second quarter), 22% preeclampsia (60% in patients with renal disease), whether it is associated with delays on fetal growth (12.7%), preterm delivery (39.4% - mainly termination for medical indications), fetal death (3.6%) or neonatal deaths (2.5%) (Cervera et al.).

The differential diagnosis of proteinuria and hematuria in pregnancy is broad and includes active lupus nephritis. Identification of the correct diagnosis often has a profound therapeutic impact on not only the mother but also the fetus.

To date, relatively few reports exist on the role of renal biopsy during pregnancy among women with systemic lupus erythematosus (SLE). We present a case series of 11 pregnant women with SLE who underwent a renal biopsy to evaluate a presumptive flare of lupus nephritis. The electronic medical record was retrospectively analyzed for pre-biopsy serum creatinine, proteinuria, hematuria, antinuclear antibodies (ANA), and antibodies to double-stranded DNA (anti-dsDNA); histologic findings on renal biopsy; and the clinical course of each mother and fetus. From 2001 to 2012, 11 pregnant women with SLE flares during pregnancy underwent a renal biopsy at an academic tertiary medical center. Among the remaining cases, there were three pre-term deliveries, one fetus with complete heart block, one fetal loss, and one maternal death. Renal biopsy is helpful at informing the management of patients with lupus nephritis during pregnancy (Chen T et al.).

The prognosis of both improved when there is an absence of an outbreak at least six months before pregnancy. Hence, it is very important family planning and therapeutic management of these patients to achieve remission of the disease prior to pregnancy (Diniz da Costa et al.).

Table 1. Scenarios high obstetric risk in pregnant women with SLE

- Related to lupus
  - Organ damage or irreversible renal failure, cardiac, pulmonary hypertension or intestinal lung diseases
  - Nephritis
  - Lupus activity previous 6 months
  - High doses of corticosteroids at the time of conception
  - Positive antiphospholipid antibodies
  - Or anti-Ro/ anti-La positive
- Not related to lupus
  - Previous obstetric complications: preeclampsia or Hellp syndrome
  - Age > 40 years

For clinical assessment must consider organ damage caused by the disease on preconception, it is important for prognosis of pregnancy itself. We know that chronic renal damage has been associated with poor control of blood pressure during pregnancy, preeclampsia and increased incidence of abortions; especially if the creatinine is above 3g/dl. We must also take account of antiphospholipid antibodies (APA) or antiRo/anti-LA, age, obstetric history or multiple gestations are factors to consider when assessing risk (Teixió et al.).

Table 2. Situations in which pregnancy should be contraindicated in patients with SLE

Situations
Severe pulmonary hypertension
Severe restrictive lung disease
Heart failure
Chronic renal failure: creatinine > 2,8 mg/dl
Stroke in the previous 6 months
Severe lupus flare previous 6 months

2.1. Follow Up and Treatment

Upon confirmation of pregnancy, patients should be monitored closely to assess and treat reactivations as soon as possible. At first visit after confirmation of pregnancy (or wish) is advisable:

- Physical examination, including blood pressure
- Renal function (glomerular filtration rate, urinalysis)
- Complete blood count
- Anti-ro/SSA and anti-La/SSB antibodies
- Lupus anticoagulant (LA) and anticardiolipin antibody assays
- Anti-double stranded DNA antibodies
- Complement
- Uric acid level

In patients with lupus and high levels of anticardiolipin antibodies or the presence of lupus anticoagulant is recommended to use low-dose aspirin and monitoring more frequently in cases of patients with only SLE.

In women having anti-Ro and/or anti-La is required a study fetal heart during pregnancy. It is advisable urine protein/urine creatinine ratio, anticardiolipin antibodies and complement too.

Anti- DNA antibodies risk posed development of heart block, although there is no treatment to prevent its progression, early diagnosis does improve development.

During last trimester of pregnancy:

- In complicated pregnancies (preeclampsia, hypertension, fetal growth restriction, fetal heart block), the fetus should be monitored at least weekly using either the biophysical profile score or non stress test (if no heart block) with amniotic fluid assessment.
- Women who show evidence of increased serologic activity but who remain asymptomatic should be monitored more closely. We do not initiate therapy for serologic finding alone.
- If fetal growth restriction is noted, the umbilical artery Doppler ultrasonography is recommended to monitor fetal well-being. Information from umbilical artery Doppler ultrasonography helps guide decision making regarding timing of delivery and has been proven to reduce perinatal mortality in this setting.

Postpartum: some women will experience exacerbations of SLE in the postpartum period. The following laboratory tests are recommended following an uncomplicated delivery:

- Urinalysis, urine protein /urine creatinine ratio
- Renal function if the urinalysis is abnormal
- Completed blood count
- Anti double stranded DNA
- Complement

Treatment of postpartum women with active SLE is the same as that of nonpregnant women.

Table 3. Drugs used in pregnant women with SLE

DRUGS	PREGNANCY	BREASTFEEDING	FDA
NSAID	yes	yes	B/D
Hydroxychloroquine	yes	yes	C
Prednisolone	yes	yes	B
Azathioprine	yes	Probably safe	D
Cyclosporine	yes	Probably safe	C
Tacrolimus	yes	Probably safe	C
Methotrexate	No	No	X
Mycophenolate	No	No	D
Cyclophosphamide	No	No	D
Rituximab	No	No	C
Belimumab	No	No	C
Aspirin	yes	yes	C
Clopidogrel	yes	yes	B
Heparin	yes	yes	C
Warfarin	No (6 -13 weeks)	yes	D

Treating active lupus during de pregnancy is associated with some unique problems. Consideration must be given to the following issues: Medications used to treat SLE may cross the placenta and cause fetal harm. Thus the risk and benefits or treatment during pregnancy must be repeatedly weighed against the risk of activity of SLE having a deleterious effect on the mother and the fetus.

Treatment of SLE depends on the severity and the affected organ. The drugs used are NSAIDs, antimalarials such as hydroxychloroquine, corticosteroids, immunosuppressants or biologic agents (monoclonal antibodies). (Schur et al)

Firstly it is very important to review the treatment that the patient is taking to identify who has a teratogenic potential in order to suspend or replace it with one that can be administered during pregnancy (Table 3). Thus if the patient is being treated with methotrexate or mycophenolate should be replaced by azathioprine and postpone pregnancy for a period of approximately 6 months. If the disease remains stable during this time, you can allow pregnancy (Teixió et al.).

2.2. Treatment

Medications that are typically used to treat patients with SLE may be divided into four categories:

- Drugs with a moderate to high risk of fetal harm.
- Drugs that may be used selectively during pregnancy
- Drugs with minimal fetal and maternal risk
- Drugs with an unknown level of risk

2.2.1 Moderated to high risk of fetal harm

Medications with a high risk of causing birth defects should be avoided during conception and pregnancy, these include: ciclophosphamide, metrotexate, warfarin. Heparin is generally safe but must be discontinued prior delivery to reduce the risk of postpartum hemorrhage.

2.2.2 Selective use allowed during pregnancy

The following drugs are potentially safe during pregnancy, but certain limitations apply to their use. NSAIDs, glucocorticoids and azathioprine are included in this category. They each have a small risk of causing fetal harm, but their use may be acceptable if needed to control manifestations of SLE during de pregnancy. Used of NSAIDs or aspirin near time of conception or during early pregnancy can interfere with implantation. Thus, these agents should be avoided during a conception cycle and early pregnancy. An exception, would be a low-dose aspirin use if needed for lupus associated antiphospholipid syndrome. Used NSAIDs in the third trimester may cause premature closure of the ductus arteriosus and inhibition of labor. Indeed, use of indomethacin is one of several approaches to inhibiting preterm labor, but use any NSAIDs for more than 48 hours should be accompanied by fetal sonographic monitoring for signs of tricuspid regurgitation that could indicate unwanted constriction of the ductus.

Glucocorticoids are relatively safe to use during the pregnancy. Maternal and fetal adverse effects of glucocorticoids are discussed in detail separately. They include: an increased risk of cleft palate in children, premature rupture of membranes, maternal hypertension, gestational diabetes o intrauterine growth restriction.

We recommend, if at all possible, control of the disease with low doses of prednisone (less than 10 mg/day). Steroid side effects in the mother may be reduced by recommending a low salt diet, an exercise program, and calcium and vitamin d supplementation (to prevent osteoporosis)

Azathioprine may be used vary cautiously.

Cyclosporine: when weighed against the risk of rejection, the risk to the fetus is generally judge to be acceptable.

2.2.3 Minimal fetal and maternal risk

NSAIDs used during the first and late pregnancy and antimalarial drug use throughout pregnancy are probably safe. NSAIDs in late first and second trimester are generally safe but should be discontinued in the last trimester of pregnancy. The safety use of antimalarial drugs is uncertain. However, data from observational studies of the infants of patients with SLE and other rheumatic disorders who received antimalarials during pregnancy suggest that these agents are safe. Patients who discontinue hydroxychloroquine prior to, or during, pregnancy are more likely to have exacerbations of SLE.

2.2.4 Unknown level of risk

Use of biologic drugs such us B cell targeted antibodies (rituximab) and T-B cell constimulation blockers (abatacept) is discouraged in part because of a lack of data on safety of their use during pregnancy (Schur et al.).

2.3. Summary

The prognosis for both mother and child is best when SLE has been quiescent for at least six months prior to the pregnancy. Renal disease should be in remission for at least six months prior conception. Patients should have their disease control maintained by use of medications compatible with pregnancy.

The incidence of SLE exacerbation with pregnancy, which may occur at any time during the pregnancy or the postpartum period, has progressively decreased in the past few decades, especially in those in remission at the beginning of pregnancy.

Pregnancy in women with lupus nephritis is associated with an increased risk of fetal loss and with worsening of renal and extra renal manifestations of SLE. Preeclampsia is a frequent complication of pregnancy in SLE; the incidence may be higher among women with active renal disease.

The rate of fetal loss is increased in pregnant women with SLE, but it has improved in the past few decades. Risk is increased in women with hypertension, active lupus or lupus nephritis and in those with hypocomplementemia, increased anti-DNA antibodies, antiphospholipid antibodies and thrombocytopenia.

Maternal SLE is also associated with an increased risk of premature delivery and intrauterine growth restriction.

Breast feeding is feasible for most women with SLE. However, some medication may enter breast milk.

3. Antiphospholipid Syndrome and Pregnancy

The antiphospholipid syndrome is an entity that has aroused more interest in recent years. Its main clinical manifestations are developing abortions and fetal deaths of repetition, and the emergence of other obstetric complications (preeclampsia, eclampsia, HELLP syndrome, intrauterine growth retardation and prematurity).

Although many patients suffering from this syndrome also have SLE, some have a primary antiphospholipid syndrome. The prevalence of antiphospholipid antibodies in the obstetric population has been estimated at 2-3%. The incidence of fetal loss in patients with untreated antiphospholipid antibodies may be up to 80-90%. These fetal losses can occur at any time during pregnancy, although up to 50% of cases occur during the second and third quarter, in contrast to what happens in the general population, which appear mainly in the first quarter due to morphological and chromosomal alterations causes not immunological. The administration of treatment, mainly aspirin and heparin, prevents over 80% of cases fetal loss, although the incidence of intrauterine growth retardation and prematurity is very high.

Antiphospholipid syndrome (APS) in women refers to a syndrome characterized by arterial or venous thrombosis or specific pregnancy complications, and laboratory evidence of antibodies to proteins bound to anionic phospholipids. The two main types of antiphospholipid antibodies of concern to obstetricians are lupus anticoagulant (LA) and anticardiolipin antibodies (aCL).

3.1. Diagnosis

In 2006, an international committee proposed the following criteria for defining pregnancy morbidity in diagnosis of antiphospholipid syndrome.

≥unexplained fetal deaths ≥10 weeks of gestation with normal morphology by prenatal ultrasound examination or direct postnatal examination.

≥1 preterm deliveries of a morphologically normal infant before 34 weeks of gestation due to severe preeclampsia, eclampsia or features consistent with placental insufficiency.

≥3 unexplained, consecutive, spontaneous pregnancy losses <10 weeks of gestation, after exclusion of maternal anatomic and hormonal abnormalities and paternal/ maternal chromosomal abnormalities.

Although the evidence described above supports an association between antiphospholipid antibodies (aPL) and pregnancy morbidity, the predictive value of these antibodies is poor. The reported prevalence of anticardiolipid antibodies in women with uncomplicated pregnancies ranges from 0 to 11 percent, with a median value of about 2 percent. Since antiphospholipid antibodies can be found in normal asymptomatic individuals, a casual relationship between these antibodies and a clinical event in any one individual is difficult to prove, particularly when the adverse obstetrical outcomes is relatively common (spontaneous abortion before 10 weeks) (Lockwood et al.).

3.2. Pathogenesis

The pathogenesis of pregnancy morbidity in APS is incompletely understood. Antiphospholipid antibodies are thought to affect platelet and endothelial cell activation, promote coagulation, and have direct effects on human placental trophoblast (Asherson et al.).

The association between recurrent early miscarriage (REM) and aPL remains inconclusive and that the findings of treatment trials are at best inconsistent and at worst misleading. More convincing data are critically needed. Studies that identify, or at least stratify, according to international consensus criteria and include standardized core laboratory testing results are crucial if we are to establish an evidence-based association between aPL and REM and treatment recommendations (Wong et al.).

Pregnancy and the puerperium are associated with an increased risk of thromboembolic disease, and this risk is particularly high in pregnant women with antiphosphlipid syndrome.

3.3. Treatment

Nonpregnant women with a definite diagnosis of antiphospholipid syndrome, based on laboratory criteria for antiphospholipid antibodies and a history of arterial or venous thrombosis, are at high risk of recurrent thrombosis and are generally treated with warfarin for an indefinite period that may be lifelong. During pregnancy these women use low molecular weight heparin (LMWH) for anticoagulation, with resumption of warfarin postpartum.

If these women also have a history of antiphospholipid syndrome, should treatment with heparin and low dose of aspirin during pregnancy rather than heparin alone.

For women with laboratory criteria for antiphospholipid antibodies and ≥1 fetal losses ≥10 weeks of gestation or ≥3 unexplained, consecutive, spontaneous pregnancy losses <10 weeks of gestations, should combined therapy with low dose of AAS (50 to 100 mg per day) and prophylactic dose of heparin (LMWH); until 6 weeks postpartum (grade 2B).

For women with laboratory criteria for antiphospholipid antibodies and ≥ one preterm deliveries of a morphologically normal infant before 34 weeks of gestation due to severe preeclampsia, eclampsia or other findings consistent with placental insufficiency it is better low dose ASA therapy rather than no therapy or heparin (grade 2c) (Balasch J et al.).

For pregnant women with the incidental finding of persistent antiphospholipid without meeting any of the clinical criteria for antiphospholipid syndrome, it should be managed low dose ASA (grade 2c) (Lockwood et al.).

4. Other Autoinmune Disorders

Other autoimmune diseases such as Sjögren's syndrome, rheumatoid arthritis, or vasculitis are rare in women of childbearing age.

In the coming years we hope to reach an increase of pregnancy in women with systemic autoimmune diseases. The best control of these diseases and the increasingly widespread that its fertility rate is not diminished can motivate greater interest on the part of patients seeking pregnancy knowledge.

It will be necessary therefore properly consider planning such pregnancies to occur at the most appropriate moments in the evolution of the disease and, moreover, once initiated pregnancy, should insist on the need for coordinated action among clinical experts in these diseases, obstetricians experienced in managing high-risk pregnancies and subsequently perinatologist pediatricians.

References

[1] Asherson RA, Cervera R, Piette JC, Shoenfeld Y. (1996). The antiphospholipid syndrome: history, definition, classification, and differential diagnosis. *The antiphospholipid syndrome*; USA: CRC Press; 3-12.

[2] Balasch J, Carmona F, López-Soto A, Font J, Creus M, Fàbregues F et al.(1993). Low-dose aspirin for prevention of pregnancy losses in women with primary antiphospholipid syndrome. *Hum Reprod*; vol 8, 2.234-2.239.

[3] Cervera R, Font J. (1999) Pregnancy and systemic autoimmune disorders. *Medicina clínica*. Vol. 113. Num 20

[4] Chen T, Gelber A, Witter F, Petri M, Fine D. (2014) Renal biopsy in the management of lupus nephritis during the pregnancy. *Lupus*

[5] Diniz da Costa, Centeno M, Pinto L, Marqués A, Mendes-Gracia L. (2013). *Acta Med Port*; 25(6):448-53.

[6] Lim W. Antiphospholipid syndromes.(2013). *Hematology Am Soc Hematol* ; 2013:675-80.Review.

[7] Lockwood CJ, Schur PH. (2014). Pregnancy in women with antiphospholipid syndrome. *Uptodate* Review.

[8] Schur PH, Bermas L. (2014). Pregnancy in women with systemic lupus erithematosus. *Uptodate* Review.

[9] Schur PH, Wallace DJ.(2014). Overview of the management and prognosis of systemic lupus erythematosus in adults. *Uptodate*

[10] Teixidó I, Masoller N, Martínez JP, Ramírez JC. (2013). Systemic lupus erythematosus and pregnancy. ICGON. Feb 2013.

[11] Wong L, Porter T, Gol J.(2014). Recurrent early pregnancy loss and antiphospholipid antibodies: where do we stand? *Lupus*; 23 (12): 1226-8.

In: Handbook for High Risk Pregnancy: Clinical Management ISBN: 978-1-63482-299-2
Editors: E. González-Mesa and D. Abehsera

Chapter 9

LIVER DISEASES IN PREGNANCY

***Araceli Sánchez-Bayton López**, MD*[1], *and Alfonso Alcalde Vargas, MD*[2]**
[1]Obstetrics and Gynecology Department, Quiron University Hospital Málaga, Spain
[2]Digestive Department, Costa del Sol Hospital, Málaga, Spain

INTRODUCTION

Liver disease may complicate 3-5% of gestations (Hay et al., 2008). Liver disorders during pregnancy include: anodyne liver enzyme abnormalities and severe liver failure. Liver disease during pregnancy may become life threatening for the mother and/or the fetus.

Examples of Liver Disease in Pregnancy:

Pregnancy-related liver diseases

- Hyperemesis gravidarum
- Intrahepatic cholestasis of pregnancy
- Pre-eclampsia and eclampsia
- HELLP síndrome
- Acute fatty liver of pregnancy

Pregnancy-unrelated liver diseases

Pre-existing liver diseases

- Cirrhosis and portal hypertension
- Hepatitis B and C
- Autoinmune liver disease
- Wilson´s disease

* Corresponding author: arabayton@hotmail.com.

Liver diseases co-incident with pregnancy

- Viral hepatitis
- Biliary disease
- Budd-Chiari síndrome
- Liver transplantation
- Drug-induced Hepatotoxicity

Physiological Changes During Gestation

During pregnancy the mother's heart rate increases, as does cardiac output; blood pressure and vascular resistance drop. These changes are similar to physiological changes observed in patients with descompensated liver disease. Blood volume increases in aproximately 50%, reaching a peak in the second trimester, although blood flow remains constant.

Telangiectasies, angiomes and palmar erithema are frequently found during pregnancy due to the increased level of estrogens. There is also an increased rate of gallstones due to this high estrogen levels. Estrogens stimulate lipoprotein receptors in the liver, causing cholesterol saturation of the bile. Bilar acid secretion is also affected by female sexual hormones. Stasis due to gallbladder hypomotility in pregnancy is also an important risk factor for the formation of cholesterol gallstones during pregnancy.

During a normal pregnancy alkaline phosphatase, cholesterol, triglicerides and alpha-fetoprotein may increase, whereas albumin decreases due to plasmatic volume expansion. Aminotranferases, bilirubin, gamma-glutamyl transpeptidase (GGT) generally do not suffer changes during pregnancy; therefore any abnormalities must be studied.

Hyperemesis Gravidarum

Nausea and vomiting are common symptoms amongst pregnant women. Nausea appears in 75% of pregnancies and vomiting in 50% during the first trimester. Although, hyperemesis gravidarum (HG) *per se* is only found in 0.3-2% of pregnancies (Joshi et al., 2010).

HG consists in severe and persistant vomiting during the first trimester, rarely during the second. Dehydration, water-electrolyte imbalance, ketosis and up to 5% weight loss may follow. HG is more commonly found amongst primigravidas, young, obese and non smoking women. Multiple gestations, psychatric disease, molar pregnancies, fetal abnomalies such as *hydrops fetalis* and Down's syndrome have also been associated to HG (Philip et al., 2003; Koch et al., 2003).

Hyperthyroidism was diagnosed in up to 60% of women suffering from HG. 94% of hypertransaminasemias during the first trimester were attributed to HG (Wong et al., 2004). Veenendaal et al. (Veenendaal et al., 2011), found that women with HG have a higher risk of concieving underweight and premature children. However, a low Apgar score, a higher incidence of congenital abnormalities or perinatal death were not attributed to HG.

Pathogenesis

The mechanism by which HG is produced is currently unknown. A multifactorial origin is the most probable cause: abnormal gastric motility, hormonal changes and autonomic nervous system disorders are thought to be involved.

Clinical Presentation

HG appears in the 4th gestational week and is resolved by the 18th. If symptoms persist beyond the 18th week a gastroscopy may be prescribed to discard an obstructive cause to vomiting. In aproximately half of the patients suffering from HG biochemical liver alterations such as: increased bilirubin levels (<4g/dL) associated to a discreat increment in aminotranferases (<200U/L) and alkaline phosphate two times above upper limit of normal (ULN) may be found. The severity of nausea and vomiting is directly related to liver enzyme augmentation. Abdominal ultrasonography does not show any specific findings in HG. Liver biopsy (general unrecommended in HG) shows necrosis, steatosis and bile blocage.

Electrolyte abnormalities such as hypokaliemia and hyponatremia may also occur. Neuropathy consequence to vitamin B6 and B12 defeciency is rare, as is Wernike's Encephalopathy (ocular alterations, ataxia and confusion) from thiamine (vitamin B1) deficiency.

Treatment

Patients suffering from HG generally require hospital in-patient care. Intravenous antiemetics, water and electrolyte replenishing and gut rest is initially prescribed. Parenteral nutrition may be necessary in extreme cases. The American College of Obstetritians and Ginecologists (ACOG), recommends as first-line treatment vitamin B6 administration (10 - 25mg/8h, oral administration) and doxalamine (25 mg at night, 12mg at breakfast and lunch if necessary, administrated orally). This treatment manages to resolve 70% of HG. As second-line treatment, metoclopramide is prescribed (10mg/6h orally admistrated). This must be suspended before the 12th week of treatment due to the risk of tardive dyskinesia. Ondasertron (4-6mg/6h) may also be prescribed. Steroids (methilprednisone 16mg/8h for 3 days, suspended after 2 weeks of treatment by progressive decrease in dose) are used in refractory cases (ACOG, 2011). In case of prolonged vomiting, thiamine is administrated in order to prevent Wernicke's Encephalopathy.

Prognosis

HG is generally a reversible condition, with no permanent damage to the liver and is rarely fatal. Fulminating liver failure due to HG has not been found. Most patients need 5-8 days of hospitalisation. Relapses during gestation and reccurence in subsequent pregnancies are common (Yost et al., 2003).

Intrahepatic Cholestasis of Pregnancy

Intrahepatic cholestasis of pregnancy (ICP) is a reversible and non obstructive form of intrahepatic cholestasis, due to incomplete bile secretion in pregnant women. Although ICP does not produce illness in the mother, the fetus may suffer severe complications (placental insuffiency, anoxia, prematurity and fetal death). There have been ICP cases reported in the second trimester (Lammert et al., 2000) although ICP occurs typically during the third trimester in 0,1-1,5% of pregnant women in Europe, United States, Canada and Australia combined (Geenes et al., 2009).

In a recent review, ICP was associated to an increased risk of hepatobiliar diseases such as: hepatitis C, cirrhosis and gallstone. Mothers with previous liver disease have an increased probability of developing ICP (Marschall et al., 2013).

Pathogenesis

Sexual hormones have known effects on cholestasis. Abnormal cholesterol metabolism and reduced bile secretion may cause ICP. In 15% of patients suffering from ICP, bile salt export protein, MDRP3 (multidrug resistant protein 3) is mutated in chromosome 7q21.1. (Trauner et al., 2007). This protein exports phospholipids to the bile canaliculi.

ICP reccurance rate is estimated 45-70% with variable intensity. Meaning exogenous factors may also play a part in ICP. Severness of ICP has also been found to change seasonally (Schneider et al., 2007).

Clinical Presentation

Severe nocturnal palmoplantar pruritus starts around the 25th-32nd week (also during the first trimester). Jaundice is found in 10-25% of patients, 2-4 weeks after itching appears. Patients may present other symptoms such as steatorrhea, malabsorption of liposoluble vitamins and weight loss. ICP seems to increase the risk in developing gasllstones and cholecystitis (Ropponen et al., 2006).

In blood analysis an increase in conjugated bilirubin (<6mg), alkaline phosphatase (<4xULN) and GGT can be found. Aminotranferases may be normal or sightly increased (<300U/L). Prothrombine time can be elongated due to vitamine K deficiency and cholestyramine use. In order to diagnose a patient of ICP, bile acids are measured in serum during fasting (>10mmol/L).

Certain studies suggest that above 40mmol/L fetal complications occur (Glantz et al., 2004). Augmented levels of bile acids in the blood increase uterus contraction, causing premature birth (in 19-60% of patients suffering from ICP), stimulate colon motility, increasing meconium (26-58%) and vasoconstrict chorionic villus, causing acute hypoxia. If untreated, 10% of ICP result intrauterus or peripartum fetal death and 0-2% preterm babies suffer the same fate. Differential diagnosis includes viral hepatitis, gallstones and other typical liver diseases in pregnant women (Table 1). However, pregnancy is a cholestasic and pruritus state, so previous chronic liver disease, such as primary sclerosing cholangitis or hepatitis C, may be revealed. The previously described clinical findings, in absence of other liver diseases, highly suggest ICP, expecially if pruritus was present in previous pregnancies and disappeared after delivery. Liver biopsy, which is generally not recommended in ICP, reveals slight cholestasis (intrahepatic cholestasis, with no parenchymal inflammation).

Fetal complications of ICP include: placental insufficency, premature delivery and fetal sudden death, probally in realtion to high biliar acid levels.

Treatment

The objective is to reduce biliar acids in the blood until pulmonary maturity has been reached. Although certain centers promote premature delivery (before 37 weeks of gestation) when biliar levels are high, no significant benefits to this practice have been found (ACOG, 2011). Pruritus and liver dysfunction are immediately resolved after delivery, therefore there is no influence on mother's mortality rate.

Vitamin K may be necessary during birth in case of severe steatorrhea and elongated prothrombin time.

Therapeutic options are the following:

- Ursodeoxycholic acid (UDCA) 15mg/Kg/24h, has been found to be effective and safefor both the mother and the fetus. UDCA releaves pruritus and reduces biliar acid, transaminases and bilirubin levels. High doses of UDCA (1.5-2.0g/24h) reduce biliar acid levels in the mother and fetus (Kondrackiene et al., 2005). UDCA is to be administered preferentially to patients with severe cholestasis (before the 33rd week) or patients with a history of fetal death.
- In case of refractory pruritus, antihistamines and opiate antgonists may be used.
- Cholestyramine (8-16g/24h), may be used to treat pruritus, although it does not affect
- biliar acid levels and may reduce vitamin K levels.
- Phenobarbital (90mg at night) can be used as an alternative to cholestyramine.
- Dexamethasone (12mg/24h for 7 days) is used for pulmonary development of the fetus and is less effective in pruritus and hypertransaminasia treatement (Glantz et al., 2005).
- S-adenosyl-L-methionine is also less effective than UDCA, but may have an synergic effect when combined (Binder et al., 2006).

In relation to fetal complications, fetal monotoring for chronic placental insufficiency is essential, although not all fetal deaths due to acute anoxia are prevented. Acute anoxia can only be prevented by delivery, which is recommended as soon as the fetus's lungs are developed

Prognosis

Cholestasis lasts as long as the pregnancy does, and is normally resolved after birth or within a maximum of 4 weeks after delivery. Rare cases of persistant cholestasis in pregnancy after childbirth have been described, contributing to the development of liver fibrosis and cirrosis (Ropponen et al., 2006). This may be indicative of previous chronic liver disease. 45-70% relapse rate in later pregnancies with variable severity (Bacq et al., 1997). Perinatal prognosis is better when pregnancy is medically terminated after lung development is completed or before in case of fetal suffering. Fetal complications in ICP are: premature delivery (in 60% of patients suffering from ICP), fetal suffering (61%) and intrauterus fetal death (1.6%) (Joshi et al., 2010). ICP does not contraindicate breast feeding.

Acute Fatty Liver in Pregnancy

Acute fatty liver of pregnancy (AFLP) was described for the first time in 1934 by Stander and Cadden as "acute yellow atrophy of the liver" (Stander et al., 1934). This rare disorder was caracterized by massive microvesicular fatty infiltration and severe repercusions for both mother and fetus, appearing almost exclusively in the third trimester. Incidence rate is of 1/6600 births. It is vital to suspect this disease early on, in order to diagnose and treat patients as soon as possible.

Pathogenesis

AFLP is produced by a mitochondrial anomaly in 3-hydroxyacyl-coenzyme A deshydrogenase, affecting fatty acid β-oxidation (Uchida et al., 1992). This mutation was also found in month old children, being a conditioning factor to non ketosic hypoglycaemia and hepatic encephalopathy, both severe conditions that may result in death if diagnosis is delayed. AFLP has also been associated to insipidus diabetes, pre-eclampsia, nutritional deficiencies, bacterial infections and tetracyclin and valproate consumption.

Clinical Presentation

Normally start the third quarter of the pregnancy (rarely at the end of the second trimester) and initial symptoms are non specific: nausea, vomiting, weight loss, asthenia and epigastrial pain. Later on, right upper quadrant pain and progressive jaundice appear; pruritus is rare. In some patients, jaundice is found in postpartum. AFLP frequently evolves towards more severe manifestations, such as hepatic encephalopathy, pulmonary edema, ascitis, pre-eclampsia, consumption coagulopathy and multi organ failure with a higher tendency to intestinal and ginecological bleeding.

Biochemical blood analysis show: an increment in alkaline phosphatase, bilirubin (<10g/dL), aminotranferases (300-500U/mL), hypoglycaemia (bad prognostic sign), hyperuricemia, hypocalcemia, lactic acidosis, hyperamilasemia, hypoalbuminemia (18-30g/L) a reduction in fibrinogen, an elongated prothrombine time and in some cases renal failure (Borwning et al., 2006). Hemogram shows: normocytic anemia, leucocytosis, thrombopenia. Viral serology is mandatory in every case. Intrauterus death may occur. About 50% of patients with AFLP suffer from pre-eclampsia or HELLP syndrome. Even though hypertension may be present, severe hypertension is normally in relation to decrease in vascular resistancce in liver failure.

Liver biopsy is not routinely used for AFLP diagnosis; it could be useful in early diagnosis of cases with mild symptoms when diagnosis is unclear. Biopsies are not possible in severe cases due to the increased risk of hemorrhaging. Microvesicular fatty acid (free fatty acid) infiltration, predominately in zone 3, with disorganised lobular architecture, portal space cholestasis and inflammation are found (Joshi et al., 2010).

In acute liver failure of the third trimester: HELLP syndome, pre-eclampsia, fulminating viral or toxic hepatitis, thrombotic thrombocytopenic pupura and uremic-hemolystic syndrome must be discarded. In comparaison with HELLP syndrome patients (Table 1), AFLP patients have a higher tendency to develop liver failure with coagulopathy, hypoglycemia, encephalopathy, disseminated intravascular coagulopathy (DIC) and renal failure (Joshi et al., 2010).

Treatment

AFLP treatment is based on stabilising the mother and in early delivery; this is the only treatment that has demonstrated to be efficient; recovery before, is not possible. Although natural delivery is possible (<24h), a caesarean section is normally programed in these cases. Compared to cesarean section, vaginal delivery has a reduced risk of intraabdominal hemorrhaging, and is therefore indicated in cases where INR=1.5 and low platelet count (<50.000 UI/mL).

After delivery, low molecular weight heparin is used in thromboembolic profilaxis. Patients are predisposed to this complication due to excessively low Antithrombin III levels. Severe hypoglucemia, requires continous IV hypertonic glucosate solutions. Sometimes, a supplementary dose of 25% glucosate is required according to daily glycemic controls. On the other hand, hyperglucemia occurs when acute pancreatitis is associated to AFLP. Profilactic antibiotics are recommended in order to prevent uterus infecction. In some cases plasmaferesis was used, showing encouraging results (Seyyed et al., 2013).

Two to three days after delivery, aminotranferases and encephalopathy improve, although intensive care is needed in order to manage the complications of liver failure (Hay et al., 2005). The majority of patients improve in 1 to 4 weeks after childbirth, even though this is a cholestasic phase with increased levels of bilirubin and alkaline phosphatase. Critically ill patients during childbirth, or patients that develop complications (severe encephalopathy, hypoglycaemia, coagulopathy) or patients which state rapidly deteriorates few days after delivery, must be sent to a reference center with liver transplant possibilities.

New borns must be screened for hypoglycaemia, liver failure, myopathy, and other diseases associated to fatty acid oxidation defects (Goodin et al., 2006).

Prognosis

Current mortality rates are between 7-18% in mothers and 9-23% in the fetus. The most frequent causes of death are cerebral edema, sepsis, renal failure, pancreatitis and digestive bleeding. Hepatic coma, prothrombin time >10%, persistant hypoglycemia resistant to treatment by glucosate and small livers with quasi normal transaminase levels (due to cytolytic depletion) are all considered to be negative prognostic factors. Survivours recover with no sequelae. Reccurence in future pregnancies is exceptional, except in patients that suffer from 3-hydroxyacyl-CoA deshydrogenase defect, in which 25% of patients develop reccurence (Yang et al., 2002). The fetus that survives with an enzyme defect is exposed to cardiac failure, fulminating liver failure and sudden death (Rinaldo 1997) if a specific diet in order to avoid episodes that ressemble Reye's syndrome is not followed.

PRE-ECLAMPSIA

Pre-eclampsia is defined by hypertension and proteinuria (>300mg in 24h) after the 20th gestational week and/or within 48h after childbirth. The presence of edemas is no longer necessary for diagnosis (Sibai et al., 2003). Pre-eclampsia is exclusive to pregnancy and in severe cases is associated to liver damage. Other organs may also be affected: kidney, central nervous system and hematopoyetic system. When pre-eclampsia evolves towards eclampsia seizures and coma appear due to hypertensive encephalopathy.

Pre-eclampsia or toxemia in pregnancy is the most severe and common disease found in pregnant women (present in 5-7% and eclampsia en 0.1-0.2% of pregnancies) (Hay et al., 2005). The risk of suffering pre-eclampsia is incresed in primiparas, multiple gestation, patients with a history of pre-eclampsia, extreme age groupes (<16 y.o >45 y.o), diabetes and hypertension (Joshi et al., 2010).

Clinical Presentation

Liver disease must be suspected when the following symptoms are present: right upper quadrant and epigastric pain, nausea and vomiting. These symptomes are common to acute cholecystitis, gallstones, peptic ulcers, hepatitis and pancreatitis.

Jaundice appears in up to 40% of cases, bilirrubin levels are generally under 6mg/dL. When levels of bilirrubin are higher, liver infarction, subcapsular hemorrhaging or liver fracture diagnosis must be taken into consideration. Aminotranferases are 5 to 100 times above ULN in 30% of pre-eclampsias and 90% of eclampsias.

Liver lesion in this context indicates severe illness; the only possible treatment at this state is immediate delivery in order to prevent eclampsia and other complications.

Fibrin deposits in periportal sinusoids, areas with hemorrhaging and thrombosis of small blood vessels are found in liver biopsies of patients suffering from pre-eclampsia (Hay et al., 2008).

Treatment

In order to prevent liver failure, treatment must be intiated as soon as possible. Mild cases are treated as outpatients: bed rest and antihypertensive treatment is recommended. Severe cases should be hospitalized. Depending on the clinical picture and fetal development, ending the pregnancy may be necessary.

The recommended treatment of hypertension in this context is as follows:

- Administration of magnesium sulfate, in order to prevent seizures (6g during 20 minutes, followed by a mantained dose of 2g/h).
- Hidralazine is used to maintain systolic blood pressure under 160 mmHg or diastolic blood pressure under 105mmHg (bolus 5mg every 15-20 minutes, maximum dose 20mg/h).

If blood pressure remains uncontrolled, labetalol may be used (20-40mg intravenous every 10-15minutes, maximum dose 220mg/h) or nifedipine (10-20mg administrated orally every 30 minutes, maximum dose 50mg/h).

HELLP Syndrome

2-12% cases of pre-eclampsia evolve towards HELLP syndrome. 'H' standing for hemolysis, 'EL' for liver enzymes, 'LP' for low platelets (Weinstein et al., 1982).

HELLP syndrome's prevalency in patiensts with pre-eclampsia is between 4-12%, with a 4-27% reccurence risk. Even though HELLP syndrome has similar symptoms to pre-eclampsia and is a consequence of severe pre-eclampsia, HELLP syndrome may occur in patients without previous symptoms of pre-eclampsia.

Pathogenesis

HELLP syndrome is a microangiopathic hemolytic anemia, associated to lesions of vascular endothelium, fibrin deposits in blood vessels and platelet activation, with consumption of plateles (Joshi et al., 2010). These alterations result in hemorrhaging and necrosis; therefore important hematomas, capsular laceration and intraperitoneal hemorrhaging.

Clinical Presentation

Signs and symptoms start before childbirth, between the 27th and 36th gestational week and 25-30% of cases appear in postpartum. These are similar to signs and symptoms of pre-eclampsia: right upper quadrant and epigastric pain (present in 63% of HELLP syndromes), nausea and vomiting (36%), head-aches (33%), hypertension (85%) and proteinuria (87%). There are therefore, no specific signs or symptoms to HELLP syndrome that distinguish it from pre-eclampsia.

The diagnosis of HELLP syndrome is based on the following:

- Hemolysis. Microangiopathic hemolytic anemia is caracteristic. Jaundice appears in 66% of patients suffering from HELLP syndrome. Bilirubin is >2mg/dL and is generally <5mg/dL, LDH >600 U/L. Differential diagnosis must be established between biliar pathology and uremic hemolytic syndrome.
- Increase in liver enzymes. LDH is the enzyme that increases the most in relation to hemolysis and liver malfunction (>600U/L). AST >70U/L and ALT increases in 2-20 times its normal value.
- Platelets <100 x 10^9 /L, <50 x 10^9 /L

Diagnosis is difficult in asymptomatic cases, which, on the other hand, are rare. Differential diagnosis includes: thrombocytopenic purpura, uremic-hemolytic syndrome, antiphospholipid syndrome and AFLP. In some cases these diseases may be co-exist with HELLP síndrome (Barton et al., 2004). The main complications of HELLP syndrome are (Sibai et al., 2004): disseminated intravascular coagulation (complicating 21% cases of HELLP syndrome), placental abruption (16%) and acute kidney failure (8%).

Treatment

Patients should be hospitalized in an intensive care unit (Barton et al., 2004), in order to stabilize hypertension and disseminated intravascular coagulation before delivery, to prevent seizures, to monitor the fetus and quickly proceed to patient intubation if necessary, since edema of the larnyx is a cause of impossible intubation and death of the mother.

Prompt delivery is the only definite treatment, this is why in pregnancies of >34 gestational weeks or if there is evidence of multiple organ failure (DIC, kidney failure, placental abruption or fetal suffering) pregnancy must be terminated (Sibai et al., 2004). It making a determination about terminating the pregnancy before 34 wk of gestation can be difficult.

Current recommendations are as following:

- Treating hypertension (use of labetalol, hydralazine, and nifedipine. Diuretics are not recommended in patients with HELLP, because they can cause utero–placental hypoperfusion), hemodynamic alterations and coagulopathy (with fresh plasma and platelet concentrates before delivery).
- <34 weeks of gestation: in non severe cases, steroides are administered in order to accelerate lung development and delivery is induced near the 34th week. Betamethasone 12mg/24h IM for 2 days or dexamethasone 6mg/12h IM during 2 days is recommended for enhancing fetal maturity. Although steroids do not reduce the number of complications or reduce mortality rate in the mother, perinatal clinical course is improved when steroids are administerd (before the 34th gestational week) in HELLP síndrome (NIH Consensus Development Panel on the Effect of Corticosteroids for Fetal Maturation on Perinatal Outcomes, 1995).

- >34 weeks of gestation: Prompt delivery must be induced, even earlier if multiple organ failure occurs and waiting is not an option (Sibai et al., 2004).

Most patients soon recover after postpartum, although some patient's state may continue to deteriorate. Postpartum HELLP syndrome's treatment is the same.

Liver transplant is indicated in persistant bleeding, liver rupture or liver failure. 88% of these patients survive 5 years after the transplant (Zarrinpar et al., 2007).

Prognosis

Mother's mortality rate is estimated between 2-8%, in relation to multiple organ failure. Perinatal death is estimated between 7-20% (Mihu et al., 2007), consequence to premature delivery, delayed intrauterus growth, placental failure or due to complications in the mother. This is why early on diagnosis and immediately terminating pregnancy is a priority.

The risk of recurrence of HELLP syndrome in subsequent pregnancies is increased (Sibai et al., 1995).

Hepatic Haematoma, Infarction, and Rupture

Infarction, haematomas and liver ruptures may occur in severe pre-eclampsia and in 80% of patients with eclampsia. Haematomas almost always appear on the anterior and superior superface of the right lobule of the liver and may result in hemoperitoneum.

Clinical Presentation

The presence of right upper quadrant pain, hypovolaemic shock and pre-eclampsia in the third trimester (although it may also appear in postpartum) indicate subcapsular hemorrhaging or liver rupture.

High increase in aminotranferases levels is to be expected (3000 UI/L) as are anemia and fever. Acute complications include: respiratory distress, acute kidney injury and hypovolaemic shock. Diagnosis is possible using paracentesis, peritoneal washing, Magnetic resonanace imaging and computerised tomography scan (Barton et al., 1996).

Brain hemorrhage is the main cause of death in the mother and the fetus. 16% of deaths are due to liver complications.

Treatment

Contained haematomas should be managed conservatively with blood transfusion and supportive measures for the mother. Infection can occur within areas of hepatic infarction. Haemodynamic instability suggests persistent active bleeding and should prompt hepatic angiography, and when required, invasive haemostatic measures by arterial embolisation of the hepatic artery or surgical exploration (Joshi et al., 2010).

Hepatectomy is only indicated in liver laceration, or when there is uncontrollable hemorrhaging. After laparotomy a caesarean must be done.

Prognosis

A 50% mortality rate in the mother has been reported for this complication, with a higher prevalency of liver rupture in patients with severe thrombopenia (Sibai et al., 1993).

Perinatal mortality rates are estimated between 10-60%, most of these deaths are related to placental abruption, intrauterus asfixia or prematurity.

Table 1. Distinguishing features of intrahepatic cholestasis of pregnancy, the HELLP síndrome and acute fatty liver of pregnancy

	HELLP	AFLP	ICP
Trimester/onset	3° or postpartum	3° or postpartum	25-32 weeks
Family history	No	Occasionally	Often
Presence of preeclampsia	Yes	50%	No
Typical clinical features	Hemolysis, Thrombocytopenia (<50.000 often)	Liver failure with coagulopathy, encefalophaty, hipoglycaemia, disseminated intravascular coagulation	Pruritus, mild jaundice, elevates bile acids, low leves of vitamin K
Aminotransferases	Mild to 10-20-fold elevation	300-500 typical but variable	Mild to 10-20-fold elevation
Bilirubin	<5 mg/dL unless massive necrosis	Often <5 mg/dL, higher if severe	<5mg/dl
Hepatic imaging	Hepatic infarcts, haematomas, rupture	Fatty infiltration	Normal
Histology	Patchy/extensive necrosis and hemorrhage	Microvesicular fat in zone 3	Normal-mild cholestasis, no necrosis
Maternal mortality	1%-25%	7%-18%	0%
Fetal/perinatal mortality	11%	9%-23%	0.4%-1.4%
Recurrence in subsequent pregnancies	4%-19%		45%-70%

References

Bacq Y, Sapey T, Bréchot MC, Pierre F, Fignon A, Dubois F (1997). Intrahepatic cholestasis of pregnancy: a French prospective study. *Hepatology*, 26: 358-364.

Barton JR, Sibai BM (2004). Diagnosis and management of hemolysis, elevated liver enzymes, and low platelets syndrome. *Clinics in Perinatology*, 31:807-833.

Barton JR, Sibai BM (1996). Hepatic imaging in HELLP síndrome (hemolysis, elevated liver enzymes, and low platelet count). *American Journal of Obstetrics & Gynecology*, 174: 1820-1825; discussion 1825-1827.

Binder T, Salaj P, Zima T, Vitek L (2006). Randomized prospective comparative study of ursodeoxycholic acid and S-adenosyl-L-methionine in the treatment of intrahepatic cholestasis of pregnancy. *Journal of Perinatal Medicine*, 34:383- 391.

Borwning MF, Levy HL, Wilkins-Haug L, Larson C, Shih VE (2006). Fetal fatty acid oxidation defects and maternal liver disease in pregnancy. *Obstetrics & Gynecology*, 107:115-120.

Geenes V, Williamson C. Intrahepatic cholestasis of pregnancy (2009). *World Journal of Gastroenteroly*, 15: 2049-2066.

Glantz A, Marschall H-U, Lammert F, Mattsson L-A (2005). Intrahepatic cholestasis of pregnancy: a randomized controlled trial comparing dexamethasone and ursodeoxycholic acid. *Hepatology*, 42:1399-1405.

Glantz A, Marschall HU, Mattsson LA (2004). Intrahepatic cholestasis of pregnancy: Relationships between bile acid levels and fetal complication rates. *Hepatology*, 40: 467–74.

Goodin B (2006). An overview of expanded newborn screening for inborn errors of metabolism. *Practical Gastroenterology*, 41:34-51

Hay JE (2008). Liver diseases in pregnanacy. *Hepatology*, 47(3):1067-76.

Joshi D, James A, Quaglia A, Westbrook RH, Heneghan MA (2010). Liver disease in pregnancy. *Lancet*, 375: 594-605.

Koch KL, Frissora CL (2003). Nausea and vomiting during pregnancy. *Gastroenterology Clinics of North America*, 32: 201-234.

Kondrackiene J, Beuers U, Kupcinskas L (2005). Efficacy and safety of ursodeoxycholic acid versus cholestyramine in intrahepatic cholestasis of pregnancy. *Gastroenterology,* 129:894-901

Lammert F, Marschall HU, Glantz A, Matern S (2000). Intrahepatic cholestasis of pregnancy: molecular pathogenesis, diagnosis and management. *Journal of Hepatology*, 33: 1012-1021.

Marschall HU, Wikström Shemer E, Ludvigsson JF, Stephansson O (2013). Intrahepatic cholestasis of pregnancy and associated hepatobiliary disease: A population-based cohort study. *Hepatology*, 58: 1385-1391.

Mihu D, Costin N, Mihu CM, Seicean A, Ciortea R (2007). HELLP yndrome—a multisystemic disorder. *Journal of Gastrointestinal and Liver Diseases*, 16: 419–24.

NIH Consensus Development Panel on the Effect of Corticosteroids for Fetal Maturation on Perinatal Outcomes (1995). Effect of corticosteroids for fetal maturation on perinatal outcomes. J*ournal of the American Medical Association*, 273: 413-418.

Philip B (2003). Hyperemesis gravidarum: literature review. *Wisconsin Medical Journal*, 102: 46-51.

Report of the National High Blood Pressure Education Program Working Group on High Blood Pressure in Pregnancy (2000). *American Journal of Obstetrics & Gynecology*, 183: S1-S22.

Ropponen A, Sund R, Riikonen S, Ylikorkala O, Aittomäki K (2006). Intrahepatic cholestasis of pregnancy as an indicator of liver and biliary diseases: a population-based study. *Hepatology*, 43: 723-728.

Royal College of Obstetricians and Gynecologists. Obstetric cholestasis (2011). London (UK): RCOG Green-top Guideline, No. 43: 7.

Schneider G, Paus TC, Kullak-Ublick GA, Meier PJ, Wienker TF, et al., (2007). Linkage between a new splicing site mutation in the MDR3 alias ABCB4 gene and intrahepatic cholestasis of pregnancy. *Hepatology*, 45:150-158.

Seyyed Majidi MR, Vafaeimanesh J. (2013) Plasmapheresis in acute Fatty liver of pregnancy: an effective treatment. *Obstetrics & Gynecology*, 2013: 615975.

Sibai BM (2004). Diagnosis, controversies, and management of the syndrome of hemolysis, elevated liver enzymes, and low platelet count. *Obstetrics & Gynecology,* 103:981-991.

Sibai BM (2003). Diagnosis and management of gestational hypertension and pre-eclampsia. *Obstetrics & Gynecology*, 102: 181–92.

Sibai BM, Ramadan MK, Chari RS, Friedman SA (1995). Pregnancies complicated by HELLP syndrome (hemolysis, elevated liver enzymes, and low platelets): subsequent pregnancy outcome and long-term prognosis. *American Journal of Obstetrics & Gynecology* 172: 125–29.

Sibai BM, Ramadan MK, Usta I, Salama M, Mercer BM et al., (1993). Maternal morbidity and mortality in 442 pregnancies with hemolysis, elevated liver enzymes, and low platelets (HELLP syndrome). *American Journal of Obstetrics & Gynecology* 169: 1000–06.

Stander H, Cadden B (1934). Acute yellow atrophy of the liver in pregnancy. *American Journal of Obstetrics & Gynecology* 28: 61–69.

Trauner M, Fickert P, Wagner M (2007). MDR3 (ABCB4) defects: a paradigm for the genetics of adult cholestatic syndromes. *Seminars in Liver Disease*, 27: 77–98.

Uchida Y, Izai K, Orii T, Hashimoto T (1992). Novel fatty acid betaoxidation enzymes in rat liver mitochondria. II. Purifi cation and properties of enoyl-coenzyme A (CoA) hydratase/3-hydroxyacyl-CoA dehydrogenase/3-ketoacyl-CoA thiolase trifunctional protein. *The Journal of Biological Chemistry*, 267: 1034–41.

Veenendaal MV, van Abeelen AF, Painter RC, van der Post JA, Roseboom TJ (2011). Consequences of hyperemesis gravidarum for offspring: a systematic review and meta-analysis. *An International Journal of Obstetrics & Gynaecology*, 118: 1302-1313.

Weinstein L (1982). Syndrome of hemolysis, elevated liver enzymes, and low platelet count: a severe consequence of hypertension in pregnancy. *American Journal of Obstetrics & Gynecology*, 142: 159–67.

Wong HY, Tan JY, Lim CC (2004). Abnormal liver function tests in the symptomatic pregnant patient: the local experience in Singapore. *Annals Academy of Medicine Singapore*, 33: 204-208.

Yang Z, Zhao Y, Bennett MJ, Strauss AW, Ibdah JA (2002). Fetal genotypes and pregnancy outcomes in 35 families with mitocondrial trifunctional protein mutations. *American Journal of Obstetrics & Gynecology*, 187: 715–20.

Yost NP, McIntire DD, Wians FH Jr, Ramin SM, Balko JA et al., (2003). A randomized, placebo-controlled trial of corticosteroids for hyperemesis due to pregnancy. *Obstetrics & Gynecology*, 102: 1250–54.

Zarrinpar A, Farmer DG, Ghobrial RM, et al., (2007). Liver transplantation for HELLP syndrome. *American Surgery,* 73: 1013–16.

In: Handbook for High Risk Pregnancy: Clinical Management ISBN: 978-1-63482-299-2
Editors: E. González-Mesa and D. Abehsera

Chapter 10

SPECIFIC DERMATOLOGICAL CONDITIONS

Jessica Martín Orlando, Evelyn García Pintor and María Micaela Fernández Abellán
Obstetric and Gynecology Department, Quirón Hospital, Málaga, Spain

Pregnant women are particularly susceptible to a group of changes in their skin that can be divided into physiological and pathological changes. These changes are due to vascular, endocrinological, metabolic and immunological modifications (Cunningham et al., 2006). Placental substances increase activity in endocrine system and alter the purification system, causing more availability of estrogens in plasma and generating a clinical impact.

In addition to physiological changes in the skin and pre-existing skin disease, it can develop specific skin diseases that are seen only during pregnancy or postpartum period. The importance of detection of these disorders lies in the possible adverse maternal and fetal outcomes.

Classification of skin diseases during pregnancy is highly controversial. Many different names have been used to define similar clinical disorders. It is very important to differentiate in a practical way the common changes from those that could have an effect on the mother and fetus. In order to differentiate the types of skin lesions we will summarize its nomenclature and semiological definition (Martínez Cabañero et al., 2007)

- Taint: change of skin colour without elevation. For example: melasma, spider nevi.
- Papule: palpable and elevated lesion which measures less than 1 centimeter.
- Nodule: papule bigger than 1 centimeter.
- Wheal: erythematous and edematous lesion with fleeting evolution.
- Vesicle: intraepidermal or subepidermal collection that contains clear liquid.
- Pustule: papule that contains necrotic remains, fibrin y polymorphonuclear leucocytes in response to a bacterial process.
- Ulcer: absence of epidermis or dermis as a result of trauma or necrosis; it heals with a scar.
- Erosion: loss of epithelium surface; it heals without scar.
- Excoriation: erosion epidermis because of scrape.

Dermatoses in pregnancy can be classified in:

1. Physiological cutaneous changes in pregnancy
2. Specific dermatoses of pregnancy
3. Other dermatoses and infections affected in pregnancy

1. Physiological Cutaneous Changes in Pregnancy

The maternal skin and related structures (hair, nails and glands) undergo numerous changes during pregnancy.

1.1. Pigmentation

The change in pigmentation occurs in 90% of women. There is increased pigmentation. The pathogenesis is not completely understood. One possibility is that estrogens and progesterone cause melanocytic stimulation and melatonin accumulation in macrophages.

This hyperpigmentation appears in localized areas. The most frequent cutaneous pigmentary change is darkening of linea alba which becomes the linea nigra. The skin around the areola also darkens (Lawley et al., 1999).

1.1.1. Melasma or Chloasma or Mask of Pregnancy

This is the characteristic hyperpigmentation of the face that is present in 70% of pregnant women. There are three clinical patterns: centrofacial, malar and mandibular. Melasma intensifies with solar irradiation, so protection from the sun is essential as preventive treatment. Melasma due to pregnancy usually regresses within one year but some areas of hyperpigmentation may never completely resolve (Gelber et al., 2004).

The overall treatment is very unsatisfactory and consists of sunscreen and topical bleaching agents such as hydroquinone creams and tretinoin. There have been reports of temporary associated cases of congenital malformations with topical tretinoin (Berlin et al., 2012). Hydroquinone is acceptable for use during pregnancy. A chemical peel can be considered, and laser treatments and dermabrasion have also been tried.

1.1.2. Nevi

During pregnancy, nevi presents bigger melanocytes but there is no evidence of malignant transformation. Although, all nevi that changes in any manner should be examined histologically. (Driscoll et al., 2007).

1.2. Vascular Changes

Pregnancy involves variations in vascular structures such as bloating and instability due to the effect of estrogens. There are numerous changes through the skin that usually regress postpartum.

Vasomotor instability causes facial flushing, hot and cold sensations and cutis marmorata. Cappilary permeability, increased sodium and water retention result in edema of extremities. Increased hydrostatic pressure and capillary fragility lead to pigmented purpura from extravasation of red blood cells.

1.2.1. Spider Angiomas

These are red rounded stains with branches extending out from a central artery. They appear in the second to fifth month of pregnancy and are most common in areas drained by superior vena cava: face, neck, chest and hands. These changes regress three months after birth.

1.2.2. Palmar Erythema

It is caused by extended vascular dilatation. There are two distributions limited to the hypothenar or thenar eminence or diffuse.

1.2.3. Varicosities

This venous dilatation is present in almost 40% of pregnant women. They appear in saphenous, vulvar and hemorrhoidal territories. Genetic predisposition plays a role but pregnancy is an aggravating factor due to increased blood volume and venous pressure in femoral and pelvis vessels from the enlarging uterus.

It is very important to recommend: leg elevation, exercise, sleeping of the left side, compression with support hose and avoidance of long periods of standing or sitting.

Jacquemier's sign refers to venous distention in the vestibule and vagina and is associated with vulvar varicosities.

Hemorrhoidal disease is most common in the last trimester of pregnancy. They are varicosities in the anal canal caused by local pressure. Symptoms include pruritus, discomfort and bleeding.

These changes usually disappear within three months postpartum.

1.2.4. Pyogenic Granulomas

This vascular tumour-like structure is also called granuloma gravidarum, pregnancy tumour or pregnancy epulis. It is an exophytic, reddish purple papues made up of granulation tissue. No infection is involved and it appears in traumatic areas as a vascular and fibrotic response most commonly on the anterior mandibular or maxillary gingiva.

1.3. Connective Tissue Changes

1.3.1. Striae Gravidarum

These stretch marks begin as pink or violet patches in the sixth to seventh month of gestation. They become linear depressions with fine wrinkles and hypopigmentation. Stretch marks are most prominent in the abdomen, breasts and thighs.

The etiology is a disminution of elastin fibers in the dermis. There is a strong familiar predisposition. They do not disappear but can lose colour and are less visible after losing weight (Nassar et al., 2007).

Treatment is not always effective. Hydration with cream that contains vitamin A and D is recommended.

1.3.2. Molluscum Fibrosum Gravidarum (or Acrocordon)

They are soft fibromas that develop on neck, axillae and inframammary area. The size is from milimeters to centimeters. Histologically composed by connective tissue covered by epidermis.

1.4. Cutaneous Adnexa Changes

1.4.1. Hirsutism

It results from increased levels of ovarian and placental androgens in the pilosebaceous unit. Its localization is most frequent in face.

1.4.2. Telogen Effluvium

This hair loss is common one to five months postpartum and resolves within fifteenth months postpartum. However, complete recovery is not always obtained. No medical intervention is necessary.

1.4.3. Nails

Nails grow faster during pregnancy and slow down postpartum. They can become dystrophic with transverse grooves and subungual keratosis. Onycholysis and fragility are frequent.

1.4.4. Hyperhidrosis

Eccrine glands show a gradual increase in activity during pregnancy. This, along with an increase in thyroid activity, results in hyperhidrosis and increased miliaria.

1.4.5. Apocrine Glands

During pregnancy there is a decrease in the apocrine glands activity and an increase in conditions such as hidradenitis suppurativa.

1.4.6. Sebaceous Glands

These glands show an increased activity in pregnancy resulting in exacerbation of pre-existing acne. Treatment is difficult because most oral or topical agents are contraindicated. Based on the severity of the acne, agents commonly prescribed include oral or topical erythomycin preparations, topical benzoyl peroxide and topical sulfur.

1.5. Pruritus

This symptom may be physiological. The common locations are scalp, anus, vulva and abdominal skin.

The etiology is multifactorial but it could be caused by hepatic disorder because of estrogens. It is very important to make different diagnosis with liver disease, thryroid disfunction, contact dermatoses and atopia. Pruritus without any underlying pathological process affects up to twenty percent of pregnant women.

The treatment is symptomatic and sometimes it is necessary the use of topic corticoids and antihistamine.

2. Specific Dermatoses of Pregnancy

2.1. Pemphigoid Gestaionis

Pemphigoid gestationis (PG) is a rare autoimmune bullous dermatoses of pregnancy. Initially described by Milton in 1872 as "herpes gestationis" but this name has been changed because there is no association with herpes virus infection.

Estimated incidence of PG is 1 in 50,000 cases. It occurs on the second or third trimester of pregnancy; about 25% of cases may have an initial presentation immediately postpartum. It usually recurs with subsequent pregnancies and occurs after oral contraceptive use in about 25%.

Causes

It appears to be an autoimmune phenomenon, it is a Type II Hypersensitivity reaction caused by an IgG antibodies blind to an antigen (180-KdA protein, BP-80) in the hemidesmosomes (attach basal cells of epidermis to the basal lamina and hence to dermis) of the dermoepidermal junction, leading to blister formation as loss of hemidesmosomes causes the epidermis to separate from dermis.

Clinical

Itching is common and often starts around the umbilicus. It starts with urticarial wheals (like hives from nettles) and large raised red patches (plaques) commonly occurring on the trunk, back, buttocks and limbs. The face, scalp and mucous membranes (mouth and genital area) are usually not involved. Large tense blisters then occur on the red patches within 1-2 weeks, and may also occur on palms and soles. The blisters contain clear fluid though occasionally this can be blood-stained. The blisters usually heal without scarring.

Diagnosis

Pemphigoid gestationis may be clinically confused with several other pruritic eruptions of pregnancy, particularly pruritic urticarial papules and plaques of pregnancy. Pemphigoid gestationis can often be distinguished because it usually begins in the periumbilical area; pruritic urticarial papules and plaques of pregnancy usually begin in the striae.

Direct immunofluorescence examination of perilesional skin is diagnostic of PG. It detects a linear band of C3 at the basement membrane zone. (Al-Fouzan et al., 2006).

Treatment

Pemphigoid gestationis can't be cured but can be suppressed with treatment. Symptoms usually resolve days or weeks after giving birth, but in some women the disease can remain active for months and may require continued treatment. Restarting periods, use of oral contraceptive therapy and further pregnancies can all cause flare-ups of the condition.

The primary aim of treatment is to relieve itching, prevent blister formation and treat any secondary infection.

Blisters may be burst (with a sterile needle) to offer relief from discomfort and dressings can be applied to weepy or raw areas of skin. Emollient creams or ointments can also be applied to reduce itching and soothe sore areas.

Topical steroid (0.1% triamcinolone acetonide cream up to 6 times/ day) can be used in mild cases if only a limited area of skin is affected. If the rash is quite extensive systemic steroid may be recommended (Black et al., 2009).

Oral antihistamines (those suitable for use during pregnancy) can be used to relieve itching.

Steroid tablets (prednisolone 0.1-1mg/kg/day, clobetasol, betamethasone)) are usually needed to control the blisters and itching. The dose of steroid tablets may need to be increased at the end of pregnancy to prevent the disease flaring after delivery.

Occasionally immuno plasmapheresis may be used if the condition is severe or does not respond to treatment with steroids.

In the post partum period, if necessary, the full range of immunosuppressive treatment may be administered for cases unresponsive to corticosteroid treatments, such as tetracyclines, nicotinamide, cyclophosphamide, ciclosporin, goserelin, azathioprine, dapsone, rituximumab, or plasmaphoresis, or intravenous immunoglobulin may sometimes be considered when the symptoms are severe.

Prognosis

PG can potentially put the mother and fetus at serious risk. Pregnant women with PG should be monitored for conditions that may affect the fetus, including, but not limited to, low or decreasing volume of amniotic fluid, preterm labour, and intrauterine growth retardation. When a pregnant mother develops PG, the risk for the development of other autoimmune diseases increases specifically Grave's disease. Prognosis of the fetus is usually good, but the rate of premature births and small-for-date babies rises. Recent studies have shown the risks are related to the severity of the disease and are not caused by the treatment with corticosteroids. PG usually reoccurs with following pregnancies, and symptoms appear earlier and more severely. With earlier onset of PG comes a greater risk of adverse pregnancy outcomes. Passive transfer of the mother's antibodies to the fetus causes some (about 10%) newborns to develop mild skin lesions, but they will usually resolve within weeks after parturition.

2.2. Polymorfhic Eruption of Pregnancy

Polymorphic eruption of pregnancy (PEP) was described by Lawley in 1979. It is the most common of the dermatoses unique to pregnancy, with an incidence of 1 in 160-240 pregnancies. It occurs predominantly in primigravidas (80%), on the third trimester of pregnancy, and less often on the other trimesters or postpartum. It is characterised by an itchy rash that commonly begins on the abdomen, particularly within stretch marks (striae).

Causes

The cause of PEP is unknown. It occurs more commonly with multiple pregnancy (twins or triplets). Previous studies have suggested a link with increased maternal weight during pregnancy, increased birth weight and sex hormones, but these have not been proven.

Clinical

The pruritic eruption starts on the abdomen and proximal thighs in 91% of cases, and 80% of patients will subsequently develop involvement of upper extremities and other areas of the trunk (lower abdomen, under the breast and limbs). The face, scalp and mucous membranes (mouth and genital area) are hardly ever affected. The lesions characteristically start on or adjacent to the abdominal striae and typically show periumbilical sparing. The lesions are usually urticarial, but the eruption often becomes polymorphous, showing vesicular, targetoid, polycyclic or purpuric lesions. Excoriations and eczematous features are common. Generalized PEP with extensive desquamation may resemble a toxic erythema. The presence of polymorphous lesions may increase with disease duration, and an association between nonurticarial morphology and disease duration of more than 6 weeks has been reported. The eruption resolves spontaneously or with delivery. (Orion, 2006).

Diagnosed

Diagnosis is usually made by a dermatologist based on the typical appearance and distribution of the rash. However, if the appearance is not typical your dermatologist may take a sample of skin and a blood test to help in making the diagnosis and rule out other causes of the rash. (Fermand et al., 2008).

Direct immunofluorescence is negative for a linear band of C3 or IgG along the skin dermoepidermal junction; however, there have been reports of deposition of IgM, C3, and IgA along the dermoepidermal junction and blood vessels on direct immunofluorescence. Differential diagnosis of PEP includes pemphigoid gestations (PG), contact dermatitis, drug eruption, and viral exanthems.

Treatment

The primary aim of treatment is to relieve itching and to reduce inflammation and redness in the skin. Treatment is symptomatic relief of pruritus with topical corticosteroids of low- to mid-potency (use of ultra-high-potency corticosteroids for an extended period of time should be avoided) and pregnancy category B antihistamines such as loratadine and cetirizine. Hydroxyzine and diphenhydramine are pregnancy category C antihistamines that have been used to relieve pruritus. In cases of severe pruritus unresponsive to conservative measures, systemic corticosteroid administration or induced delivery may be considered.

Prognosis

It is important to know that it is a benign, self-limiting condition with no risk to the unborn baby. Recurrence in subsequent pregnancies is unusual (less than 7% of cases).

2.3. Atopic Eruption of Pregnancy (AEP)

Atopic eruption of pregnancy (AEP) is a benign, self-limited pruritic disorder of pregnancy, seen in patients with a personal and/or family history of atopy, and clinically presents as eczematous lesions (also called E-type, in two-thirds of cases) or prurigo lesions (also called P-type in one-third of cases). Atopic eruption of pregnancy usually develops during the first half of pregnancy (75% before the third trimester). AEP was previously also known as "prurigo of pregnancy" but this name has been abandoned.

Causes

The pathogenesis of AEP is not fully known. In AEP there is always a personal and/or family history of atopy. This atopic background shows the impact of a possible genetic predisposition in the pathogenesis of the disease.

During pregnancy, the immune system changes considerably, which may lead to worsening of pre-existing eczema or to a first development of atopic skin changes. These changes are usually reversible after delivery; however, a small number of women may continue to have eczema in following pregnancies.

Symptoms

The main feature is itch which can be bad enough to interfere with sleeping. The severity of the rash depends on the type of AEP. If you suffer from worsening of pre-existing eczema, it is likely that your skin will be red and dry. When the eczema is very active (during a 'flare-up') you may develop small water blisters on the hands and feet or your skin may become wet and weepy. In areas that are repeatedly scratched, the skin may thicken in response - a process known as lichenification. If you experience AEP for the first time during pregnancy, the rash is usually much milder. Two third of patients suffer from red scaly itchy patches (so called eczematous type or E-type AEP) in sites typically affected by atopic eczema such as the neck, breasts, and skin creases on the elbows and knees.

The other third shows tiny red raised spots (1-2mm) or slightly larger raised skin lumps (5-10mm, at times with small open wounds (excoriations) due to scratching) on the abdomen, back, and limbs (so called prurigo type or P-type AEP).

Diagnosis

It is helpful to know the personal and/or family history of atopy and signs of the tendency to be atopic.

Worsening of already existing eczema is usually easy to diagnose by investigating your skin and taking your history. However, first manifestation may be more difficult to diagnose; it can be confused with other skin diseases.

Prognosis

Prognosis is good even in severe cases. (Ambros-Rudolph et al., 2006) Pruritus is the most distressing symptom, generally more severe at night, causing a considerable discomfort to the pregnant woman. Marked improvement occurs due to prompt treatment or the natural course of the disorder. Fetal prognosis is good, but there is a risk of developing atopic skin changes (such as atopic dermatitis, eczema, asthma…) later in infancy.

2.4. Intrahepatic Cholestasis of PregnancyAtopic Eruption of Pregnancy

In other chapter.

Table 1. Specific dermatoses of pregnancy

3. Other Dermatoses and Infections Affected in Pregnancy

The pregnancy exercises a very variable influence on the evolution of the dermatosis, already coexistent or preexisting.

In many of these diseases the impact of the gestation is unpredictable. The most frequent dermatoses coexistent with pregnancy are summarized below.

3.1. Pustular Psoriasis of Pregnancy

Pustular psoriasis of pregnancy is a newer name for impetigo herpetiformis. The former is more descriptive and avoids the implication of bacterial or viral infection, neither of which plays a role in this disease. It is debated whether pustular psoriasis of pregnancy is truly specific to pregnancy. We favour a true association as these women rarely have a history of psoriasis and the eruption resolves postpartum.

Incidence

Pustular psoriasis of pregnancy is exceedingly rare.

Clinical Manifestations and Diagnosis

The diagnosis can be made clinically, based on characteristic findings on history and physical examination. However, we suggest confirmation by histological evaluation of a biopsy specimen, given the potential consequences of the disease and its treatment to maternal and child health (e.g., side effects of systemic corticosteroids, preterm delivery).

The disease can occur anytime during pregnancy. Lesions begin as erythematous plaques with rings of pustules. The plaques then enlarge from the periphery as the center becomes eroded and crusted. There may be concentric rings of pustules. The nails may become onycholytic.

The lesions often first show in intertriginous regions. The trunk and extremities are affected, while the hands, feet, and face are usually spared, although the soles were affected in one case report. Oral and esophageal erosions may occur.

Pustular psoriasis of pregnancy is usually not pruritic, usually abates quickly postpartum, but may also flare after delivery. It recurs with subsequent pregnancies and may also recur with menses or use of oral contraceptive pills. The disease tends to be more severe and have an earlier onset with subsequent pregnancies. (Konro et al., 2013).

Treatment

Evidence for the treatment of pustular psoriasis of pregnancy is limited. We suggest systemic corticosteroids as initial therapy. High dose systemic corticosteroids, such as prednisolone up to 60 to 80 mg per day, are given for a few days and then slowly tapered as symptoms improve, with monitoring in case a flare occurs.

Hypocalcemia must be corrected, when present, and fluid and electrolyte balance should be maintained. These patients sometimes require early delivery for relief of symptoms and for fetal safety.

Prognosis

Placental insufficiency with sequelae such as miscarriage, fetal growth restriction, or stillbirth may occur. Therefore, antepartum fetal monitoring with nonstress tests or biophysical profiles and ultrasound assessment of fetal growth are indicated. (Luan et al., 2014)

3.2. Eczema

Eczema is the most common pruritic skin disorder occurring in pregnancy, and women with clinical findings consistent with eczema account for the vast majority of patients with atopic eruption of pregnancy.

This disorder often begins during the first or second trimester. Symptoms frequently present in a flexural distribution, similar to classic atopic dermatitis. However, any area of the skin may be affected. Lesions may be eczematous patches or intact or excoriated papules. The diagnosis is based upon the recognition of clinical features. Skin biopsy is not necessary in most cases, and findings are non-specific.

Treatment is similar to non-pregnant patients with eczema; these patients should be encouraged to maintain adequate skin hydration through the use of topical emollients. Low- to mid-potency topical corticosteroids (group four to six) are useful for controlling symptoms. Eczema in pregnancy has not been associated with adverse effects on the fetus.

3.3. Erithema Nodosum

Painful, erythematous nodules typically develop on the anterior surfaces of both legs, though occasionally elsewhere, and evolve into bruise-like lesions that resolve without scarring over a two- to eight-week period. Histologically, erythema nodosum (EN) is a panniculitis involving inflammation of septa in the subcutaneous fat tissue. Polyarthralgia, fever, and malaise frequently accompany the eruption, and the erythrocyte sedimentation rate is often elevated.

The diagnosis of this disorder is most often clinical, with biopsy required only in atypical cases. When biopsy is obtained, it is crucial to obtain a deep incisional biopsy.

Numerous conditions have been associated with EN. The diagnosis most frequently associated with EN is streptococcal pharyngitis; however, EN is also frequently idiopathic, and EN may precede other manifestations of diseases associated with EN by months to years.

Other conditions associated with EN include pregnancy and oral contraceptives, other medications, leprosy, systemic rheumatic diseases and vasculitides, and infections.

EN is usually self-limited or resolves with treatment of the underlying disorder. Thus, treatment is typically symptomatic.

Treatment with antibiotics is generally not warranted in patients with EN thought related to streptococcal infection, if such suspicion is based solely upon serological evidence of recent streptococcal infection or a positive throat culture in the absence of symptomatic pharyngitis. Glucocorticoids are usually not necessary for idiopathic EN. (Calonje et al., 2014)

3.4. Leprosy in Pregnancy

Immunologic reactions appear to occur more frequently in pregnant and postpartum women. In two small series, such reactions were observed in up to 38 percent of patients. Type 2 reactions were observed more frequently during pregnancy; Type 1 reactions were observed more frequently in the postpartum period.

Management of leprosy and immunologic reactions in pregnancy is the same as described for other patients. Dapsone, rifampin, clofazimine, clarithromycin, and ofloxacin are listed by the FDA as category C for use in pregnancy; minocycline is category D. Regimens of all medications must be modified appropriately if the mother is breastfeeding.

3.5. Systemic Lupus Erythematous (SLE)

The prognosis for both mother and child is best when systemic lupus erythematosus (SLE) has been quiescent for at least six months prior to the pregnancy. Renal disease should be in remission for at least six months prior to conception. Patients should have their disease control maintained by use of medications compatible with pregnancy. Care by an obstetrician experienced in the management of high risk pregnancies is particularly desirable for women with one or more of the following: a history of poor obstetric outcomes, renal or cardiac involvement, pulmonary hypertension, interstitial lung disease, active lupus, high-dose glucocorticoid therapy or use of immunosuppressives, antiphospholipid antibodies/syndrome, antibodies to Ro/La, and multiple gestation. Characteristics associated with high maternal and fetal risk have been identified. The incidence of SLE exacerbation with pregnancy, which may occur at any time during the pregnancy or the postpartum period, has progressively decreased in the past few decades, especially in those in remission at the beginning of pregnancy; this improvement may be related to a combination of factors. The frequency of exacerbation (or persistently active disease) is greater in patients with active disease at the time of conception. Pregnancy in women with lupus nephritis is associated with an increased risk of fetal loss and with worsening of the renal and extrarenal manifestations of SLE. Pregnancy outcomes following renal transplantation for lupus nephritis are similar to those of other transplant recipients. Preeclampsia is a frequent complication of pregnancy in SLE; the incidence may be higher among women with active renal disease. Laboratory testing is sometimes useful in distinguishing preeclampsia from nephritis or a lupus flare. The rate of fetal loss is increased in pregnant women with SLE, but it has improved in the past few decades. Risk is increased in women with hypertension, active lupus, or lupus nephritis and in those with hypocomplementemia, increased anti-DNA antibodies, antiphospholipid antibodies, and thrombocytopenia. Neonatal lupus is a passively transferred autoimmune disease that occurs in some babies born to mothers with anti-Ro/SSA and/or anti-La/SSB antibodies; many of these women do not have lupus or other autoimmune disease, although they frequently develop such a disease during follow-up. Maternal SLE is also associated with an increased risk of premature delivery and intrauterine growth restriction. There may be an increased risk of learning disabilities in the offspring, especially in males.

Breast feeding is feasible for most women with SLE. However, some medications may enter breast milk. (Hamed et al., 2013).

REFERENCES

Al-Fouzan AW, Galadari I, Oumeish I, Oumeish OY. 2006. Herpes gestationis (Pemphigoid gestationis). *Clinical Dermatolgy*.

Ambros-Rudolph, Christina M, Robert R, Mullegger, Samantha A. 2006. The specific dermatoses of pregnancy revisited and reclassified: Results of a retrospective two-center study on 505 pregnant patients. *Journal of the American Academy of Dermatology*:395-404.

Berlin M, Csajka C, De Santis M, Panchaud A, Schaefer C. 2012. Pregnancy outcome following exposure to topical retinoids: a multicenter prospective study. *The Journal of Clinical Farmacology*: 1844-1851.

Black M, Semkova K. 2009. Pemphigoid gestationis: current insights into pathogenesis and treatment. *European Journal of Obstetric and Gynecolgy Reproduccion Biology*: 138-44.

Calonje E. Dermatopathology:LC07-1 Panniculitis. *Patology*. Oct; 46 Suppl 2:S10. 2014.

Cunnighan S, MacDonald P. 2006. Enfermedades dermatológicas y embarazo. Obstetricia de Williams: 1249-1255.

Driscoll MS, Grant-Kels JM. 2007. Hormones, nevi and melanoma: an approach to the patient. *Journal of the American Academy of Dermatology*: 919.

Fermand V, Levy P, Regnier S, Uzan S. 2008 A case-control study of polymorphic eruption of pregnancy. *Journal of the American Academy of Dermatology:* 63–67.

Gelber J, Rao B, Victor FC. 2004. Melasma: a review. *Journal of Cutaneous Medicine and Surgery:* 97-102.

Hamed HO, Ahmed SR, Alzolibani A, Kamal MM, Mostafa MS, Gamal RM, Atallah DA, Abd-El-Aall DE. Does cutaneous lupus erythematosus have more favorable pregnancy outcomes tan systemic disease? A two-center stydy. *Acta Obstet. Gynecol. Scand.* 2013 Aug;92(8):934-42.

Kondo RN, Araújo FM, Pereira AM, Lopes VC, Martins LM. Pustular psoriasis of pregnancy (impetigo herpetiformis)-case report. *An Bras. Dermatol.* 2013 Nov-Dec; 88 (6 Suppl 1): 186-9.

Lawley TJ, Yancey KB. 1999. Skin changes and diseases in pregnancy. *Fitzpatrick´s Dermatology in General Medicine*: 1963-1969.

Luan L, Han S, Zhang Z, Liu X. Personal treatment experience for severe generalized pustular psoriasis of pregnancy: two case reports. *Dermatol. Ther.* 2014 May-Jun;27(3):174-7.

Martínez Cabañero RM, Gómez García B, González de Merlo G. 2007. Dermatopatías específicas del embarazo. *Fundamentos de Obstetricia de la Sociedad Española Ginecología y Obstetricia*:661-670.

Nassar AH, Osman H, Rubeiz N, Tamim H. 2007. Risk factors for the development of striae gravidarum. *American Journal of Obstetric and Gynecology:* 62.

Orion E, Matz H, Wolf R. 2006. Pruritic urticarial papules and plaques of pregnancy: polymorphic eruption of pregnancy. *Clinical Dermatology.*

In: Handbook for High Risk Pregnancy: Clinical Management ISBN: 978-1-63482-299-2
Editors: E. González-Mesa and D. Abehsera

Chapter 11

THROMBOTIC MICROANGIOPATHY DURING PREGNANCY: THROMBOTIC THROMBOCYTOPENIC PURPURA DURING PREGNANCY

E. Ernesto González-Mesa*, MD, PhD, and J. José Herrera-Peral, MD, PhD
Obstetrics and Gynecology Department,
Malaga University, School of Medicine, Spain

INTRODUCTION

Thrombotic thrombocytopenic purpura (TTP) is one of the microangiopathic disorders that can be diagnosed during pregnancy. These alterations are characterized by the formation of microthrombi in small vessels, leading to thrombocytopenia, microangiopathic hemolytic anemia, and multiorgan damage.

The hypercoagulability state observed during pregnancy conditions the incidence of such disorders in pregnant women compared with the general population. Specifically, these disorders comprise TTP, uremic hemolytic syndrome (HUS), preeclampsia-HELLP syndrome, and some other autoimmune diseases like catastrophic antiphospholipid syndrome (CAPS).

TTP is clinically characterized by a group of five symptoms: thrombocytopenia, microangiopathic hemolytic anemia, fever, neurological alterations and renal failure. It can exhibit a familial trait, though idiopathic TTP is the most common presentation. HUS in turn is characterized by renal failure, and although it is typically observed in children with a history of infection due to toxin-producing bacteria in the previous days or weeks, the disease occasionally has also been reported during pregnancy. On the other hand, both preeclampsia and HELLP syndrome belong to a range of disorders in which arterial hypertension is the fundamental clinical feature - HELLP syndrome being one of the most serious conditions. On the other hand, CAPS is a serious and rapidly progressive form of antiphospholipid syndrome

* Corresponding author: egonzalezmesa@uma.es.

leading to multiorgan failure. CAPS may be the first manifestation of the disease, although previous history of antiphospholipid syndrome, systemic lupus erythematosus, or in a small number of cases, Sjogren's syndrome or Systemic Sclerosis, could guide the doctor. In CAPS the activation of coagulation is caused by the presence of autoantibodies that bind to membrane phospholipids.

Although the underlying physiopathological mechanisms differ, the clinical consequences are very similar. This makes it very difficult to establish a differential diagnosis. Each disease has its own treatment particularities, and maternal and perinatal morbidity and mortality is high when treatment is not appropriate. It is therefore necessary for gynecologists to have a thorough understanding of differentiating characteristics of these disorders.

EPIDEMIOLOGY AND PRESENTATIONS

The reported incidence (Miller, 2004) of TTP in the general population is 3.8 cases per million individuals. In turn, the incidence of PPT and HUS, as disorders differentiated on the basis of laboratory test criteria, is one case in every 25,000 pregnancies (Egermen, 1996) and one case in every 198,000 pregnancies (Moatti-Cohen, 2012), respectivey.

TTP is more common in women, with a peak incidence in the fourth decade of life, and 10% of all cases occur during pregnancy (Ezza, 1996). The incidence of TTP shows a female/male ratio of 3:2, possibly because of the greater female susceptibility towards autoimmune disorders. Pregnancy triggers both the appearance of the disease and its recurrence (Battaglioli, 2006) TTP associated to pregnancy accounts for 10-30% of all cases of TTP diagnosed in adults (Scully, 2008; Fujimura, 2010).

TTP can manifest in three clinical forms. A first form is familial-hereditary congenital disease or Upshaw Schumann syndrome (SUS), which accounts for a mere 5% of all cases in the general population and 24% of all cases associated with pregnancy, while a second form is acquired idiopathic disease (the most frequent presentation), and a third form is related to use of drugs, infections, neoplasms and pregnancy. The disease often evolves in the form of outbreaks. In this sense, following remission of the initial episode, recurrences of the clinical symptoms are typically observed, particularly during the first year after the diagnosis (Peyvandi, 2008).

The inclusion in some series of pregnant women with minor forms of TTP or with probable HELLP syndrome results in reported (Vesseley, 2004) maternal mortality rates of less than 10%. However, in the absence of adequate diagnosis and treatment, the maternal and fetal mortality rate approaches 90% (DAngelo, 2010). In this context, unlike in HELLP syndrome or severe preeclampsia, there is no evidence that uterine evacuation is able to solve the problem (Natelson, 1985); a correct differential diagnosis is therefore of crucial importance.

TTP as either an initial episode or recurrence can manifest at any time during pregnancy (Trisolini, 2012), though the condition is more often diagnosed in advanced gestation, during the second or third trimester, in peripartum, or even in the puerperal period (Martin, 2008; George, 2003).

TTP was first described in 1924 by Moschovitz in a 16-year-old girl (Moschovitz, 1924) who developed hemolytic anemia, thrombocytopenia, neurological alterations and impaired renal function, followed by death due to cerebral infarction and heart failure. The autopsy revealed generalized thrombosis, particularly of the terminal arterioles. The first documented case of TTP during pregnancy was reported in 1955, in a 30-year-old woman in the eighth month of pregnancy (Miner, 1955) who died as a result of the disease.

PHYSIOPATHOLOGY

Von Willebrand factor is a multimeric glycoprotein fundamentally produced in the endothelial cells, where it accumulates in the Weibel-Palade bodies, and in megakaryocytes, conforming the so-called alpha granules. These intracellular Von Willebrand factor multimers are larger (ultra-large multimers) than those that circulate freely in plasma under normal conditions (large multimers). The ultra-large multimers are able to bind with greater affinity than the large multimers to the platelet GPIb receptors, thereby favoring platelet aggregation. Regulation of multimer size is therefore essential in order to maintain adequate function.

Von Willebrand factor also has zones for binding to the vascular endothelium and platelets, favoring their adhesion; to activated platelets, facilitating their aggregation; and to factor VIII, preventing the latter from undergoing premature degradation (Sadler, 2004).

Regulation of multimer size is mediated by a metalloproteinase known as ADAMTS-13 (A desintegrin and metalloproteinase with a thrombospondin type 1 motif, member 13) that cleaves the ultra-large multimers as they are secreted, converting them into chains that are anchored in the collagen of the vascular wall or circulate freely (Lotta, 2011).

Defects in degradation of the ultra-large Von Willebrand factor multimers give rise to the different forms of TTP. The existence of ultra-large Von Willebrand factor multimers in the plasma of patients with recurrent TTP was reported in 1982. These multimers would increase platelet adherence to the endothelium, particularly in high-flow vessels (capillaries), thereby favoring the appearance of thrombi (Moake, 1982; Moake, 1986).

In the familial forms of the disease (SUS), homozygous mutation of the gene encoding for the synthesis of ADAMTS-13 (chromosome 9) causes the protease activity to drop to below 5% of that seen under normal conditions (Moake, 2002). The familial form usually begins to manifest during childhood, though in some cases it develops later in life, and occasionally during pregnancy. Many mutations have been identified in relation to ADAMTS-13 deficiency, with variable impact in relation to the clinical severity of the condition. Approximately 90% of all patients with both homo- and heterozygous mutations present symptomatic TTP (Camilleri, 2012; Levy, 2001).

In the acquired forms, protease activity is either low or absent during the disease outbreaks, and recovers during the disease-free intervals. In these cases the existence of an anti-ADAMTS-13 IgG autoantibody has been identified. The production of autoantibodies may be transient and/or recurrent, thereby conditioning the course of acquired idiopathic TTP. Autoantibodies can be detected in approximately 31-38% of all patients with idiopathic TTP.

Increased circulating estrogen levels have been related to an increase in coagulation (Kim, 1981) factors such as factor VIII and Von Willebrand factor, as well as to a decrease in the protease activity of the enzyme ADAMTS-13 (Westerlund, 2011). This circumstance is another factor giving rise to an increased incidence of TTP among women and its occurrence or relapse during pregnancy (Kato, 2009) and is co-responsible for the hypercoagulability state seen during pregnancy (Sanchez-Luceros, 2004; George, 2004). A significant observation is the fact that 100% of all patients with SUS who do not receive prophylactic treatment initially develop the disease or experience recurrences during pregnancy, and an important percentage suffer their first episode upon becoming pregnant. On the other hand, 25% of all patients with acquired TTP develop recurrences during pregnancy or in the immediate puerperal period.

Despite knowledge of the mentioned physiopathological aspects of the disease, doubts remain regarding the existence of still unknown additional etiopathogenic factors. The fact that there have been reports of cases of acquired idiopathic TTP in which the ADAMTS-13 levels are normal, or of familial TTP characterized by a complete absence of ADAMTS-13 without clinical manifestations until adult age, points to the need for further investigation of the pathogenesis of this disease (Murrin, 2000) Quantification of ADAMTS-13 in the disease-free intervals contributes to distinguish among the different forms of the disease. In this sense, values of under 10% of normal are typical of hereditary TTP, while values above 30% are indicative of acquired TTP.

Clinical Manifestations and Diagnosis

Between 10-40% of the patients experience pseudoinfluenza syndrome in the weeks prior to diagnosis, and asthenia, malaise and fever for days or weeks, refractory to initial empirical symptomatic treatment, is occasionally observed.

The classical group of five clinical symptoms is observed in 40% of the cases, while 75% of all patients exhibit a triad in the form of microangiopathic hemolytic anemia, thrombocytopenia, and neurological symptoms such as headache, diminished consciousness or seizures (Ridolfi, 1981).

It is also possible to observe moderate renal dysfunction, with creatinine levels below 3 mg/dl, though both neurological and renal disorders are more common in the terminal stages of untreated cases. It must be also taken into account that cardiac abnormalities may be important and often unrecognized causes of mortality and morbidity in patients with TT (Hawkins, 2008). Cardiac symptoms are frequently overlooked because many patients are young, without cardiac risk factors, but angina, congestive heart failure, arrhythmias and syncope have been reported in more than 20% of TTP patients and myocardial infarctions appear in 24% of autopsies. In the absence of clear evidence for cardiac involvement, all TTP patients should be screened with a focused cardiac history, electrocardiogram, and serial cardiac enzymes and monitored (Patschan, 2006).

Because of the need for early diagnosis and adequate treatment, the five clinical characteristics regarded as crucial for diagnosing the disease have been reduced to only two: thrombocytopenia and microangiopathic hemolytic anemia. Thus, in daily practice, the presence of thrombocytopenia ($<20x10^9/L$), schistocytes representing over 1% of the global red cell population, and LDH elevation in the absence of other apparent causes suffice to diagnose TTP and start treatment (George, 2000; Lara, 1999; Thompson, 1992; Rock, 1992;

Rock, 1991). Since in this way TTP is indistinguishable from HUS, some authors include both conditions under the term TTP-HUS (Veseley, 2003).

Table 1. Clinical and laboratory findings

	TTP	HUS	HELLP
Hypertension (%	20-75	80-90	85
Proteinuria (%)	With hematuria	80-90	90-95
Fever (%)	20-50	Not reported	Absent
Nausea and vomiting (%)	Common	Common	40
Abdominal pain (%)	Common	Common	60-80
Central nervous system (%)	60-70	Not reported	40-60
ADAMST13 activity 5%	33-100	Rare	Absent
von Willebrand factor multimers (%)	80-90	90	Absent
Platelet count (mm3)	>20.000	< 20.000	< 20.000
Anemia (%)	100	100	< 50
Elevated transaminases (%)	Usually absent	Usually absent	100
Elevated lactic dehydrogenase (%)	100	100	100

Adapted from Stella CL, Dacus J, Guzman E, et al. The diagnostic dilema of thrombotic thrombocytopenic purpura/hemolytic uremis síndrome in the obstetric triage and emergency department: lessons from 4 tertiary hospitals. Am J Obstet Gynecol 2009; 200:381-386.

The role of the determination of ADAMTS-13 and ultra-large Von Willebrand factor multimers in characterizing the different microangiopathic disorders is unclear. ADAMTS-13 activity varies between 50-178% in healthy adults, though during pregnancy the variability is usually lower, and only in cases of SUS are activity values of under 5% observed. There have been reports of patients who develop an episode of TTP with ADAMTS-13 levels above 50%. In turn, some patients with activity levels under 5% remain disease-free (Furlan, 2001) and some series have reported higher mortality in cases of TTP during pregnancy than in idiopathic PTT in non-pregnant patients, independently of the ADAMTS-13 activity level (Zheng, 2004).

It should be mentioned that HELLP syndrome occurs in 0.5-0.9% of all pregnancies and affects 10-20% of all patients with severe preeclampsia. Both TTP and preeclampsia-HELLP syndrome occur more frequently in the second half of pregnancy, in the peripartum or postpartum. Establishing a differential diagnosis is therefore complicated, since the clinical manifestations are very similar. However, while the end of pregnancy contributes to treatment in cases of preeclampsia-HELLP syndrome, the clinical course of TTP or HUS is not modified. The need for an adequate differential diagnosis has caused the diagnosis of TTP-HUS to be considered in those pregnant women who beyond week 24 present microangiopathic hemolytic anemia (negative indirect Coombs' test) and thrombocytopenia in the absence of arterial hypertension and/or proteinuria, as well as in pregnant women in the first or second trimester (less than 24 weeks) in which any of the orienting symptoms are suspected, in view of the low frequency of HELLP syndrome in these gestational weeks. The shorter the interval from symptoms onset to the start of treatment, the better the perinatal outcomes (Stella, 2004).

Regarding CAPS diagnostic criteria include: 1) Evidence of involvement of three or more organs, systems and/or tissues, 2) Development of events simultaneously or in less than a week, 3) Pathologic confirmation of occlusion of small vessels in at least one organ or tissue, and 4) Laboratory confirmation of antiphospholipid antibodies (lupus anticoagulant and/or anticardiolipin antibodies) (Asherson, 2003; Cervera, 2007).

Table 2. Clinical criteria for diagnosis

Severe Preeclampsia ACOG criteria. (any of these findings)	– Systolic blood pressure of 160 mm Hg or higher, or diastolic blood pressure of 110 mm Hg or higher on two ocassions at least 4 hours apart while the patient is on bed rest – Cerebral or visual disturbances – Pulmonary edema – Trombocytopenia (platelets count less than $100x10^9/L$ – Impaired liver function as indicated by abnormally elevated blood concentrations of liver enzymes (to twice normal concentration), severe persistent right upper quadrant or epigastric pain unresponsive to medication and not accounted for by alternative diagnoses, or both – Progressive renal insuffiency (serum creatinine concentration greater than 1.1 mg/dl or a doubling of the serum creatinine concentration in the absence of other renal disease
HELLP Mississippi criteria	– Thrombocytopenia (usually $<100x10^9/L$) with a documented prenatally normal platelet count – Hepatic dysfunction: AST> 48 IU/L, ALT >24 IU/L or LDH>164 IU/L – Evidence of intravascular hemolysis, to include a decreasing hematocrit concurrent with worsening thrombocytopenia, an increase in LDH, and/or evidence of bleeding involving intravenous sites or hematuria – No evidence of another disorder primarily causative of clinical and laboratory findings

Adapted from. Pels et al., ACOG and Martin et al.

On the other hand the effects of hepatic insufficiency due to acute fatty liver of pregnancy should be considered in TTP differential diagnosis. This disorder has uncertain aetiology but inherited defects in the mitochondrial beta-oxidation of long chain fatty acids is associated. Clinical manifestations include abdominal pain, headache, nausea, vomiting, anorexia and ictericia. The 20% is associated with preeclampsia, and very often appears coagulopathy secondary to severe hepatic impairment. Transaminases are often over 300-500 IU/L (Steingrub, 2004). Typical laboratory findings in acute fatty liver of pregnancy include bilirubin >2mg/dL, Hypocholesterolemia <200mg/dL, Hypoglycemia <60mg/dL, Hypofibrinogenemia <300 md/dL, decreased Antithrombin III and prothrombin time prolongation (Vigil, 2001).

Treatment

The initial treatment of TTP-HUS during pregnancy is no different from that indicated in the non-pregnant patient (Gernesheimer, 2013). Patients with SUS benefit from prophylactic treatment with fresh plasma infusions every 2-3 weeks, according to the ADAMTS-13 activity levels (Scully, 2006).

TTP is potentially fatal, with a mortality rate of over 90% before introduction of the current treatments. The prognosis, in terms of maternal-fetal survival rates, has improved since the 1970s with the development of treatments such as plasma transfusions and plasmapheresis. The mortality rate has dropped to approximately 10-20%, with a response in up to 90% of all cases of TTP, and healing rates of up to 80%. Plasmapheresis is the most effective treatment option and should be started as soon as possible. Even when the diagnosis is uncertain, the possible complications of TTP outweigh the risks of such treatment (Ridolfi, 1981; George, 2010). Plasma administration while plasmapheresis is started may be useful (Rock, 1991). In fact, when plasma exchange cannot be started immediately, it is advisable to start the infusion of high fresh plasma doses under constant central venous pressure control in order to avoid volume overload (Coppo, 1991). Pregnancy does not appear to modify treatment response, though the effects upon the fetus have not been evaluated.

Plasmapheresis is able to eliminate circulating anti-ADAMTS-13 autoantibodies and ultra-large Von Willebrand factor multimers from plasma. The infusion of fresh plasma in turn helps restore the deficient ADAMTS-13 levels. A schematic representation of treatment for acute TTP episodes is provided in Figure 1. Corticosteroids have some effect in the treatment of TTP episodes.

Before the generalized use of plasma exchange therapy, some authors reported a favorable response in 55% of the patients with neurological disorders when using high dose corticosteroids (Bell, 1991). Subsequent studies have shown the benefit of high dose corticosteroids as adjuvant therapy (dexamethasone 10 mg/kg/day for 3 days and 2.5 mg/kg/day thereafter) (Balduini, 2010).

Although antiplatelet treatment could seem adequate from the physiopathological perspective, some studies have found it to increase bleeding risk. The administration of antiplatelet drugs is therefore not generalized. Nevertheless, some recent clinical guides suggest the administration of 75 mg/day of acetylsalicylic acid if the platelet count is over 50. $x10^9/L$ (Scully, 2012).

The risk of venous thromboembolism has never been formally quantified in acute TTP but is likely to be increased due to immobility and acute illness. Therefore routine LMWH thromboprophylaxis should be given once the plate- let count has recovered to $>50x10^9/l$ (Yarranton, 2003). Platelet transfusion should be reserved for patients with life-threatening bleeding problems, since the worsened clinical condition reported by different authors after platelet transfusion suggests that it worsens microangiopathic disorder. If platelet transfusion proves necessary, it should always be associated to plasma replacement therapy (Swisher, 2009).

In patients refractory to treatment (10-20% of all cases), and when exacerbations of the acute episode occur in under 30 days after normalization of the platelet count, a monoclonal antibody (rituximab) has been shown to be effective as second-line treatment (Ojeda-Uribe, 2010). An 88% success rate has been reported with the administration of rituximab in refractory cases (Caramazza, 2010).

This monoclonal antibody allows faster recovery of the platelet count, lowers the circulating autoantibody titers, and increases ADAMTS-13 activity (Scully, 2011). Rituximab is able to normalize the platelet count within an average of two weeks, with remission of the condition in 5 weeks, and is effective in preventing relapse during the year following treatment. The use of rituximab during pregnancy has been associated with neonatal neutropenia, though it has been administered in the first three months of pregnancy without neonatal adverse effects (Ojeda-Uribe, 2013).

Although some studies have reported benefits with other drugs, randomized studies are needed to clarify the role of agents such as vincristine, cyclophosphamide or immunoglobulins via the intravenous route in the treatment of TTP in pregnancy.

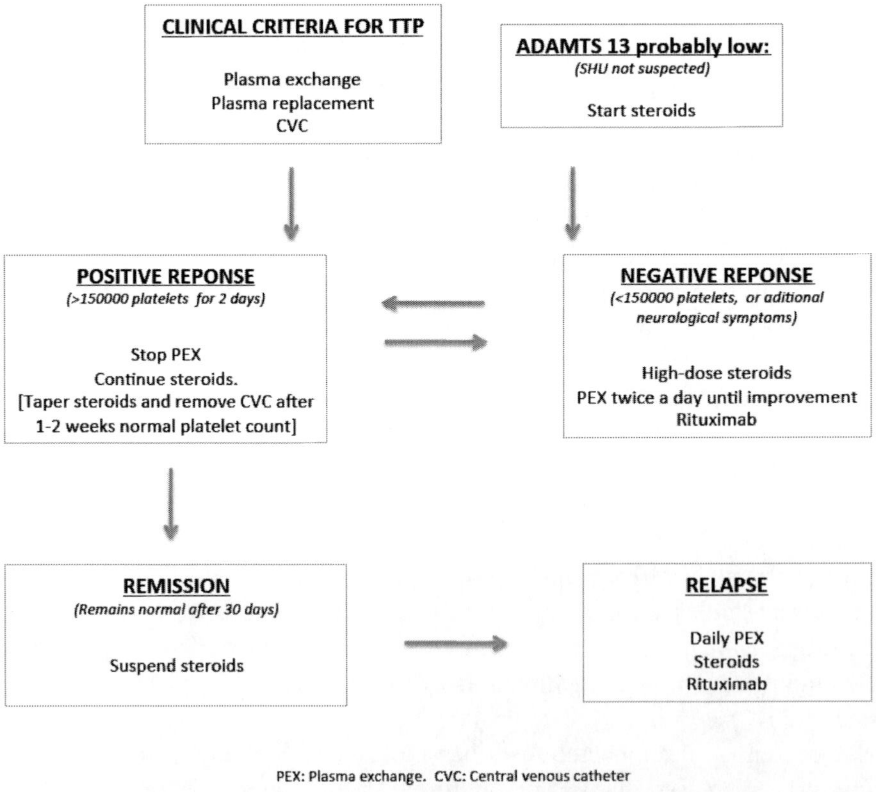

Figure 1. Schematic representation of treatment for acute TTP episodes.

Prognosis

Before the introduction of plasma exchange, maternal survival in cases of TTP related to pregnancy was very limited, with a mortality rate of over 90%. However, following the introduction of this treatment modality, the maternal mortality rate has dropped to 0-10%. At present, morbidity remains high, with neurological damage in up to 10% of all cases and renal damage in 21% (Dashe, 1987). In some series the perinatal mortality rate reaches (Weiner, 1987) 80%, and is usually related to hypoxia due to placental vascular lesions secondary to thrombotic occlusion of the decidual arterioles. No cases of idiopathic TTP to newborn infants have been reported.

Since treatment with plasmapheresis must be started urgently after the onset of symptoms, any delay in establishing the diagnosis has negative consequences. An adequate differential diagnosis must be established between TTP and HELLP syndrome, since the treatment in each case differs, and confusing the two diseases has been associated to increased maternal mortality (Proia, 2002).

The ending of pregnancy does not improve the course of TTP. It therefore should only be performed when there is evidence of fetal distress or growth retardation, concurrent preeclampsia, or in cases where plasma exchange proves ineffective. Perimortem cesarean delivery has been described in patients with TTP following irreversible cardiorespiratory arrest (González-Mesa E, 2013).

The risk of relapse in subsequent pregnancies in the case of hereditary TTP is 100% in the absence of plasma-based preventive treatment. The latter therefore must be started as soon as possible in the first trimester (Veseley, 2004). The risk of relapse in a subsequent pregnancy in women with acquired idiopathic TTP associated to severe ADAMTS-13 deficiency is relatively low (close to 20%)[49]. Therefore, with appropriate prenatal management and correct planning, future pregnancy in patients with antecedents of TTP is reasonably safe.

The general recommendation for controlling pregnancies of this kind is to closely monitor the patients during pregnancy and start prophylactic plasmapheresis every two weeks if the ADAMTS-13 activity falls to under 10% or blood smears yield unequivocal evidence of red cell fragmentation (schistocytes) suggesting the presence of hemolytic anemia[41]. Plasmapheresis is recommended before delivery.

The management of patients with TTP during pregnancy should be established on an individualized basis. As a general rule it is accepted that if a patient with a prior diagnosis of TTP becomes pregnant, a first test of ADAMTS-13 activity is useful. In this way plasma exchange can be indicated if necessary, with adoption of the necessary controls.

On the other hand, pregnant or puerperal women who develop severe thrombocytopenia ($< 50x10^9/L$) as a component of HELLP syndrome may benefit from rapid ADAMTS-13 activity testing to determine whether urgent plasma exchange could offer benefit instead of other methods, since none of the published series have found HELLP to be associated with severe ADAMTS-13 deficiency. The LDH/GOT ratio is very high in cases of TTP, since the LDH levels are far higher than in HELLP syndrome, while GOT is only slightly elevated. On the other hand, if a patient diagnosed with HELLP syndrome is unable to reach platelet counts above $25x10^9/L$ after 8-12 hours of treatment with dexamethasone 10 mg, it is prudent to assume a diagnosis of TTP.

According to the recent clinical guides (grade IA recommendation), mothers with congenital TTP should visit a specialized center to receive ADAMTS-13 through the infusion of fresh plasma on a regular basis throughout pregnancy and during puerperium if necessary. Close coordination between hematologists and obstetricians with an interest in maternal-fetal medicine is required in patients with TTP (grade IA recommendation). Counseling before conception is very important, providing information about the risks posed by pregnancy as a relapse-triggering factor (grade IIB recommendation).

REFERENCES

Asherson RA, Cervera R, de Groot P, Erkan D, Boffa MC, Piette JC, et al. Catastrophic antiphospholipid syndrome: International consensus statement on classification criteria and treatment guidelines. *Lupus.* 2003;12:530-4.

Balduini CL, Gugliotta L, Luppi M, Laurenti L, Klersy C, Pieresca C et al. High versus standard dose methylprednisolone in the acute phase of idiopathic thrombotic thrombocytopenic purpura: a randomized study. *Ann. Hematol* 2010; 89(6):591-6.

Battaglioli T, Valsecchi C, Lavoretano S, Mannucci PM, Peyvandi F, Palla R: Risk factors for recurrence of thrombotic thrombocytopenic purpura. *Blood* 2006; 108:11.

Bell WR, Braine HG, Ness PM, Kickler TS. Improved survival in thrombotic thrombocytopenic purpura- hemolytic uremic syndrome. Clinical experience in 108 patients. *N. Engl. J. Med* 1991; 325(6):398-403.

Camilleri RS, Scully M, Thomas M, Mackie IJ, Liesner R, Chen WJ, Manns K, Machin SJ. A phenotype-genotype correlation of ADAMTS13 mutations in congenital thrombotic thrombocytopenic purpura patients treated in the United Kingdom. *J. Thromb. Haemost.* 2012;10(9):1792-801.

Caramazza D, Quintini G, Abbene I, Coco LL, Malato A, Di Trapani R et al. Rituximab for managing relapsing or refractory patients with idiopathic thrombotic thrombocytopenic purpura–haemolytic uraemic syndrome. *Blood Transfus* 2010; 8(3):203-10.

Cervera R, Asherson RA. Catastrophic antiphospholipid syndrome: Therapeutic developments. *Expert Rev. Clin. Immunol.* 2007;3:277-85.

Coppo P, Veyradier A. Current management and therapeutical perspectives in thrombotic thrombocytopenic purpura. *Presse Med* 2012; 41:163-176.

DÁngelo A, Fattorini A, Crippa L. Thrombotic microangiopathy in pregnancy. *Thrombosis research* 2009; 123 (Suppl): 556-562.

Dashe JS, Ramin SM, Cunningham FG. The long-term consequences of thrombotic microangiopathy thrombotic thrombocutopenic purpura and haemolytic uremic syndrome) in pregnancy. *Obstet Gynecol* 1998; 91:662–668.

Egerman RS, Witlin AG, Friedman SA, et al. Thrombotic thrombocytopenic purpura and hemolytic uremic syndrome in pregnancy: review of 11 cases. *Am. J. Obstet. Gynecol* 1996; 175: 950–956.

Ezra Y, Rose M, Eldor A. Therapy and prevention of thrombotic thrombocytopenic purpura during pregnancy: A clinical study of 16 pregnancies. *Am. J. Hematol* 1996; 51:1- 6.

Fujimura Y, Matsumoto M. Registry of 919 pa- tients with thrombotic microangiopathies across Japan: database of Nara medical university dur- ing 1998-2008. *Intern. Med.* 2010; 49(1):7-15.

Furlan M, Lammle B. Aetiology and pathogenesis of thrombotic thrombocytopenic purpura and hemolytic uremic síndrome: The role of von Willebrand factor cleaving proteasa. *Best Pract. Res. Clin. Haematolo* 2001; 14:437-454.

George JN. How I treat patients with thrombotic thrombocytopenic purpura-hemolytic uremic syndrome. *Blood* 2000;96:1223-1229.

George JN. How I treat patients with thrombotic thrombocytopenic purpura: 2010. Blood 2010; 116:4060-4069.

George JN. The association of pregnancy with thrombotic thromcytopenic purpura-hemolyticuremic syndrome. *Curr. Opin. Hematol* 2003, 10:339–344.

George JN. The association of pregnancy with TTP-S. Curr Opin Hematol 2004; 92:1320-6

Gernesheimer T, james AH, Stasi R. How I treat thrombocytopenia in pregnancy. *Blood* 2013; 121:38-47.

González-Mesa E, Narbona I, Blasco M, Cohen I. *Journal of Medical Case Reports* 2013, 7:119.

Hawkins BM, Abu-Fadel M, Vesely SK, George JN. Clinical cardiac involvement in thrombotic thrombocytopenic purpura: a systematic review. *Transfusion.* 2008 ;48(2):382-92.

Kato R, Shinohara A, Sato J. ADAMTS 13 deficincy, an important cause of thrombocytopenia during pregnancy. *International Journal of Obstetetric Anesthesia* 2009; 18:73-77

Kim HC, Kemmann E, Shelden RM, Saidi P. Responso of blood coagulation parameteres to elevated endogenous 17 beta estradiol level induced by human menopausal gonadotropins. *Am. J. Obstet. Gynecol* 1981; 140:807-810.

Lara PN Jr, Coe TL, Zhou H, et al. Improved survival with plasma exchange in patients with thrombotic thrombocytopenic purpura-hemolytic uremic syndrome. *Am. J. Med.* 1999;107:573-579.

Levy GA, Nichols WC, Lian EC, Foroud T, McClintick JN, McGee BM, Yang AY, Siemieniak DR, Stark KR, Gruppo R, Sarode R, Shurin SB, Chandrasekaran V, Stabler SP, Sabio H, Bouhassira EE, Upshaw JD Jr, Ginsburg D, Tsai HM: Mutations in a member of the ADAMTS gene family cause thrombotic thrombocytopenic purpura. *Nature* 2001, 413:488-494.

Lotta LA, Lombardi R, MarianiM, et al. Platelet reactive conformation and multimeric pattern of von Willebrand factor in acquired thrombotic thrombocytopenic purpura during acute disease and remission. *J. Thromb. Haemost.* 2011; 9:1744-51.

Martin JN, Bailey A, Rehberg JF, et al. Thrombotic thrombocytopenic purpura in 166 pregnancies-2006. *American Journal of Obstetrics and Gynecology* 2008; 199:98-104.

Martin JN, Blake PG, Perry KG, McCaul JF, Hess LW, Martin RW. The natural history of HELLP síndrome: patterns of disease progression and regression. American Journal *Obstetrics and Gynecology1991*; 164: 1500-1513.

Miller D, Kaye JA, Shea K, et al. Incidence of Thrombotic Thrombocytopenic Purpura/Hemolytic Uremic Syndrome. *Epidemiology* 2004; 15: 208-215.

Miner PF, Nutt RL, Thomas ME. Thrombotic thrombocytopenic purpura occurring during pregnancy. *Am. J. Obstet. Gynecol.* 1955; 70:611-617.

Moake JL, Rudy CK, Troll JH, Weinstein MJ, Colamino NM, Azocar J, et al. Unusually large plasma factor VIII: vonWillebrand factor multimers in chronic relapsing thrombotic thrombocytopenic purpura. *N. Eng. J. Med.* 1982; 307;1432-1435.

Moake JL, Turner NA, Stathopoulos NA, Nolasco LH, Hellums JD. Involvement of large plasma von Willebrand factor multimers and usually large VWF forms derived from endotelial cells in shear stress-induced platelet aggregation. *J. Clin. Invest.* 1986; 78: 1456-1461.

Moake JL. Thrombotic microangiopathies. N. Engl. J. Med. 2002; 347:589-600.

Moatti-Cohen M, Garrec C, Wolf M, et al. Unexpected frequency of Upshaw-Schulman syndrome in pregnancy-onset thrombotic thrombocytopenic purpura. *Blood* 2012; 119: 5888-5897.

Moschovitz E. Hyaline thrombosis of the terminal arterioles and capilliaries: a a hitherto undiscribed disease. *Proc. NY Pathol. Soc.* 1924; 24.21-4.

Murrin RJA, Murray JA. Thrombotic Thrombocytopenic purpura: aetiology, pathophysiology and treatment. Blood Reviews.2000; 20:51-60.

Natelson EA, White D. Recurrent thrombotic thrombocytopenic purpura in early pregnancy: Effect of uterine evacuation. *Obstet. Gynecol* 1985; 66:45s 54s..

Ojeda-Uribe M, Afif N, Dahan E, Sparsa L, Haby C, Sibilia J, Ternant D, Ardizzone M. Exposure to abatacept or rituximab in the first trimester of pregnancy in three women with autoimmune diseases. *Clin. Rheumatol.* 2013; 32(5):695-700.

Ojeda-Uribe M, Federici L, Wolf M, Coppo P, Veyradler A: Successful long-term rituximab maintenance for a relapsing patient with idiopathic thrombotic thrombocytopenic purpura. *Transfusion* 2010; 50:733-735.

Patschan D, Witzke O, Dührsen U, Erbel R, Philipp T, Herget-Rosenthal S. Acute myocardial infarction in throm- botic microangiopathies—clinical characteristics, risk factors, and outcome. *Nephrol Dial Transplant* 2006;21: 1549-54.

Pels SG, Paidas MJ. Microangiopathic Disorders in Pregnancy. *Hematol Oncol Clin N Am* 2011; 25: 311-322.

Peyvandi F, Lavoretano S, Palla R, et al. ADAMTS 13 and anti-ADAMTS 13 antibodies as markers for recurrence of acquired thrombotic thrombocytopenic purpura during remission. *Haematologica* 2008; 93: 232-239

Proia A, Paesano R, Torcia F, Annino L, Capria S, Ferrari A, Ferrazza G, Pacifici E, Pantalissi A, Meloni G: Thrombotic thrombocytopenic purpura and pregnancy: a case report and a review of the literature. *Ann. Hematol.* 2002, 81:210-214.

Ridolfi RL, Bell WR. Thrombotic thrombocytopenia purpura: Report of 25 cases and a review of the literatura. *Medicine* 1981;60:413 28.

Ridolfi RL, Bell WR. Thrombotic thrombocytopenic purpura. Report of 25 cases and review of the iterature. Medicine (Baltimore) 1981; 60(6):413-28.

Rock G, Shumak K, Kelton J, et al. Thrombotic thrombocytopenic purpura: outcome in 24 patients with renal impairment treated with plasma exchange. *Transfusion* 1992;32:710-714.

Rock GA, Shumak KH, Buskard NA, et al. Com- parison of plasma exchange with plasma infusion in the treatment of thrombotic thrombocytopenic purpura. *N. Engl. J. Med.* 1991;3 25(6):393-397.

Rock GA, Shumak KH, Buskard NA, et al. Comparison of plasma exchange with plasma infusion in the treatment of thrombotic thrombocytopenic purpura. *N. Engl. J. Med.* 1991;325:393-397.

Sadler JE, Moake JL, Miyata T, George JN. Recent advances in thrombotic thrombocytopenic purpura. *Hematology Am. Soc. Hematol Educ. Program.* 2004:407-23.

Sanchez-Luceros A, Farias CE, Amaral M, et al. Von Willebrand factor cleaving proteasa (ADAMTS 13) activity in normal non-pregnant women, pregnant and postdelivery women. *Thromb Haemost* 2004; 2:1320-26.

Scully M, Hunt BJ, Benjamin S, Liesner R, et al. Guidelines on the diagnosis and management of thrombotic thrombocytopenic purpura and other thrombotic microangiopathies. *British Journal of Haematology* 2012, 158, 323–335.

Scully M, McDonald V, Cavenagh J, Hunt BJ, Longair I, Cohen H et al. A phase II study of the safety and efficacy of rituximab with plasma exchange in acute acquired thrombotic thrombocytopenic purpura. *Blood* 2011; 118(7):1746-53.

Scully M, Starke R, Lee R: Successful management of pregnancy in women with a history of thrombotic thrombocytopenic purpura. *Blood Coagul Fibrinolysis* 2006, 17:459-463.

Scully M, Yarranton H, Liesner R, et al. Regional United Kingdom TTP registry: correlation with laboratory ADAMTS13 analysis and clinical fea-tures. *Br. J. Haematol* 2008;142(5):819-826.

Shamseddine A, Chehal A, Salem Z, et al. Thrombotic Thrombocytopenic Purpura and Pregnancy: Report of four cases and literatura review. *Journal of clinical Apheresis* 2004; 19:5-10.

Steingrub J. Pregnancy associated severe liver dysfunction. Crit. Care Clin. 2004;20:763-776

Stella CL, Dacus J, Guzman E, et al. The diagnostic dilema of thrombotic thrombocytopenic purpura/hemolytic uremis síndrome in the obstetric triage and emergency department: lessons from 4 tertiary hospitals. *Am. J. Obstet. Gynecol* 200 Steingrub J. Pregnancy associated severe liver dysfunction. Crit Care Clin 2004;20:763-7769; 200:381-386.

Swisher KK, Terrell DR, Vesely SK, Kremer Hovinga JA, Lammle B, George JN. Clinical outcomes after platelet transfusions in patients with thrombotic thrombocytopenic purpura. *Transfusion* 2009;49(5):873-87.

Task Force on hypertension in Pregnancy. The American College of Obstetricians and Gynecologists. Hypertension in Pregnancy. *Practice Guideline* WQ 244. ISBN 978-1-934984-28-4.

Thompson CE, Damon LE, Ries CA, Linker CA. Thrombotic microangiopathies in the 1980s: clinical features, response to treatment, and the impact of the human immunodeficiency virus epidemic. *Blood* 1992; 80:1890-1895.

Trisolini SM, Capria S, Gozzer M, et al. Thrombotic thrombocytopenic purpura in the first trimester and successful pregnancy. *Ann. Hematol.* 2009; 88:287–289.

Veseley S, George J, Lammle B, Studt J, Alberio L, El-Harake M, Raskob G. ADAMTS-13 activity in TTP-HUS: a prospective cohort of 142 patients uremic syndrome: relation to presenting features and clinical outcomes. *Blood* 2003; 102:60-68.

Veseley S, Li X, McMinn J, Terrell D, George J. Pregnancy outcomes after recovery from thrombotic thrombocytopenic purpura-hemolytic uremic syndrome. *Transfusion* 2004; 44:1149-1158.

Veseley S, Li X, McMinn J, Terrell D, George J. Pregnancy outcomes after recovery from thrombotic thrombocytopenic purpura-hemolytic uremic syndrome. *Transfusion* 2004; 44:1149-1158..

Vigil De Gracia P, Lavergne J. Acute fatty liver of pregnancy. *Int. J. Gynecol. Obstet* 2001;72:193-195.

Weiner CP. Thrombotic microangiopathy in pregnancy and in the postpartum period. *Sem Hematol.* 1987; 24:119–129.

Westerlund E, Antovic A, Hovatta O, Eberg KP, Blomback M, Wallen H, Heriksson P. Changes in von Willebrand factor and ADAMTS 13 during IVF. *Blood coagulation and fibrinolysis* 2011; 22:127-131.

Yarranton, H., Cohen, H., Pavord, S.R., Benjamin, S., Hagger, D. & Machin, S.J. (2003) Venous thromboembolism associated with the manage- ment of acute thrombotic thrombocytopenic purpura. *British Journal of Haematology*, 121, 778–785.

Zheng, Kaufman RM, Goodnough LT, et al. Effect of plasma Exchange on plasma ADAMTS 13 metalloprotease activity, inhibitor level, and clinical outcome in patients with idiopathic and non-idiopathic thrombotic thrombocytopenic purpura. *Blood* 2004, 103:4023-4049.

In: Handbook for High Risk Pregnancy: Clinical Management ISBN: 978-1-63482-299-2
Editors: E. González-Mesa and D. Abehsera

Chapter 12

NEUROLOGICAL DISEASE AND PREGNANCY

Rocio Revello Alvarez*
Obstetrics and Gynecology Department,
La Paz University Hospital. Madrid, Spain

INTRODUCTION

Neurological symptoms and conditions are frequently observed in women in reproductive age. Most of them are caused by exacerbation of pre-existing disorders, others are pregnancy related disorders. Understanding the physiological changes during pregnancy is mandatory for the management of these conditions.

Currently almost all of these neurological diseases are compatible with successful pregnancy outcome. However, neurological diseases contribute to maternal mortality, with stroke and epilepsy accounting for the majority of deaths from neurologic causes (Wilkinson, 2011). Several other disabling neurologic conditions, ranging from multiple sclerosis to migraine, present both medical and obstetric challenges to clinicians unfamiliar with their management within the context of pregnancy. All these patients have specific therapies and risks that the physician should know.

1. MIGRAINE

The most common primary headache disorder is migraine (both with and without aura) (Melhado, Maciel & Guerreiro, 2007). These headaches may start during pregnancy, but most often a woman has a previous headache disorder that may be exacerbated especially by the first trimester of pregnancy. However, women who present with a headache that is different from their usual headache or women presenting with new-onset headache in pregnancy need a neurological assessment in order to look for a potential secondary cause for the headache (Digre, 2013).

* Correspondence: rociorevello@hotmail.com.

Many studies have shown that pregnancy reduces the frequency and severity of migraines (Aegidius, Zwart, Hagenv & Stovner, 2009; Kvisvik, Stovner, Helde, Bovim & Linde, 2011). In general, women with migraine without aura seem to do better than those who experience migraine with aura (Evans & Loder, 2003). Among pre-existing primary headaches, migraine is more sensitive to ovarian hormones. Increased estrogen levels and the lack of hormonal fluctuations are associated with an amelioration of migraines without auras (Evans & Loder, 2003; Haider & Von Oertzen, 2013). However, if the headache is no better after the first trimester, there is evidence to suggest that it may not improve further; and one should consider more aggressive treatment (Digre, 2013; Scharff, Marcus, & Turk, 1997). After delivery, as estrogen levels fall, migraines may return (Marcus, Scharff & Turk, 1999). Nevertheless, it has been claimed that breastfeeding may delay the return of migraines (Wall, 1992; Rukmini & Bushnell, 2008).

Migraine with aura during pregnancy has been shown to be more problematic (Digre, 2013; Torelli, Allais & Manzoni, 2010). Aside from the concern for secondary causes of the aura, the auras may be more complicated, with involvement of speech as well as sensory symptoms (Lipton, Bigal, Steiner, Silberstein & Olesen, 2004). Untreated, the headache and associated symptoms can last for 2–3 days.

Although generally it is thought that migraine does not appear to affect pregnancy outcome, an increasing body of evidence supports an association between migraine and complications such cerebrovascular diseases, myocardial infraction, pulmonary embolus and thrombophilia (Bushnell, Jamison, & James, 2009; Adeney, Williams, Miller, Frederick, Sorensen & Luthy, 2005). One study reported a strong association between migraines and ischemic stroke with a population database of 33,956 women with migraines (Bushnell, Jamison, & James, 2009). This study could not, however, identify whether migraine preceded or followed ischemic stroke, therefore some migrainous headache must have been caused by the stroke itself. Migraine has also been identified as a risk factor for pregnancy-induced hypertension, and preeclampsia. A case-control study compared women with preeclampsia with normotensive women and reported an increased risk of preeclampsia in those women with a history of migraine (Adeney, Williams, Miller, Frederick, Sorensen & Luthy, 2005).

Although these findings suggest a strong association between migraine during pregnancy and increased risk of vascular disease, further research is necessary to identify the relationship between and migraine with or without aura and pregnancy outcome.

To avoid the potential for drug-related effects on pregnancy, it is important to minimize drug exposure in any woman who is planning pregnancy. If possible, prophylactic medication should be discontinued and strategies for the management of acute attacks discussed. However, when headaches are more frequent than twice weekly, it seems to be reasonable to prescribe some preventive medication. If prophylaxis is indicated during pregnancy or lactation, the lowest effective dose of propranolol is the first line recommendation (McGregor, 2012). In general, we should avoid anticonvulsants; if one is to be used, the woman should of course be supplemented with folate. We would avoid Valproate during pregnancy if possible. Topiramate is also a category D drug because of the possibility of increased birth defects (Digre, 2013).

Current effective treatment of an acute migrainous attack has reduced the need for chronic migraine prophylaxis. In particular, the use of the serotonin 5-HT1 agonist sumatriptan during the first trimester appears to be safe and is often effective (McGregor, 2012; Evans & Lorber, 2008). Triptans are also an option.

The use of nonsteroidal anti-inflammatory drugs (NSAID) should be avoided during the third trimester of pregnancy as it has been shown that it can lead an increase musculature within the fetal patent ductus arteriosus leading a pulmonary hypertension (Koren, Florescu, Costei, Boskovic & Moreti, 2006). For severe attacks, a regime of opioids – codeine, morphine or pethidine with antiemetics is often effective. Regular maternal opioid use must be avoided to prevent dependence and neonatal withdrawal.

2. Epilepsy

Epilepsy is the most common chronic neurological disorder affecting 0.7% of the population. The incidence will be lower in pregnancy as peak incidence occurs in early life and in older age (Hirtz et al. 2007). Nevertheless, after headaches, seizure disorders are the second most common neurological diagnosis in pregnancy (Hirtz et al., 2007). An understanding of the disease is essential for obstetricians.

2.1. Effects of Pregnancy on Epilepsy

There is no consensus on changes in seizure frequency and pregnancy. According with some studies, among all pregnant women with epilepsy one third will have a change in seizure frequency, approximately half have an increase in seizure frequency and half have a decrease in seizure frequency (Haider & Von Oertzen, 2013). To the best of our knowledge, seizure frequency in the preceding 9- 12 months before pregnancy seems to be a good predictor of seizure activity in pregnancy (Kamyar & Varmer, 2013). Some studies have shown that no seizures in the year before pregnancy are associated with seizure freedom during pregnancy (Kamyar & Varmer, 2013; Harden & Sethi, 2008). Status epilepticus is relatively rare, less than 2% of pregnancies, with approximately one-third presenting as convulsive episodes and two thirds presenting as non-convulsive episodes (Haider & Von Oerzten, 2013). The risk of status epilepticus is not significantly increased in pregnancy (Haider & Von Oerzten, 2013).

The seizure pattern may be influenced by variations in ovarian hormones, blood levels of antiepileptic drugs (AEDs) and metabolic changes. Renal function and glomerular filtration rate are increased in pregnancy, leading to increased losses from the body of drugs which are cleared mainly by renal excretion in un-metabolised form, for example, gabapentin (Eadie, 2014) Increased clearances occur as well for drugs whose first stage of metabolism is through cytochrome P450 activity or glucuronidation. Overall, drugs cleared by glucuronidation as a Phase I mechanism, for example, lamotrigine, show the greatest changes (Eadie, 2014).

During pregnancy, epilepsy has associated neurological comorbidities, the most common being migraines and sleep disorder (Kamyar & Varmer, 2013). There are also the remote possibilities of maternal death during seizures and of sudden unexpected death in epilepsy (SUDEP) that can occur in those with epilepsy (Eadie, 2014). The cause of this phenomenon is unknown, but it is thought to occur more commonly in patients who are noncompliant or patients whose epilepsy is refractory to medications and most occur at the time of seizure and may be due to cardiac mechanisms (Harden & Varmer, 2013). Women who suffer more than one generalized seizure per month are at an annual risk of SUDEP of 1% or higher (Langan, Nashef & Sander, 2005).

2.2. Effects of Epilepsy on Pregnancy

The relationships among epilepsy, the drugs used to treat epilepsy, and the risks for major congenital malformations (MCM) and poor neurodevelopment in the offspring are difficult to define.

Some studies have shown that the offspring born to epileptic women who did not take anticonvulsant drugs had the same risk of birth defects as the infants born to nonepileptic women (Holmes et al., 2001; Fried, Kozer, Nulman, Einarson & Koren, 2004). These studies report a MCM rate of 6.1% in offspring of epileptic women who were treated with AEDs, 2.8% among children of women with untreated epilepsy, and 2.2% in the healthy control group.

Many AEDs are associated with an increased risk of certain fetal malformations (particularly neural tube defects) (Cohen et al., 2011). However, given the potential adverse maternal and fetal impacts of uncontrolled seizures, continued use of AED in pregnancy is generally advised. There have been inconsistencies between some of the findings for fetal hazard rates for particular antiepileptic drugs. Recently published data suggests that maternal epilepsy, regardless of any treatment taken, may increase the risk of foetal malformations (Cassina et al., 2013). Nevertheless, for most marketed antiepileptic drugs teratogenesis is an uncommon event though valproate has emerged as a significant teratogen (Eadie, 2014).

Regarding the neurocognitive development among the offspring of epileptic women, has been argued that intrauterine exposure to antiepileptic drugs is associated with decreased motor skills and some delay in aspects of the intelligence of these children (Cohen, 2011). The intellectual shortcomings appear to be associated with intrauterine exposure to valproate but not to the other commonly used antiepileptic drugs except, perhaps, carbamazepine (Eadie, 2014). However maldevelopment of the fetal central nervous system could have a genetic etiology and it is therefore possible that either the genetics of epilepsy or the fetal environmental circumstances of poorly controlled epilepsy could cause central nervous system maldevelopment, resulting in impaired cognitive development. Thus in the last years some evidence had appeared claimed that the adverse fetal outcomes observed among offspring of women with epilepsy taking antiepileptic drugs could be due to the epilepsy per se and not the drug treatment (Holmes, 2001)

Regarding recent studies, the offspring born to epileptic mothers are twice has likely to have intrautereine growth restriction (IUGR) as compared with controls. It seems to be related with the use of AED more that with the epilepsy itself as this increased risk was not found in women with epilepsy not taking AED (Kamyar & Varmer, 2013). It has been reported that the AED which most increase the risk is carbamacepina (Kamyar & Varmer, 2013). Serial ultrasounds should be performed to evaluate fetal weight and amniotic fluid volume controls.

Epilepsy has been related as well with an increased risk of preeclampsia. A recent study (Borthen, Eide, Daltveit & Gilhus, 2011) shows that women with epilepsy using AED had an increased risk of severe preeclampsia, bleeding in early pregnancy, induction and cesarean section.

This increase on the cesarean delivery rate seems to be multifactorial and can be explained by the relative increased likelihood of the concurrent obstetric complications such as fetal anomalies, preeclampsia or IUGR.

2.3. Treatment

Unfortunately, all the presently used AED are either known teratogens or are agents for which the present pregnancy data are too limited to offer a definitive statement on the associated pregnancy risk. It has often been stated that the risk of teratogenesis is enhanced if mothers take two or more antiepileptic drug simultaneously (Kamyar & Varmer, 2013). Therefore, the most efficacious AED monotherapy with the smallest risk of teratogenic effects needs to be determined before pregnancy, with multidrug therapy reserved for patients with persistent seizures or unacceptable side effects. However, some studies (Vajda et al., 2010; Mawwer et al., 2010) have shown that the increase malformation risk applies only when the drug combination includes valproate, which in its own right is the most significant teratogen among currently used antiepileptic drugs. It seems like AEDs including lamotrigine, carbamazepine or levetiracetam in monotherapy have the lowest teratogenic risk profile (Haider & Von Oertzen, 2013)

In general, Valproate is thought to be the most teratogenic of the AED (Eadie, 2014; Kamyar & Varmer, 2013). The use of Valproate has been shown to increase the risk of MCM especially during the first trimester of pregnancy although its effect has become increasingly identified as clearly dose-related (Eadie, 2014). The most common MCM are neural tube defects, congenital heart defects, skeletal abnormalities, orofacial clefts, and hypospadias (Kamyar & Varmer, 2013).

Certain studies have demonstrated that foetal malformations are more frequent at higher carbamazepine and lamotrigine doses (Tomson et al., 2011; Morrow et al., 2006) but other reports (Vajda et al. 2010; Vajda et al., 2012) sought and failed to find evidence for such a relationship in the case of lamotrigine, which is generally considered among the safest of the major antiepileptic drugs from the foetal point of view.

Of special note is the fact that many antiepileptic drugs (AED) interfere with synthesis of the vitamin K-dependent clotting factors II, VII, IX and X directly, therefore is the risk of hemorrhagic disease of the newborn secondary to vitamin K deficiency (Digre, 2013). In order to prevent that risk the standard treatment is 1mg of vitamin K to be given intramuscularly to the newborn.

Thus, since there is no consensus as to which AED is most or least teratogenic, the AED that controls seizures in a given patient is the one that should be used. When possible, however, the use of valproate or the use of multiple AED should be avoided during pregnancy or in women planning a pregnancy.

All epileptic women with reproductive potential who require AED therapy should receive folic acid supplementation. Supplemental use of 5 mg folic acid per day prior to conception and during at least the first trimester of pregnancy in women on AEDs reduces the risk of neural tube defects (Digre, 2013).

3. MULTIPLE SCLEROSIS

Multiple sclerosis (MS) is a complex inflammatory and demyelinating disorder of the central nervous system which results in initially intermittent, and later, often, progressive neurological impairment (Houtchens, 2013). MS shows a strong female predominance and affects young adults, making the typical patient a young woman of childbearing age (Coyle, 2012). The etiology of this disease is considered heterogeneous but unfortunately, it remains unknown. The risk of MS with a first-degree relative with the disease becomes a little higher, 2% to 4% versus 0.2% (Lee, 2006). However it seems that MS is not an inherited disease; there is no gene that passes on MS.

3.1. Effects of Pregnancy on MS

Pregnancy is a major concern for many MS patients. Before 1960s, patients with MS were actively discouraged from becoming pregnant as it was thought that pregnancy could be related with severe postpartum exacerbations or increasing the risk of long disability (Schapira, Poskanzer &Newell, 1966). After forwards, most of the studies published failed to demonstrate any definite adverse effect of pregnancy on the course of the disease and no convincing evidence of a harmful effect has been uncovered (Confavreux, Hutchinson, Hours, Cortinovis- Tourniaire & Moreau, 1998) More recent studies report that long-term prognosis is more favorable in patients who become pregnant (Runmarker & Andersen 1995; D'hooghe, Nagels & Uitdehaag, 2010). This is in contradistinction to some disorders such as neuromyelitis optica (NMO) and radiologically isolated syndrome (RIS) whereby attacks may occur during later pregnancy. Some studies (Kim, Kim & Nakashima, 2012) have shown that NMO symptom onset is more likely to occur during the postpartum year than during pregnancy and that the risk of relapse increases in the first 3 to 6 months postpartum. In women with RIS, the asymptomatic precursor of MS, preliminary evidence suggests that pregnancy may accelerate time to MS symptom onset (Lebrun, Le Page & Kantarci 2012). MS disease onset is unusual during pregnancy (Coyle, 2012)

Pregnancy is a state of immune tolerance; it is recognized to induce changes in maternal immune system toward immune tolerance, so the mother will not reject the semi allogeneic fetus. Cell-mediated immunity is down regulated while humoral immunity is enhanced (Lashley, van der Hoorn & van der Mast, 2011; Neuteboom, Verbraak & Wierenga-Wolf 2010). Multiple immunoregulatory factors are at play during pregnancy, leading to reduced MS activity both clinically and on MRI, which is most marked during the last trimester (Van Walderven, Tas & Barkhof, 1994). Some effects of pregnancy on the course of the MS are well accepted, whereas others require further studies.

Pregnancy itself is thought to be beneficial to MS patients in terms of relapse. The Pregnancy in Multiple Sclerosis study (PRIMS) has provided the best largescale, prospective published data on this issue (Vukusic et al., 2004). This trial demonstrated a 70% reduction in relapse risk in the third trimester of pregnancy in MS patients. Relapse rate increased during the first 3 months postpartum, then returned to prepregnancy levels. The subsequent formal 2-year postpartum follow-up found that factors increasing the likelihood of postpartum relapse for any patient include a high relapse rate in the prepregnancy year, increased relapse rate during pregnancy and a higher MS disability score prior to pregnancy. The study conclude that most patients with MS could expect an improvement in their MS during pregnancy despite having to withdraw from their usual MS treatment as it was reported that benefit during pregnancy is greater than that seen with currently available standard therapies for MS. However, the postpartum increase in relapse frequency remains a concern and means that overall pregnancy is probably neutral in terms of relapse risk.

After delivery, about 30% of relapsing MS women have a postpartum relapse. (Coyle, 2012). Recent studies have pointed out some factors like breastfeeding, particularly the biologically distinct state of exclusive breastfeeding, as modifiable risk factors of postpartum MS relapses. Two groups had reported reduced postpartum relapse rate in MS mothers who breast fed for at least 2 months postpartum (Confavreux, Hutchinson, Hours, Cortinovis-Tourniaire& Moreau, 1998; Langer-Gould, Huang & Gupta, 2009) These studies suggest that exclusive breastfeeding which results in high prolactin levels, low and non-pulsatile luteinizing hormone (LH) levels and ovarian suppression (lack of ovulation and post-menopausal levels of estradiol and progesterone) might be protective (Langer-Gould & Beaber, 2013). In the much larger PRIMS study, breastfeeding was ultimately considered to have no effect on postpartum relapses or disability (Vukusic et al., 2004).

3.2. Effects of MS on Pregnancy

In the last years, multiples studies have demonstrated no significant increase in spontaneous abortion rates, or major obstetric or neonatal complications for patients with MS compared with women without the disease (Tsui & Lee, 2011). Therefore, the decision regarding the mode of delivery is usually based on obstetrical rather than neurological factors.

With regard to anesthesia, according to recent publications, all forms of anesthesia are considered safe for pregnant women with MS (Coyle, 2011). In the PRIMS study no impact of epidural anesthesia was observed (Vukusic et al., 2004).

3.3. Treatment

Current guidelines establish that the MS disease-modifying therapies (DMTs) should not be used in patients who are trying to become pregnant, who are pregnant, or who are breastfeeding although there are no convincing data that the MS DMTs are teratogenic (Coyle, 2012; Houtchens, 2013).

Patients suffering from at least one relapse per year are usually offered DMTs with an injectable interferon-beta (IFNb) or glatiramer acetate, which reduce relapse rates by, on average, 30% (Tsui & Lee, 2011). Studies of IFNb and glatiramer acetate in pregnancy have also failed to demonstrate significant adverse effects following early exposure, although longer-term effects are not well documented. Therefore, in practice, many physicians discuss the risks of relapse off DMT with the relative absence of evidence of risk of harm of DMT exposure during early pregnancy and often, patients with very active disease may elect to stay on interferons or glatirimer acetate for the duration of pregnancy (Houtchens & Kolb, 2012).

Patients with MS not responding to standard DMT or with very aggressive disease may be on natalizumab or Fingolimod. The safety of these drugs has not been established in pregnancy. Patients are therefore currently advised to stop the drug between 2and 3 months prior to conception. Other newly approved DMD is Teflunomide. This drug has been clasificated as category X by FDA and teratogenic. Indeed, this drug is contraindicated to pregnant women and women of childbearing age (Houtchens & Kolb, 2012).

Regarding the management of relapses during pregnancy, glucocorticoids can be used, typically methylprednisolone for 3 to 7 days depending on relapse severity. Intravenous gammaglobulin is considered safe to use during pregnancy (Coyle, 2012).

During postpartum the risk of relapse is high. The therapy options during this period depend on breastfeeding. In general, breastfeeding is a contraindication to using MS-specific therapy, so, If choice is made to not breastfeed DMT need to be resumed quickly after delivery since these medications have a delayed onset of action and most postpartum relapses occur in the first 4 months postpartum. In the other hand, if choice is made to breastfeeding, intravenous immunoglobulins and pulse intravenous methylprednisolone could be used.

4. Strokes

Pregnancy and the postpartum period are associated with an increased risk of ischemic stroke and cerebral hemorrhage contributing to more than 12% of all maternal deaths (Treadwell, Thanvi & Robinson, 2008). According the incidence from several studies, the rate of stroke is estimated to be 25 to 34 cases per 100,000 deliveries, whereas the incidence of stroke in nonpregnant woman aged 15 to 44 years of age is 11 per 100,000 women (James, Bushnell, Jamison & Myers, 2005).

Several physiologic and pathophysiologic changes during pregnancy make the cause of both ischemia and hemorrhage different from those in nonpregnant women. Hypercoagulability, venous stasis and vascular endothelial injury are a triad of risk factors described by Virchow for the development of venous thromboembolism (Anning, 1957) and all may occur during the course of normal pregnancy. However, much like nonpregnant women and men, many recent studies indicate that most cerebral infarctions in pregnant are due to arterial occlusions (Jaigobin & Silver, 2000; Grear & Kushnell, 2013).

Epidemiologic studies show that both ischemic and hemorrhagic events in the first and second trimesters are minimal, but their frequency increases in the third trimester and closer to delivery, during delivery, and postpartum (Sidorov, Feng & Caplan, 2011; Jaigobin & Silver, 2000).

Regarding the risk factors, hypertensive disorders have been implicated to play a role in stroke in pregnancy. Women with hypertension complicating pregnancy, compared with those without hypertension, are much more likely to have stroke (Lanska & Kryscio, 2000). Other risk factors that have been reported for pregnancy related stroke include age more than 35 years, black ethnicity, heart disease, smoking, diabetes, lupus, sickle cell disease, migraine headaches, alcohol and substance abuse, fluid and electrolyte disorders, thrombophilia, multiple gestation, greater parity and postpartum infection (James, Bushnell, Jamison & Myers, 2005).

Interestingly, cesarean delivery has been associated with peripartum stroke, although a causal relationship has not been well established (Lin SY, Hu CJ & Lin HC, 2008). Many of the strokes in pregnancy are secondary to cerebral vein thrombosis (CVT), mainly due to hypercoagulability, such as venous stasis and it can result in both venous ischemic and hemorrhagic infarctions. The hemorrhage arises from the venous congestion as a result of backflow of blood from the occlusion of a major sinus (Grear & Kushnell, 2013). Most of them occur during puerperium (Treadwell, Thanvi & Robinson, 2008). CVT concerns abnormal venous drainage and increase in intracranial pressures related to venous obstruction and usually results in headache, vomiting and papilloedema (Treadwell, Thanvi & Robinson, 2008). The rate of death from all-cause CVT is 2–10% (Treadwell, Thanvi & Robinson, 2008) usually as a result from secondary intracranial haemorrhage. For diagnosis of CVST, MRI and magnetic resonance venogram are the most reliable tools. Regarding the treatment, the first choice is anticoagulation with heparin or heparin analogs (Tettenborn, 2012) although it can be a difficult issue when there is hemorrhagic conversion of a venous infarct.

Subarachnoid hemorrhage (SAH) is the third leading cause of non-obstetric-related maternal death (Treadwell, Thanvi & Robinson, 2008). Most of them are due to ruptured cerebral aneurysms or traumatic injuries, and usually presents with intense headache. The same as CVT, SAH usually occurs in last trimester of gestation or postpartum period, as result from all the hemodynamic changes during pregnancy that contribute to aneurysm instability and increased risk of SAH. The diagnosis is based in neuroimaging or cerebrospinal fluid analysis and it has been claimed that surgical treatment after aneurysmal SAH during pregnancy improves both maternal and fetal outcome (Dias, 1994). In the last decades, cesarean delivery has been recommended for women with hemorrhagic stroke to avoid potential risks during labor and delivery (Cohen-Gadol, Friedman, Friedman, Tubbs, Munis & Meyer, 2009). However, some studies have reported that outcomes of vaginal and cesarean delivery are probably equivalent after hemorrhagic stroke (Treadwell, Thanvi & Robinson, 2008).

The reversible cerebral vasoconstriction syndrome (RCVS) is another important cause of stroke in pregnant and puerperal women. It applies to a group of disorders which are characterised by reversible multifocal vasoconstriction of the cerebral arteries and present as sudden headache (so called thunderclap headache). Radiological features include multifocal segmental narrowing of the cerebral arteries, with reversibility and complete resolution 4–6 weeks later (Treadwell, Thanvi & Robinson, 2008) although some of them can progress to brain infarctions and subarachnoid hemorrhages. Patients may, rarely, develop a fulminant course with poor outcome and death (Tate & Bushnell, 2011; Sidorov, Feng & Caplan, 2011). The pathophysiology of PCA remains unclear and it usually occurs a few days after delivery in patients with a history of uncomplicated pregnancy and delivery.

In general, the management of women with stroke during pregnancy should be similar to the approach to stroke in young adults. The benefit of intravenous and intra-arterial thrombolysis with intravenous tissue plasminogen activator (tPA) or mechanical clot removal in acute ischaemic stroke is well established (DeKeyser, Gdovinova, Uyttenboogaart, Vroomen & Luijckx, 2007).

Despite the fact that there are no clinical trials to evaluate the use of rtPA in pregnant women with acute stroke; it is known that it does not cross the placenta and there has been no evidence of teratogenicity in animal studies (DeKeyser, Gdovinova, Uyttenboogaart, Vroomen & Luijckx, 2007). Nevertheless, further evaluation with regard to maternal and fetal risk is warranted. There are no clear guidelines for medical treatment of intracranial hemorrhage in pregnancy. Drugs like mannitol for increased intracranial pressure or nimodipine for vasospasm must be used with caution.

REFERENCES

Adeney KL, Williams MA, Miller RS, Frederick IO, Sorensen TK & Luthy DA. (2005). Risk of preeclampsia in relation to maternal history of migraine headaches. *Journal of Maternal and Fetal Neonatal Medicine*, 18 (3), 167–72.

Aegidius K, Zwart JA, Hagen K & Stovner L. (2009). The effect of pregnancy and parity on headache prevalence: the Head-HUNT study. *Headache*, 49, 851–859.

Anning ST. (1957). The historical aspects of venous thromboembolism. Medical History, 1, 28–37.

Borthen I, Eide M, Daltveit A & Gilhus NE. (2011). Obstetric outcome in women with epilepsy: a hospitalbased, retrospective study. *British Journal of Obstetrics and Gynecology,* 118, 956–965.

Bushnell CD, Jamison M & James AH. (2009). Migraines during pregnancy linked to stroke and vascular diseases: US population based case-control study. *British Medical Journal,* 10, 338.

Cassina M, Dilaghi A, Di Gianantonio E, Cesari E, De Santis M, Mannaioni G, Pistelli A & Clementi M. (2013). Pregnancy outcome in women exposed to antiepileptic drugs: teratogenic role of maternal epilepsy and its pharmacologic treatment. *Reproductive Toxicology,* 39, 50-7.

Cohen-Gadol AA, Friedman JA, Friedman, Tubbs RS, Munis JR & Meyer FB. (2009). Neurosurgical management of intracranial lesions in the pregnant patient: a 36-year institutional experience and review of the literature. *Journal of Neurosurgery*, 111, 1150–1157.

Cohen MJ, Meador KJ, Browning N, Baker GA, Clayton-Smith J, Kalayjian LA, Kanner A, Liporace JD, Pennell PB, Privitera M & Loring DW. (2011). Fetal antiepileptic drug exposure: motor, adaptive, and emotional/behavioral functioning at age 3 years. *Epilepsy Behavior*, 22, 240–248.

Confavreux C, Hutchinson M, Hours M.M, Cortinovis- Tourniaire P & Moreau T. (1998). Rate of pregnancy-related relapse in multiple sclerosis. Pregnancy in multiple sclerosis group. *New England Journal of Medicine*, 339, 285–291.

Coyle, PK. (2012). Pregnancy and Multiple Sclerosis. *Neurologic Clinics*, 30, 877–888.

D'hooghe MB, Nagels G & Uitdehaag BM (2010). Long-term effects of childbirth in MS. *Journal of Neurology, Neurosurgery and Psychiatry*, 81, 38–41.

DeKeyser J, Gdovinova Z, Uyttenboogaart M, Vroomen PC & Luijckx GJ. (2007). Intravenous alteplase for stroke. Beyond the guidelines and in particular clinical situations. *Stroke,* 38, 2612–2618

Dias MS. (1994). Neurovascular emergencies in pregnancy. *Clinical Obstetrics and Gynecology,* 37, 337–54.

Digre K. (2013). Headaches during Pregnancy. *Clinical Obstetrics and Gynecology*, 56 (2), 317-329.

Eadie MJ. (2014). Treating epilepsy in pregnant women. Expert Opinion in Pharmacotherapy, 15 (6), 841-850.

Evans EW & Loder KC. (2003). Migraine with aura during pregnancy. *Headache,* 43, 80–84.

Evans EW & Lorber KC. (2008) Use of 5-HT1 agonists in pregnancy. *Annals of Pharmacotherapy*, 42 (4), 543–9).

Fried S, Kozer E, Nulman I, Einarson TR & Koren G. (2004). Malformation rates in children of women with untreated epilepsy: a metaanalysis. *Drug Safety*, 27(3), 197–202.

Grear K & Kushnell CD. (2013). Stroke and Pregnancy: Clinical Presentation, Evaluation, Treatment, and Epidemiology. *Obstetrics and Gynecology*, 56, 350-359.

Harden CL & Sethi NK. (2008). Epileptic disorders in pregnancy: an overview. *Current Opinion in Obstetrics and Gynecology*, 20, 557–562.

Haider B & Von Oertzen J. (2013). Neurological disorders. Best Practice & Research Clinical *Obstetrics and Gynecology,* 27, 867–875.

Hirtz D, Thurman DJ, Gwinn-Hardy K, Mohamed M, Chaudhuri AR & Zalutsky R. (2007). How common are the "common" neurologic disorders? *Neurology,* 68, 326–37.

Holmes LB, Harvey EA, Coull BA, Huntington KB, Khoshbin S, Hayes AM & Ryan LM. (2001). The teratogenicity of anticonvulsant drugs. *New England Journal of Medicine*, 344 (15), 1132–8.

Houtchens MK & Kolb C. (2012). Multiple sclerosis and pregnancy. Therapeutic considerations. *Journal of Neurology*, 260, 1202-14.

Houtchens, MK (2013). Multiple Sclerosis and Pregnancy. *Clinical obstetrics and gynecology,* 56, 342–349.

Jaigobin C, Silver FL. (2000). Stroke and pregnancy. *Stroke*, 31, 2948–51.

James AH, Bushnell CD, Jamison MG & Myers ER. (2005). Incidence and risk factors for stroke in pregnancy and the puerperium. *Obstetrics and Gynecology*, 106, 509–516.

Kamyar M & Varmer M. (2013). Epilepsy in pregnancy. *Clinical Obstetrics and Gynecology*, 56 (2), 330-341

Kim W, Kim S.H & Nakashima I. (2012). Influence of pregnancy on neuromyelitis optica spectrum disorder. *Neurology*, 78, 1264–1267.

Koren G, Florescu A, Costei AM, Boskovic R & Moreti ME. (2006). Nonsteroidal anti-inflammatory drugs during third trimester and the risk of premature closure of the ductus arteriosus: a meta-analysis. *Annals of Pharmacotherapy*, 40, 824–9.

Kvisvik EV, Stovner LJ, Helde G, Bovim G & Linde M. (2011). Headache and migraine during pregnancy and puerperium: the MIGRA-study. *Journal of Headache and Pain*, 12, 443–451.

Langan Y, Nashef L & Sander JW. (2005). Case-control study of SUDEP. *Neurology*, 64 (7), 1131–3.

Langer-Gould A, Beaber B.E. (2013). Effects of pregnancy and breastfeeding on the multiple sclerosis disease course. *Clinical Inmunology,* 149, 244–250.

Langer-Gould A, Huang SM & Gupta R (2009). Exclusive breastfeeding and the risk of postpartum relapses in women with multiple sclerosis. *Archives Neurology*, 66,958–963.

Lanska DJ & Kryscio RJ. (2000). Risk factors for peripartum and postpartum stroke and intracranial venous thrombosis. *Stroke*, 31, 1274–1282.

Lashley L, van der Hoorn ML & van der Mast BJ. (2011). Changes in cytokine production and composition of peripheral blood leukocytes during pregnancy are not associated with a difference in the proliferative immune response to the fetus. *Human Immunology*, 72, 805–11.

Lebrun C, Le Page E & Kantarci O. (2012). Impact of pregnancy on conversion to clinically isolated syndrome in a radiologically isolated syndrome cohort, *Multiple Sclerosis*, 18, 1297–1302.

Lee M & O'Brien P. (2006). Multiple sclerosis and pregnancy. *Journal of neurology Neurosurgery and Psychiatry*, 79, 1308–11.

Lin SY, Hu CJ & Lin HC. (2008). Increased risk of stroke in patients who undergo cesarean delivery: a nationwide population-based study. *American Journal of Obstetrics and Gynecology,* 198(4), 391-394.

Lipton RB, Bigal ME, Steiner TJ, Silberstein SD & Olesen J. (2004). Classification of primary headaches. *Neurology,* 63 (3), 427–35.

MacGregor EA. (2012). Headache in Pregnancy. *Neurologic Clinic*, 30, 835–866.

Marcus DA, Scharff L & Turk D. (1999). Longitudinal prospective study of headache during pregnancy and postpartum. *Headache,* 39, 625–32.

Mawwer G, Briggs M, Baker GA, Bromley R, Coyle H, Eatock J, Kerr L, Kini U, Kuzmyshcheva L, Lucas SB, Wyatt L & Clayton-Smith J; Liverpool & Manchester Neurodevelopment Group. (2010). Pregnancy with epilepsy: obstetric and neonatal outcome of a controlled study. *Seizure*, 19, 112-19.

Melhado EM, Maciel JA Jr & Guerreiro CA. (2007). Headache during gestation: evaluation of 1101 women. *Canadian Journal of Neurology Science*, 34,187–192.

Morrow J, Russell A, Guthrie E, Parsons L, Robertson I, Waddell R, Irwin B, McGivern RC, Morrison PJ & Craig J. (2006). Malformation risk of antiepileptic drugs in pregnancy: a

Neuteboom RF, Verbraak E & Wierenga-Wolf AF. (2010). Pregnancy-induced fluctuations in functional T-cell subsets in multiple sclerosis patients. Multiple Sclerosis, 16, 1073–8.

Rukmini M & Bushnell CD. (2008). Headache and pregnancy. *Neurologist,* 14, 108–19.

Runmarker B & Andersen O (1995). Pregnancy is associated with a lower risk of onset and a better prognosis in multiple sclerosis. *Brain,* 118, 253–61.

Schapira K, Poskanzer DC &Newell DJ. (1966). Pregnancy and multiple sclerosis. *Brain*, 89, 419–428.

Scharff L, Marcus DA & Turk DC. (1997). Headache during pregnancy and in the postpartum: a prospective study. *Headache*, 37, 203–210.

Sidorov EV, Feng WF & Caplan LR. (2011) Stroke in pregnant and postpartum women. *Expert Review of Cardiovascular Therapy*, 9:1235–47.

Tate J & Bushnell C. (2011). Pregnancy and stroke risk in women. *Women´s Health*, 7, 363–74.

Tettenborn B. (2012). Stroke and Pregnancy. *Neurology Clinical*, 30, 913-924.

Tomson T, Battino D, Bonizzoni E, Craig J, Lindhout D, Sabers A, Perucca E & Vajda F; EURAP study group. (2011). Dose-dependent risk of malformation with antiepileptic drugs: an analysis of data from the EURAP epilepsy and pregnancy registry. *Lancet Neurology,* 10, 609-17.

Torelli P, Allais G & Manzoni GC. (2010). Clinical review of headache in pregnancy. *Neurology Science*, 31 (1), 55–58.

Treadwell SD, Thanvi B & Robinson TG. (2008). Stroke in pregnancy and the puerperium. *Posgraduate Medical journal*, 84, 238–245.

Tsui A & Lee M.A. (2011). Multiple sclerosis and pregnancy. *Current Opinion in Obstetrics and Gynecology,* 23, 435–439.

Vajda FJE, Hitchcock A, Graham J, O'Brien TJ, Lander CM & Eadie MJ. (2010). The teratogenic risk of antiepileptic drug polytherapy. *Epilepsia*, 51, 805-10.

Vajda FJE, Graham JE, Hitchcock AA, O'Brien TJ, Lander CM & Eadie MJ. (2010). Is lamotrigine a significant human teratogen? *Observations from the Australian Pregnancy Register. Seizure,* 19, 558-61.

Vajda FJE, Graham J, Roten A, Lander CM, O'Brien TJ & Eadie M. (2012). Teratogenicity of the newer antiepileptic drugs - the Australian experience. *Journal of Clinical Neuroscience*, 19, 57-9.

Van Walderven MA, Tas MW & Barkhof F (1994). Magnetic resonance evaluation of disease activity during pregnancy in multiple sclerosis. *Neurology,* 44,327–9.

Vukusic S, Hutchinson M, Hours M, Moreau T, Cortinovis-Tourniaire P, Adeleine P & Confavreux C. The Pregnancy In Multiple Sclerosis Group (2004). Pregnancy and multiple sclerosis (the PRIMS study): clinical predictors of post-partum relapse. *Brain,* 27,1353-60.

Wall VR. (1992). Breastfeeding and migraine headaches. *Journal of Human Lactation*, 8, 209–12.

Wilkinson H. (2011). Saving mothers' lives: reviewing materal deaths to make motherhood safter. *British Journal of Obstetrics and Gynecology*, 118 (11), 1402-1403.

In: Handbook for High Risk Pregnancy: Clinical Management ISBN: 978-1-63482-299-2
Editors: E. González-Mesa and D. Abehsera

Chapter 13

PRETERM LABOR

Rosa López López, MD[1], María José Bravo Zurita, MD[1*] and María Auxiliadora Armenteros Pérez, MD[2]

[1]Obstetrics and Gynecology Department,
Quiron University Hospital, Málaga, Spain
[2]Obstetrics and Gynecology Department,
Malaga Regional University Hospital, Spain

INTRODUCTION

Preterm Labor (PTL) is one of the leading cause of perinatal morbidity and mortality (70%-85%). The incidence rate of premature birth has not declined but increased over the last years, due to the use of assisted reproductive technology associated to the rise of multiple pregnancies, obstetric interventions and a better record of premature infants at lower gestational ages than in previous decades.

New challenges are emerging with the definition of *fetal viability* as its gestational age is being discussed, but it is currently accepted to be around 24 weeks. However, either in a short or long term period the morbidity and mortality as well as the economic and emotional cost for the families increase in extremely premature infants.

The specific trigger of PTL is largely unknown and its prevention is difficult due to different reasons like medical conditions affecting the mother or fetus in which continuation of pregnancy is hazardous.

Definitions

The threatened preterm labor is defined as the symptomatic clinical state in women with a non-effective treatment or under no treatment at all, which may lead to a delivery before the 37th completed week of gestation (ACOG, 2013).

[*] Corresponding author: mariajobz@hotmail.com.

Incidence and Significance

- USA: 13%
- Europe: 7%
- Spain 7.5%

Classification

According to the gestational age (Lumley):

- Extremely preterm birth: before 28 weeks gestation (10%)
- Very preterm birth: between 28 and 31 weeks gestation (10%)
- Late preterm birth: from 32 to 36 weeks gestation (80%)

According to the birthweight:

- Low birthweight (LBW): less than 2,500 grams
- Very low birthweight (VLBW): less than 1,500 grams
- Extremely low birthweight (ELBW): less than 1,000 grams

The relationship between the gestational age and infant mortality decreases exponentially towards full-term infant.

A direct relation exists between morbidity and prematurity: any disability may occur in a 60% of the births at 26 weeks gestation and in a 30% of the births in the 31 weeks. However, there has been major improvements in the neonatal cares and therefore, perinatal results have also improved.

Clinical Settings

- Spontaneous Labor with Intact Membranes: 40-50%
- Preterm Premature Rupture of the Membranes (PPROM): 30-40%
- Iatrogenic preterm labor or labor induction for maternal or fetal indications: 20%

Intraamniotic infection has been recorded either in threatened preterm labor with intact membranes or preterm premature rupture of the membranes and the 20-25% of the etiology of PTL can be explained based on this.

Clinical Risk Factors

The identification of the risk factors of PTL could permit an early intervention to prevent it. However, it is difficult to identify the triggers of it and in most of the cases PTL occurs to women at low risk for preterm labor.

Demographic factors (affecting a 13% of the risk of PTL)

Race and ethnicity: African American women present a higher risk of PTL (17.4% against the 6.7% in white women). The ethnic differences related to polymorphisms of the cytokines and genes in the immune system in pregnant women may be reflected in the percentage of PTL. Research is now focused on this field.

Maternal age: Teenagers and women older than 35 years old are at a higher risk for PTL. However, it is not clear if these differences are due to biological mechanism related to the age or other characteristics associated with pregnancies at extreme ages (socioeconomic position, higher medical-obstetrical complications in older ages, the use of assisted reproductive technology…).

Socioeconomic position: According to maternal characteristics such as education, job and family income. The literature shows an increase in the risk of threatened preterm labor among women in the lowest family income category.

Use of drugs: Cocaine and smoking.

Low maternal body-mass index.

High levels of personal stress and poor working conditions.

Prior obstetrical history

1. Clinical history of previous preterm labors (the risk increases in 3-4 times): The risk of recurrent preterm birth rises with the number of previous preterm births, being the last PTL the most influential. Another factor to consider is the gestational age of the previous PTL.
2. Vaginal bleeding: The metrorrhagia occurred in the first trimester doubled the risk of PTL and the percentage increases if it is presented in the second and third trimester of gestation, with or without intact membranes.

Uterine factors

1. Twin gestation: Twin gestation, in which uterine distension and PPROM are important factors to consider, has a five to six times greater risk (12% of the premature infants).

Multiple gestations are at greater risk of prematurity.

2. Polyhydramnios
3. Uterine distortion
4. Submucosal Uterine Fibroids
5. Cervical incompetence
6. Trauma
7. UID
8. Exposure to diethylstilbestrol

Fetal factors

1. Fetal death.

2. Congenital anomalies. The reason why the fetal anomalies trigger the labor is not clear.

Genetic factors. Genetic polymorphisms in FNT-alpha and IL-6.
Infections:

1. Urinary tract infections: Asymptomatic bacteriuria or pyelonephritis.
2. Cervicovaginal infections: The mass colonization of the lower genital tract and the subsequent inflammatory response.
3. Chorioamnionitis: Infected amniotic fluid can trigger PTL, either with intact membranes or PPROM.
4. Maternal infections: Hematogenous spread.

Preterm labor mechanisms

1. Mymetrial and membranes overdistension
2. Decidual bleeding
3. Premature fetal endocrine activation
4. Intrauterine infection or inflammation

Diagnosis

Standard diagnosis of threatened preterm labor is based on uterine contractions accompanied by cervical change with or without PPROM or genital bleeding (Simhan et al., 2007).

Uterine contractions There are no firm criteria about the number of contractions necessary for PTL. Nevertheless, uterine contractions which are considered as an evidence of PTL occur with a frequency of at least 4 every 20-30 minutes or 8 every 60 minutes and are painful, palpable and last more than 30 seconds. Most of the case does not present specific symptoms (menstrual-like cramps, abdominal pain, increased blood flow…)

Cervical change is a strong predictor of threatened preterm labor. It is necessary to perform a bimanual vaginal examination to evaluate dilation, effacement, position and consistency of the uterine cervix as well as fetal station (Bishop Score).

Digital assessment of the cervix is subjective as it has high inter-observer variability and underestimates the true cervical length. However, these parameters have shown low sensitivity and specificity to predict PTL. Therefore, it is important to consider other markers:

Transvaginal Ultrasound Cervical Assessment

Transvaginal ultrasound is an easy, reproducible, non-invasive and low cost technique to assess cervix length. This technique is performed after bladder emptying with a probe placed into the vagina, avoiding undue pressure on the cervix, so the whole length of the cervical canal is identified and is measured from the outer to the inner cervical os. It is necessary to describe the presence of funneling (appreciation of the membranes in the canal) and its depth (To et al., 2000; Glanc et al., 2011; Berghella et al., 2013).

The average length of the uterine cervix in the second trimester is 35mm and effacement begins at the internal cervical os and progresses caudally. Threatened preterm labor is clearly identified by a cervix with a length of 25mm, with a negative predictive value of 94% (Berghella et al., 2013).

As the length of the cervix changes along the pregnancy, it is necessary to establish a cervical length cut-off value to predict low-risk of PTL (Palacio et al., 2007).

- <32weeks: 25mm. More sensibility, to avoid morbidity in PTL (<FN)
- >32weeks: 15mm. More specificity, to avoid unnecessary treatment or hospitalization (<FP)

Potential benefits of this marker need to be studied in further research.

Biochemical Markers

Fetal fibronectin (FFN) is an extracellular matrix glycoprotein produced at the maternal-fetal interface of the amniotic membranes, between the chorion and decidua. Fetal fibronectin in high concentrations (≥50ng/ml) at or after 22 weeks is associated with an increased risk of PTL (Lockwood et a, 1991). The diagnostic utility of FFN for preventing threatened PTL is really in its high NPV. In women with a negative FFN result confers a reduced risk of PTL with a <1% chance of delivery within two weeks of sampling (Goldenberg et al., 1998; Hams et al., 1998). Either fetal fibronectin or vaginal ultrasound are two accurate techniques to determine negative PTL due to the high NPV obtained. Therefore, both techniques are useful to prevent unnecessary treatments and hospitalizations (levels of evidence IIb). Nonetheless, due to the low PPV they become inaccurate to assess asymptomatic patients (Berghella et al., 2008; Kurtzman et al., 2009)).

A Cochrane 2008 review (Berghella et al., 2008) of fetal fibronectin test concludes that preterm birth less than 37 weeks was significantly decreased (15.6%) versus control (28.6%). However, no other neonatal morbidity and mortality outcomes were available for meaningful analysis. Nevertheless, some clinical guidelines include fibronectin test in combination with cervix length, when it is 20-30mm long, for improving the risk prediction of PTL (ACOG and USPS Task Force).

Inhibition of Uterine Contractions or Tocolysis

The administration of tocolytics to stop the threatened preterm labor in patients with continuous contractions in combination with cervical changes at 22-24 weeks gestation and up to 34+6 weeks, due to the need of an effective treatment with corticosteroids for fetal lung maturity. Patients at 35 weeks gestation will follow a less aggressive therapy and it can be managed with bed rest and an evaluation of the need of tocolytics. At 36 weeks no tocolytics therapy will undergo.

If there is no uterine activity, tocolytics therapy is not recommended. In those patients with a shorten cervix and without uterine activity, different possible strategies can be followed (see next section).

Initial Clinical Assessment:

- Anamnesis: markers and symptoms for possible threatened PTL.
- Blood pressure, temperature and heartbeat.
- Spec and bimanual vaginal exam.
  - ✓ Vaginal-rectal culture for group B streptococcus.
  - ✓ Vaginal or cervical swab for Chlamydia.
- Cardiotopographic monitoring.
- Transvaginal ultrasound.
- Abdominal ultrasound: fetal position, biometry, amniotic fluid and placenta.
- Urine test and urine culture.
- Hemogram, coagulation profile and CRP blood test.

In case of probable amniotic infection, an amniocentesis may be performed.

Contraindications

In those gestations in which the prolongation is not recommendable, the administration of tocolytics is contraindicated.

- Advanced labor. Tocolytics could be administered to allow enough time for a corticosteroid therapy.
- Evidence of fetal compromise with no uterine activity.
- Fetal death (singleton gestations).
- A severely anomalous fetus.
- Severe preeclampsia or eclampsia.
- Obstetric complications.
- Intrauterine infection.
- Maternal hemorrhage with hemodynamic instability (placenta previa, placental abruption).
- It is not recommended to administer indomethacin at 32-34 weeks gestation due to the risk of premature closure of ductus arteriosus.

Tocolytics

Tocolytic drugs are effective in delaying from 48 hours to even 7 days the delivery and although the preterm labor rate has not decreased, they allow the administration of corticosteroids, reduce the risk of respiratory distress syndrome, necrotizing enterocolitis, intraventricular bleeding, perinatal death (Level of evidence Ia). Furthermore, they give

rug	Mechanism	Dose	Side effects	Contraindications
itodrine	Beta2-adrenergic agonist	Initial dose: 50-100mcg/min Increased by 50mcg every 10mins Until a max. of 300mcg/min	Hypotension Maternal tachycardia Arrhythmia Hypokalemia Hyperglycemia	Hypotension Maternal tachycardia Arrhythmia Hypokalemia hyperglycemia
domethacin	Nonsteroidal anti-inflammatory analgesics (NSAIDs)	Initial dose: 50-100mg either oral or retal route Then 25-50mg every 6 hours. Oral route Or 100 every 12 hours. Either vaginal or retal routes,	Gastrointestinal bleeding Vomiting Maternal postpartum bleeding	Before 32 weeks of pregnancy kidney disease Peptic ulcer Problems with blood clotting Asthma Intolerance to ASA

roids

Corticosteroid treatment should commence after a tocolytic therapy between the 22-24 to -6 weeks gestation. It is administered for accelerating fetal lung maturity and for reducing incidence and severity of respiratory distress syndrome (level of evidence Ia) and inatal morbidity and mortality (approx. 50% of the cases). The corticosteroids used are amethasone and dexamethasone. However, betamethasone has recently shown a higher ciency.

Dosage:

- Betamethasone: 12mg intramuscularly, 2 doses 24 hours apart.
- Dexamethasone: 6mg intramuscularly, 4 doses 12 hourly.

The benefits of the corticosteroid treatment are found after 18 hours of the first dose and sually takes about 48 hours for the treatment to be fully effective (ACOG 2008; RCOG 2).

Intrauterine corticosteroids are contraindicated due to the high risk of chorioamnionitis, erculosis and porphyria.

tibiotics

In threatened PTL with intact membranes, the administration of antibiotics is not icated for routine practice except for the following cases (King et al., 2002; ACOG, 2009):

- Positive vaginal culture.
- Patients with vaginal colonization of group B streptococcus should always be treated (intravenous ampicillin, initial bolus 2gr and then 1gr every 6 hours).
- Urine infection or asymptomatic bacteriuria.
- Threaten PTL with cervical dilation and prominent gestational sac as well as patients with a positive Gram stain in amniotic fluid.

enough time to transfer the patient to a hospital with neonatal intensive care ı et al., 2006; Simhan et al., 2007; Haas et al., 2009).

The most effective tocolytic drugs nowadays are:

- Oxytocin antagonist: Atosiban.
- Calcium channel blockers (CCBs): Nifedipino.
- Nonsteroidal anti-inflammatory analgesics: Indomethacin.
- Beta2-adrenergic agonist: Ritodrine.

No tocolytic agen has been identified as the best first-line option, as the should be effective, cheap, with few side effects and an easy administratic 2009). Several studies have tried to compare the different drugs available no' et al., 2007; Haas et al., 2009; ACOG, 2012).

The Obstetricians and Gynecologists society of Spain recommends atosi safety profile with fewer side effects even if it is the most expensive. Atosił administered for multiple gestations and patients who suffer diabetes and (Romero et al., 2000; Elenady et al., 2014). However, the American College ‹ and Gynecologists, in which country atosiban does not have FDA approval, personalized medication based on maternal state, gestational age and side eff al., 2007). Recent studies on the efficacy and safety of Nifedipino have shown tocolytic agent with the same efficacy as atosiban but cheaper. However, it effects and a compassionate use for PTL (Simhan et al., 2007; Haas et al., Agudelo et al., 2011; Elenady et al., 2014).

Finally, ritodrine is as efficient as the others but it has a more restricted high rate of side effects and therefore, a higher percentage of treatment interrı et al., 2014). Indomethacin is only used before the 32 weeks gestation due to premature closure of the ductus arteriosus and IFA and doppler tests are requiı 2009). A thorough estimation of the gestational age as well as the possi threatened PTL is needed before undergoing a tocolytic therapy. Continue tocolytic therapy has little or no value still proved (Di Renzo et al., 2006; Ly Papatsonis et al., 2013; Naik et al., 2013).

Drug	Mechanism	Dose	Side effects	Contraindi
Atosiban	Oxytocin antagonist	Setp 1: 0.9ml intravenous bolus Step 2: 24ml/hour for 3 hours Then 8ml/hour for 3.5hours Step 3: 8ml/hour for up to 45 hour	Nausea Headache	Allergy to
Nifedipino	Calcium channel blockers (CCBs)	Initial dose: 5-10mg every 20 minutes. Oral route Then 10-20 every 6-8 hours Until a max of 160mg per day	Transient hypotension Headache Flushing Nausea	Heart disea Kidney dis Liver disea Basal Hyp Adjunctive antihyperte medication ritrodine oı sulfate

enough time to transfer the patient to a hospital with neonatal intensive care units (Di Renzo et al., 2006; Simhan et al., 2007; Haas et al., 2009).

The most effective tocolytic drugs nowadays are:

- Oxytocin antagonist: Atosiban.
- Calcium channel blockers (CCBs): Nifedipino.
- Nonsteroidal anti-inflammatory analgesics: Indomethacin.
- Beta2-adrenergic agonist: Ritodrine.

No tocolytic agen has been identified as the best first-line option, as the ideal tocolytic should be effective, cheap, with few side effects and an easy administration (Haas et al., 2009). Several studies have tried to compare the different drugs available nowadays (Aiham et al., 2007; Haas et al., 2009; ACOG, 2012).

The Obstetricians and Gynecologists society of Spain recommends atosiban as it has a safety profile with fewer side effects even if it is the most expensive. Atosiban is normally administered for multiple gestations and patients who suffer diabetes and heart diseases (Romero et al., 2000; Elenady et al., 2014). However, the American College of Obstetricians and Gynecologists, in which country atosiban does not have FDA approval, recommends a personalized medication based on maternal state, gestational age and side effects (Simhan et al., 2007). Recent studies on the efficacy and safety of Nifedipino have shown that it is a good tocolytic agent with the same efficacy as atosiban but cheaper. However, it has some side effects and a compassionate use for PTL (Simhan et al., 2007; Haas et al., 2009; Conde-Agudelo et al., 2011; Elenady et al., 2014).

Finally, ritodrine is as efficient as the others but it has a more restricted use due to the high rate of side effects and therefore, a higher percentage of treatment interruption (Neilson et al., 2014). Indomethacin is only used before the 32 weeks gestation due to a higher risk of premature closure of the ductus arteriosus and IFA and doppler tests are required (Haas et al., 2009). A thorough estimation of the gestational age as well as the possible causes for threatened PTL is needed before undergoing a tocolytic therapy. Continued maintenance tocolytic therapy has little or no value still proved (Di Renzo et al., 2006; Lyell et al., 2008; Papatsonis et al., 2013; Naik et al., 2013).

Drug	Mechanism	Dose	Side effects	Contraindications
Atosiban	Oxytocin antagonist	Setp 1: 0.9ml intravenous bolus Step 2: 24ml/hour for 3 hours Then 8ml/hour for 3.5hours Step 3: 8ml/hour for up to 45 hour	Nausea Headache	Allergy to the drug
Nifedipino	Calcium channel blockers (CCBs)	Initial dose: 5-10mg every 20 minutes. Oral route Then 10-20 every 6-8 hours Until a max of 160mg per day	Transient hypotension Headache Flushing Nausea	Heart disease Kidney disease Liver disease Basal Hypotension Adjunctive use of antihypertensive medications, nitroglycerin, ritrodine or magnesium sulfate

Drug	Mechanism	Dose	Side effects	Contraindications
Ritodrine	Beta2-adrenergic agonist	Initial dose: 50-100mcg/min Increased by 50mcg every 10mins Until a max. of 300mcg/min	Hypotension Maternal tachycardia Arrhythmia Hypokalemia Hyperglycemia	Hypotension Maternal tachycardia Arrhythmia Hypokalemia hyperglycemia
Indomethacin	Nonsteroidal anti-inflammatory analgesics (NSAIDs)	Initial dose: 50-100mg either oral or retal route Then 25-50mg every 6 hours. Oral route Or 100 every 12 hours. Either vaginal or retal routes,	Gastrointestinal bleeding Vomiting Maternal postpartum bleeding	Before 32 weeks of pregnancy kidney disease Peptic ulcer Problems with blood clotting Asthma Intolerance to ASA

Steroids

Corticosteroid treatment should commence after a tocolytic therapy between the 22-24 to 34+6 weeks gestation. It is administered for accelerating fetal lung maturity and for reducing the incidence and severity of respiratory distress syndrome (level of evidence Ia) and perinatal morbidity and mortality (approx. 50% of the cases). The corticosteroids used are betamethasone and dexamethasone. However, betamethasone has recently shown a higher efficiency.

Dosage:

- Betamethasone: 12mg intramuscularly, 2 doses 24 hours apart.
- Dexamethasone: 6mg intramuscularly, 4 doses 12 hourly.

The benefits of the corticosteroid treatment are found after 18 hours of the first dose and it usually takes about 48 hours for the treatment to be fully effective (ACOG 2008; RCOG 2012).

Intrauterine corticosteroids are contraindicated due to the high risk of chorioamnionitis, tuberculosis and porphyria.

Antibiotics

In threatened PTL with intact membranes, the administration of antibiotics is not indicated for routine practice except for the following cases (King et al., 2002; ACOG, 2009):

- Positive vaginal culture.
- Patients with vaginal colonization of group B streptococcus should always be treated (intravenous ampicillin, initial bolus 2gr and then 1gr every 6 hours).
- Urine infection or asymptomatic bacteriuria.
- Threaten PTL with cervical dilation and prominent gestational sac as well as patients with a positive Gram stain in amniotic fluid.

An ORACLE study has shown that in patients with PPROM, the use of antibiotics was associated with a significant decrease of chorioamnionitis and other morbidity markers indicated a beneficial use of it (Kenyon et al., 2008).

Neuroprotection with Magnesium Sulfate

Antenatal magnesium sulfate therapy is used for fetal neuroprotection to prevent cerebral palsy with a NNT of 63 (Marret et al., 2008; Rouse et al., 2008; Doyle et al., 2009).

It is administered in cases of active PTL or medical conditions affecting the mother or fetus in which continuation of pregnancy is hazardous between 24+0 to 31+6 weeks (Rouse et al., 2008; Sahen et al., 2011; Magee et al., 2011)

The contraindications are the indicated for the drug.

Adjunctive use of tocolytics with magnesium sulfate is only recommended to complete fetal lung maturity. There are no previous cases of the use of atosiban with magnesium sulfate, therefore it is not recommended. Magnesium sulfate administered together with ritodrine and nifedipino increases the risk of side effects and some studies do not approved it. However, Canadian and American Guidelines (Shane et al., 2011; Magee et al., 2011) do not consider this circumstance as a contraindication. Therefore, for patients before 32 weeks gestation eligible for tocolytics, indomethacin is the most recommendable. Before neuroprotection it is more urgent the fetal lung maturity with a tocolytic therapy.

If the treatment will not have a successful effect because the labor is due in less than two hours, an advanced cervical dilation of more than 8cms is presented or important fetal anomalies are found, patients should be excluded.

Two different dosages could be administered (ACOG 2010; Magee et al., 2011; Shane et al., 2011):

- Bolus 4g magnesium sulfate IV over 30 minutes, followed by bolus with magnesium sulfate 1g/hr IV until birth or up to 24 hours (SEGO).
- Bolus 6g magnesium sulfate IV over 30 minutes, followed by bolus with magnesium sulfate 2g/hr IV for 12 hours.

Over the magnesium sulfate treatment, a strict vigilance and a patient safety checklist must be carried out. Moreover, it is necessary the consent from patients assuming its compassionate use.

The treatment should not be longer than 24 hours and the repetition of it is not recommendable.

In case of scheduled extraction like elective cesarean, it is recommended to start the perfusion at least 4-6 hours before the deliver.

Other Strategies for Preventing Preterm Labor

Three management protocols for patients with a history of previous spontaneous PTL and short cervix have shown a reduction of the rate of PTL before 34 weeks gestation. These protocols are cerclage, progesterone and cervical pessary, although more studies are needed to determine which is the most efficient (Vidaeff et al., 2009, Society for Maternal-Fetal Medicine with Berghella, 2012; Conde-Agudelo et al., 2013; Alfirevic et al., 2013)

Cerclage

Cerclage has been demonstrated to be an effective intervention in patients who are at particularly high risk of spontaneous preterm birth (women who had more than two previous preterm birth in the second trimester) and have any potential cervical risk factor or progressive cervical shortening checked by ultrasound in the current pregnancy. Further studies are needed to clarify the role of the cerclage in short cervix (Owen et al., 2009; Simcox et al., 2009).

Prophylactic cerclage: indicated in asymptomatic women with a history of previous PTL. No significant decrease of the rate of pregnancy loss or PTL.

Therapeutic cerclage: indicated in asymptomatic women with short cervix. No significant decrease of the rate of pregnancy loss or PTL before 28 and 34 weeks gestation (CIRCLE trial).

Emergency cerclage: PTL symptoms (uterine contractions, progressive cervical dilation or presence of protruding membranes) managed with tocolytics between the 15 and 28 weeks. It is when it has been shown to be useful (Drakeley et al., 2003).

Progesterone

Progesterone reduces the risk of PTL in patients with a history of prior PTL (10%) and with short cervix between 24 to 34 weeks gestation. No evidence that indicated that this compound prevents preterm birth in multiple pregnancies (Fonseca et al., 2009; Tita et al., 2009; Hassan et al., 2011; Dodd et al., 2013).

The STOPPIT study concludes that trigger mechanism is different for multiple and singleton pregnancies. Perhaps stretching of uterine muscle has a substantial role in PTL in multiple pregnancies, and infection and inflammation a role in singletons (Norman et al., 2009).

Dosage: Vaginal micronized progesterone 200mg/24 hour at around 20-24 weeks and up to 34 week gestations, except for those patients with a history of previous PTL or with shorten cervix after a ultrasound in an earlier gestational age (Romero et al., 2014).

Cervical Pessary

A cervical pessary is a silicon ring-shape device which has been used for about 50 years as an option for delaying preterm births.

A pessary bends the cervix backward, not only elongating the cervix but also changing the uterocervical angle, which may strengthen the cervical canal and help preserve vaginal integrity (Arabin et al., 2013).

A recent Cochrane review determines that further studies are needed to assess the use of cervical pessary for preventing PTL (Abdel:Aleem et al., 2013).

The trial study PECEP concludes that it is a safe, inexpensive and reliable method for preventing preterm birth in a population of appropriately selected at-risk women previously screened for cervical length assessment at the midtrimester scan (Goya et al., 2012).

Premature Birth

It has not been shown benefits of cesarean section versus vaginal labor and experts determine that cesarean sections are not the only mechanism for delivering extremely premature infants (Skupski et al., 2009).

Vacuum assisted vaginal deliveries are not recommended for deliveries before the 34 weeks gestation or for babies with an average weigh of 2,500grams due to a higher risk of fetal intraventricular bleeding in premature newborns.

Contradicted results were found for the use of prophylactic forceps operation against spontaneous labor.

References

Abdel-Aleem H, Shaaban OM, Abdel-Aleem MA. (2013) Cervical pessary for preventing preterm birth (review). *Cochrane Database Systs Rev.*, 5: CD 007873.

Alfirevic Z, Own J, Carreras E, Sharp A, Szychowski J et al. (2013) Vaginal progesterone, cerclage or cervical pessary for preventing preterm birth in asymptomatic singleton pregnant women with a history of preterm birth and a sonographic short cervix. *Ultrasound in Obstetrics & Gynecology*, 41: 146-151.

American Collegue Obstetricians and Gynecologists (2009) Committee Opinion No. 445: antibiotics for preterm labor. *Obstetrics and Gynecology*, 114: 1159.

American Collegue of Obstetricians and Gynecologists Committee on Obstetrics Practice. (2008) Committee Opinion N° 402: Antenatal corticosteroid therapy for fetal maduration. *Obstetrics and Gynecology*, 111(3):805-7.

American College of Obstetricians and Gynecologists Committee on Practice Bulletins-Obstetrics. (2012). ACOG practice bulletin no.127: Management of preterm labour. *Obstetrics and Gynecology,* 119 (6):1308-17.

American College of Obstetricians and Gynecologists. (2010). Committee Opinion no. 455: Magnesium sulphate before anticipated preterm birth for neuroprotection. *Obstetrics and Gynecology, 115* (3): 669-671.

American College of Obstetricians and Gynecologists. Committee Opinion No 579. (2013) Definition of term pregnancy. *Obstetrics and Gynecology,* 122:1139.

Arabin B, Alfirevic Z. (2013). Cervical pessaries for prevention of spontaneous pretermbirth: past, present and future. *Ultrasound in Obstetrics & Gynecology*, 42, 390–399.

Berghella V, Baxter JK, Hendrix NW. (2013) Cervical assessment by ultrasound for preventing preterm delivery. *Cochrane Database of Syst. Rev.*, 1, CD 007235.

Berghella V, Hayes E, Visintine J, Baxter JK. (2008) Fetal fibronectin testing for reducing the risk of preterm birth. *Cochrane Database of Syst. Rev.* (4): CD006843.

Conde-Agudelo A, Romero R, Kusanovic JP. (2011). Nifedipine in the management of preterm labor: a systematic review and metaanalysis. *American Journal Obstetrics and Gynecology, 204* (2): 134. e 1-20.

Conde-Agudelo A, Romero R, Nicolaides K, Chaiworapongsa T, O'Brien JM, et al. (2013) Vaginal progesterone versus cervical cerclage for the prevention of preterm birth in women with a sonographic short cervix, previous preterm birth, and singleton gestation: a systematic review and indirect comparison metaanalysis. *American Journal of Obstetrics and Gynecology*, 208:42.e1-18.

Di Renzo GC, Roura LC; European Association of Perinatal Medicine-Study Group on Preterm Birth. (2006). Guidelines for the management of spontaneous preterm labor. *Journal Perinatal Medicine,* 34 (5): 359-66.

Dodd JM, Jones L, Flenady V, Cincotta R, Crowther CA. (2013). Prenatal administration of progesterone for preventing preterm birth in women considered to be at risk of preterm birth. *Cochrane Database Syst. Rev.,* 7: CD 004947.

Doyle L, Crowther C, Middleton P, Marret S, Rouse D. (2009) Magnesium sulphate for women at risk of preterm birth for neuroprotection of the fetus. *Cochrane Database of Systematic Review* 21; (1).

Drakeley AJ, Roberts D, Alfirivc Z (2003) Cervical stitch (cerclage) for preventing pregnancy loss in women. *Cochrane Database of Syst. Rev.*, 1: CD 003253.

Flenady V, Reinebrant HE, Liley HG, Tambimuttu EG, Papatsonis DN. (2014). Oxytocin receptor antagonists for inhibiting preterm labour. *Cochrane Database Syst. Rev.* 6: CD 004452.

Flenady V, Wojcieszek AM, Papatsonis DN, Stock OM, Murray L, et al. (2014). Calcium channel blockers for inhibiting preterm labour and birth. *Cochrane Database of Syst. Rev.* 6: CD 002255.

Fonseca E, Bittar R, Damiao R, Zugaib M. (2009). Premarurity prevention: the role of progesterone. *Current Opinion in Obstetrics and Gynecology* 21 (2):142-7.

Fonseca EB, Celik E, Parra M, Singh M, Nicolaides KH. (2007). Progesterona and the risk of preterm birth among women with a short cervix. *New England Journal of Medicine*, 357 (5): 462-9.

Glanc P, Andreotti RF, Lee SI, Dejesus Allison SO, Bennett GL, et al. (2011) ACR Appropriateness Criteria assessment of gravid cervix. *Ultrasound Q*, 27 (4): 275-80.

Goldenberg RL, Iams JD, Mercer BM. (1998). The preterm prediction study: the value of new vs standard risk factors in predicting early and all spontaneous preterm births. NICHD MFMU Network. *American Journal Public Health*, 88: 233.

Goya M, Pratcorona L, Merced C, Rodó C, Valle L, et al. (2012). Cervical pessary in pregnant women with a short cervix (PECEP): an open-label randomised controlled trial. *Lancet*, 379 (9828): 1800-1806.

Haas DM, Imperiale TF, Kirkpatrick PR, Klein RW, Zollinger TW, et al. (2009)Tocolytic therapy. *A meta-analysis and decision analysis,* 113(3):585-94.

Hassan SS, Romero R, Vidyadhari D, Fusey S, Baxter JK et al. (2011). Vaginal progesterone reduces the rate of preterm birth in women with a sonographic short cervix: a multicenter randomized, double blind, placebo-controlled trial. *Ultrasound obstetrics and Gynecology*, 38 (1): 18-31.

Iams JD, Goldenberg RL, Mercer BM. (1998). The Preterm Prediction Study: recurrence risk of spontaneous preterm birth. National Institute of Child Health and Human Development Maternal-Fetal Medicine Units Network. *American Journal of obstetrics and Gynecology*, 178: 1035.

Kenyon S, Pike K, Jones DR. (2008) Childhood outcomes after prescription of antibiotics to pregnant women with spontaneous preterm labour: 7-year follow-up of the ORACLE II trial. *Lancet,* 372: 1319.

King J, Flenady V. (2002) Prophylactic antibiotics for inhibiting preterm labour with intact membranes. *Cochrane Database Syst. Rev.*; CD 000246.

Kurtzman J, Chandiramani M, Briley A, Poston L, Das A, et al. (2009) Quantitative fetal fibronectin screening in asymptomatic high-risk patients and the spectrum of risk for recurrent preterm delivey. *American Journal of Obstetrics and Gynecology*, 200(3): 263.e1-6.

Lockwood CJ, Senyei AE, Dische MR. (1991). Fetal fibronectin in cervical and vaginal secretions as a predictor of preterm delivery. *New England Journal of Medicine*, 325: 669.

Lumley J. (2003). Defining the problem: the epidemiology of preterm birth. *British Journal of Obstetrics and Gynaecology*, 110 suppl 20: 3-7.

Lyell DJ, Pullen KM, Mannan J, Chitkara U, Druzin ML, et al. (2008). Maintenance Nifedipine tocolysis compared with placebo. A randomized controlled Trial. *Obstetrics and Gynecology*, 112(6): 1221-1226.

Magee L, Sawchuck D, Synnes A, von Dadelszen P. (2011). SOGC Clinical Practice Guideline. Magnesium sulphate for fetal neuroprotection. *Journal Obstetrics and Gynaecology Canadian,* 33 (5): 516-29.

Marret S, Marpeau L, Follet-Bouhamed C, Cambonie G, Astruc D, et al. (2008). Effect of magnesium sulphate on mortality and neurologic morbidity of the very-preterm new born with two-year neurologic outcome: results of the prospective PREMAG trial. *Gynecol. Obstet. Fertil.,* 36 (3): 278-288.

Naik Gaunekar N, Raman P, Bain E, Crowther CA. (2013). Maintanance therapy with calcium channel blockers for preventing preterm birth after threatened preterm labour (Review). *Cochrane Database of Syst. Rev.* 10: CD 004071.

Neilson JP, West HM, Dowswell T. (2014) Betamimetics for inhibiting preterm labour. *Cochrane Database Syst. Rev.* 2: 004352

Norman JE, Mackenzie F, Owen P, Mactier H, Hanretty K, et al. (2009). Progesterone for the prevention of preterm birth in twin pregnancy (STOPPIT): a randomised, double-blind, placebo-controlled study and meta-analysis. *Lancet* 13; 373 (9680):2034-40.

Owen J, Hankins G, Iams JD, Berghella V, Sheffield JS et al. (2009) Multicenter randomized trial of cerclage for preterm birth prevention in high-risk women with shortenend midtrimester cervical length. *American Journal Obstetrics and Gynecology*, 201 (4): 375.e 1-8.

Palacio M, Sanin-Blair J, Sánchez M, Crispi F, Gómez O, et al. (2007). The use of variable cut-off value of cervical length in women admitted for preterm labor before and after 32 weeks. *Ultrasound in Obstetrics and Gynecology*, 29 (4):421-6.

Papatsonis DN, Flenady V, Liley HG. (2013) Maintanance therapy with oxytocin antagonists for inhibiting preterm birth after threatened preterm labour (Review). *Cochrane Database of Syst Rev*, 10: CD 005938.

Romero R, Sibai BM, Sanchez-Ramos L, Valenzuela GJ, Veille JC et al. (2000) An oxytocin receptor antagonists (atosiban) in the treatment of preterm labor: a randomized, double-blind, placebo-controlled trial with tocolytic rescue. *American Journal Obstetrics and Gynecology* 182(5); 1173-83.

Romero R, Yeo L, Chaemsaithong P, Chaiworapongsa T, Hassan S. (2014). Progesterone to prevent spontaneous preterm birth. *Seminars in Fetal & Neonatal Medicine* 19: 15-26.

Rouse D, Hirtz D, Thom E, Varner M, Spong C, et al. (2008). A randomized controlled trial of magnesium sulphate for the prevention of cerebral palsy. *New England Journal of Medicine,* 359 (9): 895-905.

Royal Collegue of Obstetricians and Gynaecologists. (2012). Antenatal corticosteroids to reduce neonatal morbidity and mortality. *Greentop Guideline* No 7. London.

Shane AR, Gibbs RS, Steven LC. (2011). Magnesium for fetal neuroprotection. *American Journal of Obstetrics and Gynecology*. 204 (3): 202. e 1- 4.

Simcox R, Seed PT, Bennett P, Teoh TG, Poston L, et al. (2009) A randomized controlled trial of cervical scanning vs history to determine cerclage in women at high risk of preterm birth (CIRCLE trial). *American Jounal of Obstetrics and Gynecology,* 200 (6):623.e.1-6.

Simhan HN, Caritis SN. (2007). Prevention of Preterm delivery. *New England Journal of Medicine,* 357(5):477-87.

Skupski DW, Greenough A, Donn SM, Arabin B, Bancalari E, et al. (2009). Delivery mode for the extremely premature fetus: a statement of the prematurity working group of the World Association of Perinatal Medicine. *Journal of Perinatal Medicine*, 39: 583-6.

Society for Maternal-Fetal Medicine Publications Committee with the assistance of Berghella V. (2012). Progesterone and preterm birth prevention: translating clinical trials data into clinical practice. *American Journal of Obstetrics & Gynecology*,206 (5):376-386.

Tita AT, Rouse DJ. (2009). Progesterone for preterm birth prevention: an evolving intervention. *American Journal of Obstetrics and Gynecology*, 200 (3):219-24.

To MS, Skentou C, Cicero S, Nicolaides KH. (2000). Cervical assessment at the routine 23-weeks´scan: problems with transabdominal sonography. *Ultrasound Obstetrics and Gynecology,* 15:292.

Vidaeff AC, Ramin SM. (2009) Management strategies for the prevention of preterm birth. Part I: Update on progesterone supplementation. *Current Opinion in Obstetrics and Gynecology,* 21 (6): 480-4.

In: Handbook for High Risk Pregnancy: Clinical Management ISBN: 978-1-63482-299-2
Editors: E. González-Mesa and D. Abehsera

Chapter 14

HEMATOLOGICAL DISORDERS DURING PREGNANCY

Laura Sotillo Mallo, MD*
Obstetrics and Gynecological Department,
La Paz University Hospital, Madrid, Spain

THROMBOCYTOPENIA

1.1. Introduction

Thrombocytopenia is the most common blood disorder during the pregnancy after anemia.

Thrombocytopenia defined as a platelet count <150 x 10^9/L has a prevalence at the end of the pregnancy between 6.6% and 11%. However, counts <100 x 10^9/L, which is the definition for thrombocytopenia adopted by an International Working Group, are observed in only 1% of the pregnancy.

1.2. Classification

- Mild: 150-100 x 10^9 /L.
- Moderate: 100-50 x 10^9 /L.
- Severe: < 50 x 10^9 /L.

1.3. Diagnosis

1.3.1. Basic Evaluation

- History:
    - Obstetric history.

* Correspondence: sotillo2@hotmail.com.

- Family history of uncommon bleeding: in this case is important investigate causes of congenital thrombocytopenia.
- Drugs prescription or non-prescription:
    - Analgesics: aspirin, acetaminophen, indomethacin.
    - Antibiotics: ampicillin, penicillin, trimethoprim-sulfamethoxazole.
    - Others: heparin, methyldopa cyclosporine.

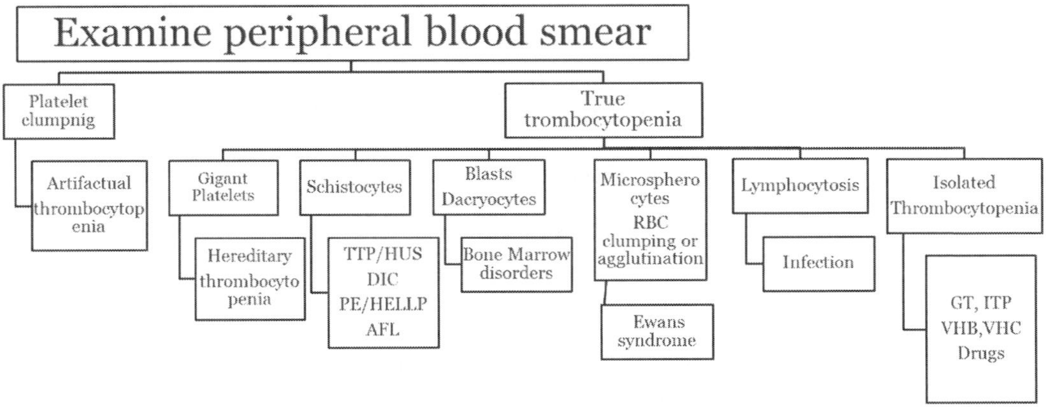

Figure 1. Peripheral blood smear for the differential diagnosis of thrombocytopenia.

- Physical examination.
- Complete blood count with reticulocyte count and screening for coagulation abnormalities (prothrombin time, activated partial thromboplastin time, fibrinogen, D-dimer).
- Liver and thyroid function test.
- Quantitative immunoglobulins (Ig): if the medical history suggests frequent infections, low immunoglobulins levels may reveal a previously undiagnosed disorder, for example Common variable immune deficiency.
- Direct antiglobulin test (Coombs test) is necessary to rule out autoimmune thrombocytopenia (Evans syndrome) if hemolytic anemia is present.
- Patients should be screened for VIH, VHB, VHC and CMV.
- Peripheral blood smear.

1.3.2. Test to Consider If Clinically Indicated

- Antiphospholipid antibodies (lupus anticoagulant, anticardiolipin and β-2-glycoprotein IgG and IgM antibodies) and antinuclear antibody, specifically in women with a history of previous miscarriage, abruption placentae o intrauterine growth restriction.
- Type 2B von Willebrand disease should be discarded, especially in women with a personal history of uncommon bleeding, or if the therapy for ITP is ineffective.
- Helicobacter pylori testing.

1.3.3. Tests Which Are Not Recommended

- Bone marrow biopsy.
- Antiplatelet antibody testing, because platelet associated immunoglobulin may be elevated in both immune and non-immune thrombocytopenia.
- Thrombopoietin (TPO) levels.

1.4. Causes

- Gestational thrombocytopenia (GT) (70-80%).
- Pre-eclampsia (15-20%).
- Immune thrombocytopenic purpura (ITP) (1-4%).
- Spurious-EDTA-induced platelet aggregation.
- Hemolysis, Elevated Liver enzymes and Low PLatelets (HELLP) (<1%).
- Acute fatty liver of pregnancy (<1%).
- Drugs (<1%).
- Thyroid disorders (<1%)
- Hemolytic uremic syndrome (HUS)/ thrombotic thrombocytopenic purple (TTP) (<1%).
- Systemic lupus erythematosus (SLE) and antiphospholipid syndrome (APS) (<1%).
- Infections such as HIV, viral hepatitis, EBV, CMV, H. pylori (<1%).
- Type 2B von Willebrand disease (<1%).
- Congenital thrombocytopenia (Wiskott-Aldrich syndrome, Bernard-Soulier syndrome…)
- Folate deficiency.
- Disseminated intravascular coagulation.

1.4.1. Gestational Thrombocytopenia (GT)

- Introduction:

GT is the leading cause of thrombocytopenia during the pregnancy because it accounts for 70-80% of causes of thrombocytopenia in pregnancy.

- Clinical features:

Thrombocytopenia is typically mild to moderate, typically remaining greater than 70 x 10^9/L, with approximately two-thirds of cases having platelet counts about 130-150 x 10^9/L, and it occurs in the mid late of second and third trimester.

Patients are asymptomatic and have no bleeding.

For the thrombocytopenia to be consistent with GT, women should have no past history of thrombocytopenia and typically resolves within six weeks postpartum, but may recur with subsequent pregnancies (in about 20%).

GT is not associated with neonatal thrombocytopenia.

- Diagnosis:

Examine peripheral blood smear: isolated thrombocytopenia, no shistocytes.

The main differential diagnosis is with ITP, but in some cases is very difficult the differential diagnosis between a severe GT and a mild ITP, and the diagnosis is not possible until 1-2 months after delivery when the thrombocytopenia resolved spontaneously and the newborn has no thrombocytopenia in the GT.

- Treatment:

In general is not necessary any treatment during the pregnacy.

1.4.2. Immune Thrombocytopenia in Pregnancy (ITP)

- Epidemiology:

ITP occurs in approximately 2 of 1000 pregnancies.

ITP accounts for 5% of cases of pregnancy-associated thrombocytopenia but it is the most common cause of isolated thrombocytopenia before 20 weeks.

- Pathogenesis:

Autoantibodies against platelet glycoproteins such as glycoprotein IIb/IIIa, or less commonly glycoproteins Ib/IX or Ia/IIa, cause peripheral platelet destruction by the reticle-endothelial system, particularly by the spleen. More recently, increasing evidence suggests concomitant immune-mediated decreased platelet production.

- Clinical features:

Around two-thirds of patients with ITP in pregnancy have pre-existing disease, whereas only one-third is diagnosed in pregnancy.

ITP that predates pregnancy may either remain quiescent or worsen during the pregnancy.

There is no lymphadenopathy or splenomegaly.

- Diagnosis:

Examine peripheral blood smear: isolated thrombocytopenia, no shistocytes.

The diagnosis of ITP is one of exclusion.

- Management:

Pregnant women with ITP require careful monitoring, and should be seen monthly in the first and the second trimester, every two weeks after 28 weeks and once a week after 36 weeks.

- Treatment:

The different treatments have not been found to affect the neonatal platelet count, for that we only use these drugs with the aim of increasing maternal platelet counts. Treatment indications:

- Until 36 weeks: <20.000-30.000 platelets/μl and/or bleeding.
- Regional anesthesia: ≥ 80.000-100.000 platelets/μl.
- Delivery o invasive procedure: ≥ 50.000 platelets/μl.
- For patients who have not required therapy during gestation but have less than 80.000 platelets/μl, can be started with prednisone 1-2 weeks before delivery.

Table 1. Treatments for thrombocytopenia during pregnancy

First-Line Therapy	Second-Line Therapy	Third-line Therapy	Not recommended but use in pregnancy described	Contraindicated
Corticosteroids	Splenectomy	Anti-D	Rituximab	Danazol
Intravenous immunoglobulin		Azathioprine	Thrombopoietin receptor agonist	Mycophenolate mofetil
				Cyclophos-phamide

- First-line therapy:

  - *Corticosteroids:* oral prednisone or prednisolone may be started at a low dose (10-20 mg/day, which could be increased to 1 to 1.5 mg/kg/day (based on the pre-pregnancy weight) if needed.

The mechanism of action of glucocorticoid is to block the production of antibodies and to reduce the phagocytosis of antibody-coated platelets in the spleen.

A response occurs within 3 to 7 days, and the platelet counts reach their maximum in 2 to 3 weeks.

Maternal side effects include osteoporosis, immunosuppression, hypertension and osteoporosis with the long-term use.

Withdrawal of corticosteroids in postpartum must be carefully monitored and dosage tapered to avoid a rapid drop in the platelet count and the precipitation of adrenal crisis.

  - *Immunoglobulins (Ig):* can be used for a rapid increase in platelet count or to maintain safe platelet counts when women are not responsive to steroids or there are poorly tolerated side effects.

The treatment dose is 2 g/kg divided over 2-5 days.

The immunoglobulins quickly raise the platelet count over several days, but the effects are transient (1- 4 weeks).

The disadvantages of Ig are that are more expensive that the corticosteroids, require intravenous access and Ig is a blood product with a theoretic risk of blood-borne infections.

Maternal side effects are: headache, that is very usual, and renal failure and thrombosis.

In a subset of patients who fail to respond to corticosteroids or Ig intravenous (iv) alone, is possible use these agents in combination (methylprednisolone 1 g + Ig 1-2 mg/Kg).

- Second-line therapy:
    - *Splenectomy:* This surgery may be useful for patients who remain refractory to the therapy or who experience significant toxicity with other therapies.

When the splenectomy is necessary it is best carried out in the second trimester and may be performed laparoscopically.

Transplacental passage of maternal antiplatelet antibodies and the risk of neonatal thrombocytopenia are not affected by the splenectomy.

After splenectomy pregnant women require vaccination against Hemophilus influenzae, Streptococcus pneumoniae and Neisseria meningitides.

- Third-line treatment:
    - *Anti-RhD:* Only use in non-splenectomized RhD positive pregnant women in the second and third trimester.

Anti-Rh D immunoglobulin binds to maternal red blood cell, when they are presented to Fc receptors in the spleen results in preferential splenic phagocytosis of the red cell rather than platelets.

The dose is 50-75 μg/kg.

Response occurs in 75% of patients within 1 to 2 days after the administration, with peak effect in 1-2 weeks and duration up to 4 weeks.

Common side effects are fever, chills and hemolytic anemia, but the limited of number of cases reported to date suggests anti-RhD is effective and safe.

If anti-Rh D is administered during the pregnancy, the neonate should be monitored for a positive direct antiglobulin test, anemia and jaundice.

-
    - *Azathioprine (Imurel®):* may be considered as another option for patients who fail to other therapies. The fetus is thought to be protected from teratogenic effects, because it lacks the enzyme that is necessary to convert azathioprine to the active metabolite 6-mercaptopurine.

- Platelet transfusion: is generally not recommended except in cases of severe hemorrhage or immediately before surgery or delivery.
- Delivery.

Cesarean section is only required for obstetric indications, because there is not conclusive evidence that the cesarean section reduces the incidence of intra-cerebral haemorrhage.

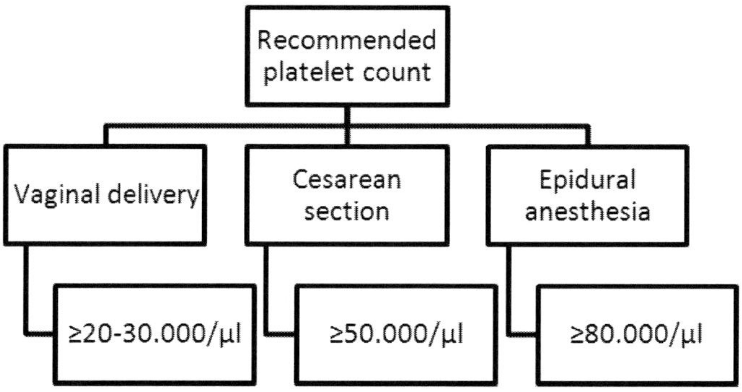

Figure 2. Recommended platelets counts during pregnancy for different procedures.

We must avoid: instrumental delivery (forceps, vacuum), fetal scalp electrode/samples and percutaneous blood sampling (PUBS).

PUBS and fetal scalp blood sampling is not helpful in predicting neonatal thrombocytopenia and present a potential hemorrhagic risk to the fetus, thus these procedures are not recomended.

- *Neonate:* a history of thrombocytopenia in a previous affected sibling appears to be the best predictor of thrombocytopenia in the neonate, only in this case the cesarean section may be more prudent than vaginal delivery.

However fetal platelet count does not correlate with:

- Maternal platelets count.
- Maternal antibodies count.
- Maternal response to treatment.
- History of splenectomy.
- Previous history of PTI or gestational debut.

- Neonatal risks: 10% of newborns of mothers with ITP have platelet counts <50 $x10^9$/L. and platelet count <20 $x10^9$/l occurs in only 5% of cases.

Mortality is rare (<1%) and the incidence of intracranial hemorrhage in the neonate is 0-1.5%. Most hemorrhagic events in neonates occur between day 2 and 5 after delivery at the nadir of the platelet count.

Neonatal ITP accounts for only 3% of all cases of thrombocytopenia at delivery, the most frequent cause of neonatal thrombocytopenia is neonatal alloimmune thrombocytopenia.

- Puerperium

Women with ITP should not be discouraged from breastfeeding.

Women with ITP are at an increasing risk of venous thromboembolism, for that thromboprophylaxis in the postpartum should be considered.

1.5. Differential Diagnosis

Table 2. Differential diagnosis of gestational thrombocytopenia versus ITP

	GESTATIONAL THROMBOCYTOPENIA	INMUNE THROMBOCYTOPENIA
Onset during the pregnancy	Mild-late of second trimester and third trimester	Anytime
Platelet count, x 10^9/L	>70	<70
Thrombocytopenia outside pregnancy	NO	POSSIBLE
Treatment	NO	YES
Neonatal thrombocytopenia	NO	POSSIBLE
Postpartum resolution	YES	POSSIBLE

2. Anemia

2.1. Introduction

Anemia in pregnancy is defined, by the Centers for Disease Control and Prevention, as hemoglobin and hematocrit lower than 11g/dl and 33% in the first trimester, 10,5g/dl and 32% in the second trimester, and 11g/d1 and 33% in the third trimester.

During pregnancy there are different changes to prepare for the blood loss that occurs at delivery. Blood volume increases nearly about 50%, which occurs from an expansion of plasma volume and red cell mass. The plasma volume increases more and more quickly than red cell mass, and that explains the physiologic anemia during the pregnancy.

Table 3. Types of hemoglobin

Types of hemoglobin	Polypeptide chains	Time
Hb Gower	$\zeta_2\varepsilon_2$	Embryonic period
Hb Fetal	$\alpha_2\gamma_2$	>12 weeks of gestation
Hb A	$\alpha_2\beta_2$	Adult
Hb A2	$\alpha_2\delta_2$	Adult (less than 3.5%)

This disproportionate increase is greater during the second trimester, because the plasma volume increase between the 6 and the 32 weeks of gestation, and the red cell mass increase is greater during the last month.

A hemoglobin molecule consists of a central non-protein heme group with four globin protein chains. The structure for these protein chains varies from the embryonic to the adult.

2.2. Classification

Anemia may be classified by the underlying causative mechanism, by whether they are acquired or inherited, by clinical presentation (acute versus chronic), but red cell morphology classification is the most widely used. Mean corpuscular volume (MCV) is used to differentiate these anemias. In this classification anemias are divided into: macrocytic (MCV >100fL), normocytic (MCV: 80-100 fL) and microcytic MCV (<80fL).

2.2.1. Macrocytic Anemia

Macrocytic anemia can be divided by non megaloblastic, which includes aplastic anemia, hypothyroidism, alcoholism, liver disease, splenectomy, and megaloblastic which includes folate and vitamin B12 deficiency and pernicious anemia.

Megaloblastic anemia is the second most common nutritional anemia during pregnancy, after iron deficiency anemia.

Folate deficiency is more frequent than deficiency of cyanocobalamin (Vitamin B12).

- Folate deficiency: this anemia is more frequent in women with diets lacking fresh vegetables, legumes or animal proteins. Also this anemia is more frequent if the woman is taking folate antagonists such as sulfasalazine or anticonvulsive drugs.

These women may have white blood cells and platelet counts decreased.
Pregnancy causes a 10-20-fold increase in folic acid requirements (from 50μg to 400μg)
The treatment recommended is 1 mg oral folate daily.

- Vitamin B12 deficiency: the most common causes of this anemia are pernicious anemia, total o partial gastric resection or malabsorption syndrome (for example after the surgery for Crohn´s disease). Treatment is 1 mg intramuscular every day for a weak, followed by once a week for one month and then once a month.

These women may present neurologic defects from damage to the posterior columns of spinal cord.

2.2.2. Normocytic Anemia: some causes of this type of anemia are: spherocytosis, anemia of chronic disease, autoimmune hemolytic anemia…

2.2.3. Microcytic Anemia: the most common causes or this anemia are the iron deficiency anemia and the hemoglobinopathies (sickle cell disease and thalassemia).

2.3. Iron deficiency anemia

2.3.1. Introduction

Iron deficiency anemia accounts for 75% of all anemias in pregnancy.

2.3.2. Risk Factors

- Diet poor in iron-rich foods such as liver, beef, lentils, beans…
- Short interpregnancy interval.
- Gastrointestinal disease affecting absorption.
- Diet poor in iron absorption enhancers such as lemon or orange juice.

Table 4. Differential diagnosis between iron deficiency anemia and thalassemia minor with laboratory tests

Laboratory	Iron defiency	Thalassemia minor
MVC	Decreased	Decreased
Iron level	Decreased	Normal
Ferritin	Decreased	Normal
Total iron-binding capacity (Transferrin)	Increased	Normal
Transferrin saturation	Decreased	Normal
Hemoglobin	Normal	Abnormal

2.3.3. Laboratory Test and Differential Diagnosis

- The first index to become uncommon is MCV, but this has the problem that may be normal when the stores become depleted.
- Ferritin level provides the most useful and easily available parameter for assessing iron deficiency.

Table 5. Normal values of the parameters ferrous

Laboratory Test	Normal Value
Plasma iron level	40-175μg/dl
Plasma total iron-binding capacity	216-400 μg/dl
Transferrin saturation	16-60%
Ferritin	<10 μg/dl

2.3.4. Clinical Effects

- Fetal: iron deficiency is associated with preterm delivery and low birthweight.
- Maternal: iron deficiency increases the risk of maternal infections and has been associated with postpartum depression and poor work capacity.

2.3.5. Prevention

- Women may be iron deficient despite having a normal MCV and hemoglobin level.
- In women at risk of iron depletion although they have normal hemoglobin level, serum ferritin should be checked. If the ferritin is <30μg/l, 65 mg elemental iron daily should be offered.
- Indications for assessment of serum ferritin are: hemoglobinopathy, previous anemia, multiparity (≥3), short interpregnancy interval (<1 year), vegetarians, teenagers, Jehovah´s witnesses and recent history of bleeding.
- Hb and serum ferritin is required after 8 weeks of treatment to confirm response.

2.3.6. Treatment

- In general, women should be given 100 mg elemental iron daily if hemoglobin is greater than 9 mg/dl and 200 mg if it is less.

- Ferrous iron salts are the preparation of choice, which should be on an empty stomach, 1 hour before meals, with ascorbic acid. Other medications should not be taken at the same moment.
- Hb is required after 2 weeks of treatment to confirm diagnosis and response to treatment.
- Side effects of oral iron include nausea, diarrhea, vomiting and constipation.
- The incidence of side effects is directly related to the dose of iron taken.
- In these patients with important side effects, parenteral therapy with intravenous iron sucrose is an alternative.

2.4. Sickle-Cell Disease

2.4.1. Introduction

- Sickle-cell disease (SCD) is the most frequently inherited blood disorder. And SCD is a group of inherited single-gene autosomal recessive disorders cause by the "sickle gene" that results in the production of the abnormal hemoglobin S.
- It´s estimated that there are 100-200 pregnancies in women with SCD each year in the UK.

2.4.2. Classification

The term SCD include:

- Sickle cell anemia (SCA): includes homozygous sickle cell anemia (Hb SS), the most common and severe of the sickle hemoglobinopathies, and the heterozygous conditions of hemoglobin S and other hemoglobinopathies, for example the combination with Hb C, D, E or β-thalassemia.
- Sickle trait (ST): is the combination of Hb S with the normal hemoglobin (Hb A). ST is asymptomatic, except for a possible increased risk of hematuria and urinary tract infecctions.

2.4.3. Pathogenesis

- Hb S is a variant of the β-chain of hemoglobin where glutamic acid is replaced by valine at the sixth position from the N terminus. Hb S will form polymers in low-oxygen conditions, which leads to the formation of rigid and fragile red cell.
- These cells have a greatly reduced life span and this causes hemolytic anemia and vaso-occlusions in the small blood vessels.

2.4.4. Clinic

All patients with SCA have hemolytic anemia and hyposplenism.

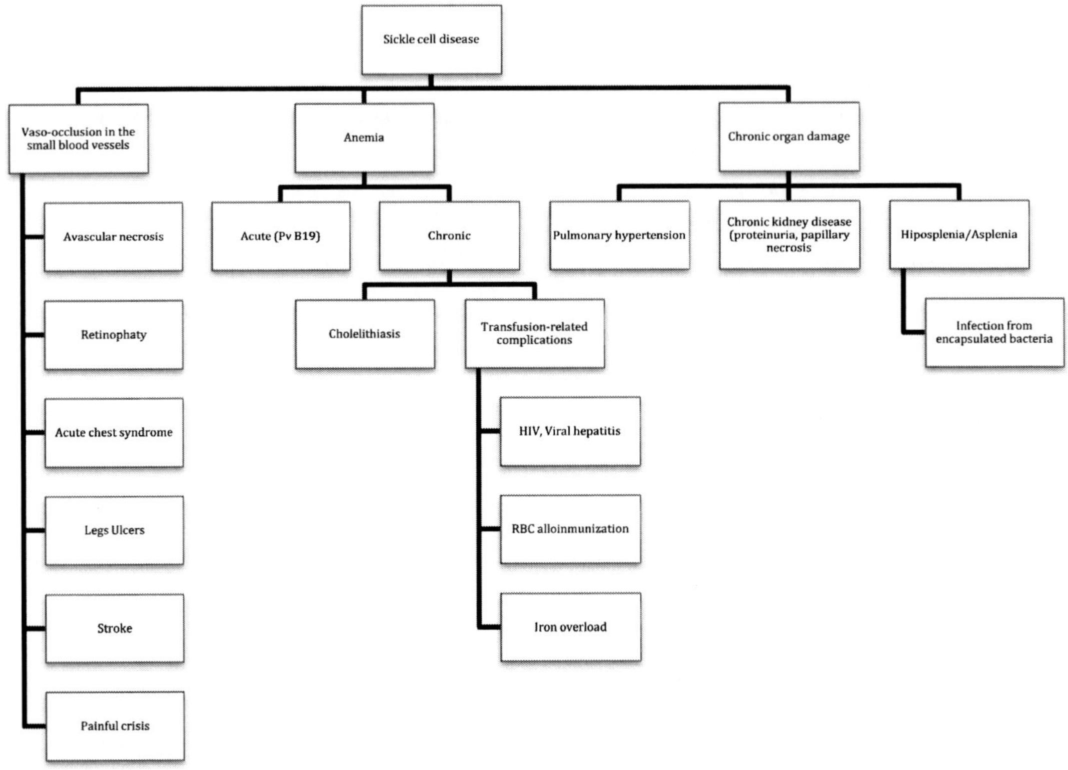

Figure 3. Clinic of sickle cell disease.

2.4.5. Preconception Care

All patients should take 5 mgrams folic acid daily for one month before conception and throughout pregnancy.

- Drugs:

Hydroxiurea is used in SCD to decrease the incidence of acute chest syndrome and acute painful crisis, but it is teratogenic for that it should be stopped three months before the conception.

Iron chelation agents (for example deferoxamine) should be stopped before the pregnancy.

The use of ACE inhibitors and angiotensin receptor II blockers in patients with proteinuria should be stopped before pregnancy.

Nom-steroidal anti-inflammatory are not recommended before 12 weeks and after 28 weeks.

Women with SCA are hyposplenic and have more risk of infection from encapsulated bacteria, for that they have to receive daily penicillin prophylaxis.

- Vaccines:

Hepatitis B vaccination is recommended.

The influenza vaccine should be recommended if it has not been administered in the previous year.

Pneumococcal C vaccine should be given to all patients with SCD every 5 years.

- Genetic counseling

Partners of women with SCD disease or trait should be screened prior to pregnancy in order to give couples an accurate estimate of the risk of having an affected baby. The risk of the child having Hb SS is 50% is the partner is sickle cell trait.

2.4.6. Antepartum Care

- Patients should have a review in a specialist clinic annually.
- Patients with SCA may have renal damage, thus blood pressure, urinalysis should be perform at each visit.
- Proliferative retinopathy is more common in women with SCA. Before pregnancy, retinal screening should be performed.
- In patients con SCA is more usually pulmonary hypertension (PH) and it is associated with increased mortality. All women with SCA should have echocardiography performed in the last year before pregnancy.
- In women who have been multiply transfused in the past is very important to assets the iron overload and screens of red cell antibodies.
- SCD is associated with an increased incidence of maternal and fetal complications:

Table 6. Maternal and fetal complications in SCD

Maternal complications	Fetal complications
Painful crises	Spontaneous miscarriage
Pre-eclampsia	Premature labour
Infections (urinary, pneumonia)	Fetal growth restriction
Thromboembolic events	Perinatal mortality
Cesarean section	
Antepartum hemorrhage	
Postpartum infection	
Maternal mortality (2.5%)	

- Acute pain episodes are the most frequent complication seen during the pregnancy in women with SCD If possible, precipitating factors such as dehydration, infections, stress and cold, should be avoided.
- A fetal monitor will be held a week from the week 38.

2.4.7. Treatment During Pregnancy

- Low dose of aspirin take from 12 weeks can decrease the risk of preeclampsia.
- Iron supplementation should not be given routinely to women with SCD, only if there is a laboratory evidence of iron deficiency.

- There is evidence from observational studies that the risk of venous thromboembolism is increased in women with SCD. For that them should be advised to receive prophylactic low-molecular-weight heparin during hospital admissions.

2.4.8. Intrapartum Care

- It is important to reduce the risk of vaso-occlusive crisis maintain good hydration, good control pain and good oxygen saturation, oxygen should be given if the oxygen saturation is less than 94-95%. But there is not evidence that the use prophylactic of antibiotics decrease the complications.
- It is recommended the continuous fetal monitoring during labour.
- Delivery is recommended between 38-40 weeks.
- The indication for cesarean should be based on obstetrical indications.

2.4.9. Postpartum-Care

Breast-feeding should be encouraged but hydroxiurea is transferred into breast-milk for that this drug is contraindicated.

An increased risk for thrombosis has been found in SCA, for that reason low-molecular-weight heparin should be administered.

2.5. Thalassemia

Thalassemia is a group of autosomal recessive disorders that are characterized by a reduced synthesis of globin chains that cause microcytic anemia.

Thalassemia is the most common monogenetic disease in the world.

Screening for thalassemia carriers is effective and simple with mean corpuscular hemoglobin (MCH less than 27 pg) and mean corpuscular volume (MCV less than 81 fL). Often this patient haven´t anemia and have a normal MCHC (as a distinct form iron deficiency when all indices are reduced)

The diagnosis is confirmed by globin chain synthesis studies, DNA analysis or in the case of β-thalassemia, raised concentrations of Hb F and Hb A2 (more than 3.5%).

Thalassemias are classified according to the globin chain affected, α-thalassemia in which one to four of the α-genes are deleted and β-thalassemia, where one or two of the β-globin genes are defective.

2.5.1. Alpha-Thalassemia

The alpha globin chain synthesis is determined by two genetic loci of each chromosome 16, thus four alleles in total.

The greater number of affected allele, the more severe the clinical manifestations of the disease.

When only one allele is affected there are not clinical symptoms and laboratory tests are normal.

Deletion of two α-globin genes causes α-thalassemia trait with a mild microcytic hypochromic anemia. These patients are at an increased risk for having a child with a more severe form of thalassemia.

When three alleles are affected the production of alpha globin chain is significantly reduced, and the beta chains form the hemoglobin H (β4), which is usually associated with mild to moderate hemolytic anemia.

When all alleles are affected, α-thalassemia major, there in not alpha globin chain, and the gamma chains for the hemoglobin Bart, this is associated with anemia and hydrops fetalis, cardiomegaly, thickened placenta, preeclampsia and are not compatible with life.

2.5.2. Beta-Thalassemia

Beta-thalassemia (βT) is accused by a mutation in the β-globin gene in the chromosome 11[0,0]that causes deficient or absent β-chain which produces absence of Hb A.

- Classification:

    - Minor (carrier or trait) or heterozygous state: causes mild to moderate microcytic anemia. Mean corpuscular volume and mean corpuscular hemoglobin are low and Hb A2 is increased (≥3.5%).
    - Major or homozygous thalassemia or Cooley´s anemia: is characterized by severe transfusion-dependent anemia with extramedullary erythropoiesis, delayed sexual development and short stature with bone deformation.

In these women, chronic hypertransfusion leads to iron overload, transmission of infections (HIV, hepatitis B and C) and risk of alloimmunization.

Iron overload may produce endocrinopathies (hypogonadotropic hypogonadism, diabetes, osteoporosis, hypothyroidism and hypoparathyroidism), cardiomyopathy and hepatic dysfunction.

Pregnancy is very rare in these women but now is more likely because actually there is more adequate iron chelation therapy.

- B-thalassemia intermedia: sometimes the mutations causing moderate impairment of beta chains productions. These women present later and moderate anemia and only require blood transfusions in some situations.

- Preconception care:

In the women who intended to conceived is very important:

- Perform an echocardiography, an electrocardiogram and a T2 cardiac MRI.
- FerriScan or Liver T2 to know the liver iron concentration.
- Gall bladder and liver ultrasound to detect cirrhosis, cholelithiasis…
- Screening for viral infections.
- Optimization of diabetic control.
- Thyroid function.
- Determining red cell antibodies.
- Know group genotype of partner.
- Bone density scan.

– Medications:

  - Iron chelators: deferasirox and deferiprone should be discontinued three months before conception, the women can use deferoxamine.
  - Bisphosphonates should be discontinued three months before pregnancy.
  - We have to change the oral hypoglycemic agent by insulin.
  - Preconceptional folic acid supplementation (5 mg) for three months before pregnancy is indicated.
  - All women have to maintain normal vitamin D levels, for that some women have to take calcio and vitamin D.

- Antepartum care:

During pregnancy, hemoglobin levels should be maintained at or near 10 g/dl with regular transfusions.

Women with betathalassemia have a higher risk of hypertension, preeclampsia and abruption placentae.

Fetal growth should be monitored with serial fetal ultrasound every four weeks from 24 weeks of gestations, because maternal anemia predisposes to intrauterine growth restriction.

Deferoxamine should be avoided in the first trimester, but it has been used safely in the second and third trimester.

Aggressive iron chelation before pregnancy can reduces the complications related to iron overload, for example endocrinopathies and/or cardiomyopathy.

- Intrapartum care.

Active management of the third stage is recommended to minimize blood loss.

Cesarean section should be performed only for obstetric indications.

- Postpartum care:

An increased risk for thrombosis has been found in women with alpha-thalassemia, beta-thalassemia major and intermedia for that thromboprophylaxis should be considered in the postpartum period.

Breast-feeding is recommended. Deferoxamine is secreted in breast milk, however is not orally absorbed, for that is safe to the newborn.

References

Adams TM, Allaf MB, Vintzileos Am. Maternal thrombocytopenia in pregnancy: diagnosis and management. *Clin. Lab. Med.* 2013;33(2):327- 41.

American College of Obstetricians and Gynecologists. Anemia in pregnancy. ACOG Practice Bulletin No. 95 *Obstet. Gynecol.* 2008;112(1):201-7.

American College of Obstetricians and Gynecologists. Hemoglobinopathies in pregnancy. ACOG practice Bulletin No.78. *Obstet. Gynecol.* 2007;109:229-37.

Andemariam B, Browning SL. Current management of sickle cell disease in pregnancy. *Clin. Lab. Med.* 2013;33(2):293-310.

Bashiri A, Burstein E, Sheiner E, Mazor M. Anemia during pregnancy and treatment with intravenous iron: review of the literature. *Eur. J. Obstet. Gynecol. Reprod Biol* 2003;110(1):2-7.

Boeckenstedt PL. Thrombocytopenia in pregnancy. *Hematol. Oncol. Clin. North Am.* 2011;25(2):293-310.

Cooper N. Intravenous inmunoglobulin and anti-RhD therapy in the management of immune thrombocytopenia. *Hematol Oncol. Cli. North Am.* 2009;23(6):1317-27.

Corwin EJ, Murray-Kolb LE, Beard JL. Low hemoglobin level is a risk factor for postpartum depression. *J. Nutr.* 2003;133(12):4139-42.

Cuker A, Cines DB. Inmune thrombocytopenia. *Hematology Am. Soc. Hematol. Educ. Program.* 2010:377-84.

Ekiz C, Agaoglu L, Karakas Z, Gurel N, Yalcin I. The effect of iron deficiency anemia on the function of the immune system. *Hematol. J.* 2005;5:579-83.

Gernsheimer T, James AH, Stair R. How I treat trombocitopenia in pregnancy. *Blood.* 2013;121(1):38-47.

Gernsheimer T, McCrae K. Inmune trombocytopenic purpura in pregnancy. *Curr. Opin Hematol.* 2007;14:574-580.

Gernsheimer T. Thrombocytopenia in pregnancy: is this inmune thrombocytopenia or…?

Gladwin MT, Sachdev V, Jison ML, Shizukuda Y, Plehn JF, Minter K, et al. Pulmonary hypertension as a risk factor for death in patients with sickle cell disease. *N. Engl. J. Med.* 2004;350:886-95.

Haas JD, Brownlie T. Iron deficiency and reduced work capacity: a critical review of the research to determine a causal relationship. *J. Nutr.* 2001 Feb;131(2S-2):676S-688S.

Hematology *Am. Soc. Hematol. Educ. Program.* 2012:198-202.

Horowitz KM, Ingardia CJ, Borgida AF. Anemia in pregnancy. *Clin. Lab. Med.* 2013;33(2):281-91.

Howard J, Oteng-Ntim E. The obstetric management of sickle cell disease. *Best Pract Res. Clin. Obstet. Gynaecol.* 2012;26(1):25-36.

Kawaguchi K, Matsubara K, Takafuta T, Shinzato I, Tanaka Y, Iwata A, et al. Factors predictive of neonatal thrombocytopenia in pregnant women with immune thrombocytopenia. *Int. J. Hematol.* 2014;99(5):570-6.

Koh MB, Lao ZT, Rhodes E. Managing haematological disorders during pregnancy. *Best Pract. Res. Clin. Obstet. Gynaecol.* 2013;27(6):855-65.

Leung KY, Cheong KB, Lee CP, Chan V, Lam YH, Tang M. Ultrasonographic prediction of homozygous alpha0-thalassemia using placental thickness, fetal cardiothoracic ratio and middle cerebral artery Doppler: alone or in combination? *Ultrasound Obstet. Gynecol..* 2010;35(2):149-54.

Leung TN, Lau TK, Chung TK. Thalassaemia screening in pregnancy. *Curr. Opin Obstet. Gynecol..* 2005;17(2):129-34.

Leung TY, Lao TT. Thalassaemia in pregnancy. *Best Pract Res. Clin. Obstet Gynaecol.* 2012;26(1):37-51.

Modell B, Khan M, Darlison M. Survival in β-thalassaemia major in the UK: data from the UK Thalassemia Register. *Lancet*2000;355:2051-52.

Naik RP, Lanzkron S. Baby on board: what you need to know about pregnancy in the hemoglobinopathies. *Hematology Am. Soc. Hematol. Educ. Program.* 2012;2012:208-14.

Nicolescu A, Vladareanu AM, Voican I, Onisai M, Vladareanu R. Therapeutic options for immune thrombocytopenia (ITP) during pregnancy. *Maedica* 2013;8(2):182-188.

Pavord S, Myers B, Robinson S, Allard S, Strong J, Oppenheimer C UK guidelines on the management of iron deficiency in pregnancy. *Br. J. Haematol.* 2012;156(5):588-600.

Polifka JE, Friedman JM. Teratogen uptodate: azathioprine and 6-mercaptopurine. *Teratology* 2002;65:240-61.

Provan D, Stasi R, Newland AC, Blanchette VS, Bolton-Maggs P, Bussel JB, et al. International consensus report on the investigation and management of primary immune thrombocytopenia. *Blood.* 2010;115(2):168-86.

Rajasekhar A, Gersnsheimer T, Stasi R, James AH. Clinical Practice Guide on thrombocytopenia in pregnancy. American Society of Hematology.2013.

Rasmussen K. Is There a Causal Relationship between Iron Deficiency or Iron-Deficiency Anemia and Weight at Birth, Length of Gestation and Perinatal Mortality? *J. Nutr.* 2001;131(2S-2):590S-601S.

Recommendations to prevent and control iron deficiency in the United States. Centers for Disease Control and Prevention. *MMWR Recomm Rep.* 1998 Apr 3;47(RR-3):1-29.

Royal College of Obstetricians and Gynaecologists. Management of sickle cell disease in pregnancy. RCOG Grenn—top guideline 61. London:RCOG; 2011.

Royal College of Obstetricians and Gynaecologists. Management of Beta Thalassaemia in Pregnancy. RCOG Grenn—top guideline 66. London:RCOG; 2014.

Ryan K, Bain BJ, Worthington D, James J, Plews D, Mason A, et al.. Significant haemoglobinopathies: guidelines for screening and diagnosis. *Br. J. Haematol.* 2010;149(1):35-49.

Sankaran S, Robinson S. Inmune trombocitopenia and pregnancy. *Obstet Med.* 2011;4:140-6.

Sieunarine K, Shapiro S, Al Obaidi M, et AL. Intravenous anti-D immunoglobulin in the treatment of resistant immune thrombocytopenic purpura during pregnancy. *BJOG* 2007;114(4):505-7.

Singer ST, Vichinsky EP. Deferoxamine treatment during pregnancy: is it harmful? *Am. J. Hematol.* 1999 ;60(1):24-6.

Stavrou E, McCrae K. Inmune thrombocytopenia in pregnancy. *Hematol. Oncol. North Am.* 2009;23(6):1299-1316.

Surbek DV, Glanzmann R, Nars PW, Holzgreve W. Pregnancy and lactation in homozygous beta-thalassemia major. *J. Perinat. Med.* 1998;26(3):240-3.

Vichinsky EP. Alpha thalassemia major--new mutations, intrauterine management, and outcomes. *Hematology Am. Soc. Hematol. Educ.* Program. 2009:35-41.

In: Handbook for High Risk Pregnancy: Clinical Management ISBN: 978-1-63482-299-2
Editors: E. González-Mesa and D. Abehsera

Chapter 15

RESPIRATORY DISEASE: ASTHMA, PNEUMONIA AND BRONCHIECTASIS

Ignacio Brunel[1], Estefanía Moreno[2], Antonio Piñera[2] and Daniel Abehsera[3,*]

[1]Obstetrics and Gynecology Department, QuirónUniversity Hospital Madrid, Spain
[2]Obstetrics and Gynecology Department, La Paz University Hospital, Madrid, Spain
[3]Obstetrics and Gynecology Department, QuirónUniversity Hospital, Málaga, Spain

1. INTRODUCTION

Pregnancy involves several changes in the pregnant's cardio respiratory system that lead to changes in the clinical expression as well as in proper therapeutic approach of each respiratory disease.

Overall, these changes involve a decrease in the respiratory reserve, which normally doesn't involve any pathological implication, but might be crucial in patients with previous respiratory diseases or if a new one is developed during pregnancy.

Respiratory diseases are an important cause of maternal morbidity and mortality, so it is essential to know their proper management during pregnancy for the best maternal and fetal prognosis to be granted.

2. PHYSIOLOGICAL CHANGES IN THE RESPIRATORY SYSTEM DURING PREGNANCY

Upper respiratory airways undergo an increase in vascularization secondary to increased plasma volume. This makes the mucosa more hyperemic, edematous and friable. That explains why rhinitis, nasal congestion and epistaxis are frequently found in pregnant women.

* Corresponding author: danielabehsera@hotmail.com.

The thorax diameter is increased by 5 to 7 cm while the diaphragm goes 4 cm up from its normal position.

These anatomical changes will lead to a decrease in both the volume and the residual capacity. These changes are more pronounced at the end of the pregnancy and in supine position. However, the increase in the diameter of the thorax will allow the vital capacity to remain stable throughout pregnancy, while only total lung capacity will decrease. (Figure 1)

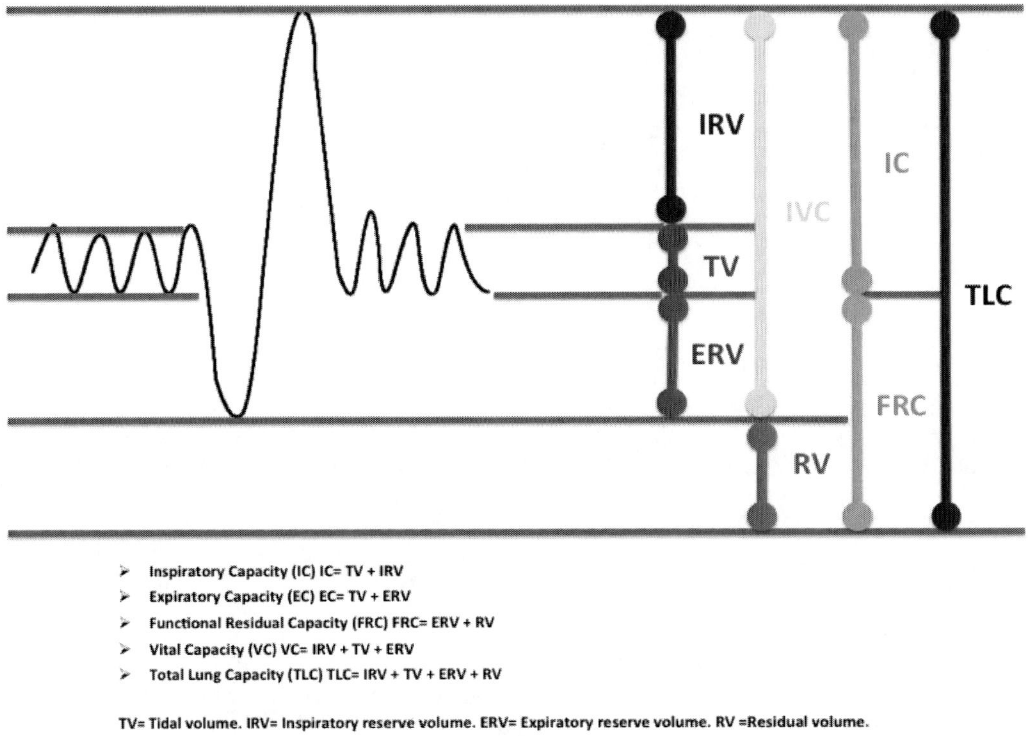

Figure 1. Lung capacity during pregnancy.

The tidal volume increases about 40%, causing an increase in minute volume. The respiratory rate remains stable until the last trimester, when it can slight increase.

This increase in ventilation causes a decrease in arterial carbon dioxide tension (PaCO2), which normal values in the pregnant women is around 30mmHg, producing respiratory alkalosis compensated with an increase in renal bicarbonate excretion.

In addition there is also an increase in arterial oxygen tension (PaO2), which is around 100-105 mmHg, probably due to an increase in cardiac output leading to an improvement in the ventilation/perfusion rate. Through these changes the increase in oxygen needs can be covered. This increase, which is around 20%, is mainly due to de needs of the fetus and the placenta, but also related with an increase in maternal renal metabolism. However, hypoxemia may occur mainly related to supine position which causes a decrease in residual capacity.

At last, there are no changes in respiratory flows, so spirometrycal parameters are mostly the same among pregnant and non-pregnant women.

3. Asthma and Pregnancy

Asthma is a chronic respiratory disease characterized by an hyper-responsiveness of the respiratory airway causing reversible bronchial bronchoconstriction, generally triggered by different stimuli like cold, exercise or allergens.

Asthma is thought to affect about 3-8% of all pregnant women (Murphy, Gibson, Smith, & Clifton, 2005), although a prevalence as high as 13% has been published, (Kurincsuk, Parsons, Dawes V., & Burton, 1999). This makes it the most frecuent respiratory disease among pregnant women.

3.1. Effects of Pregnancy on Asthma

The severity of asthma during pregnancy varies from one woman to another, so it is difficult to predict the course that asthma will follow. During pregnancy, asthma can worsen, improve or remain stable with the same probability.

Nevertheless, some patterns have been observed.

Among women whose asthma worsens, the increase in symptoms is often seen between weeks 29 and 36 of pregnancy, while symptoms are generally less severe during the last 4 weeks of pregnancy. This improvement might be due to the rise of endogenous cortisol that occurs at the end of gestation (Powrie R. O., 2010).

On the other hand, among women whose asthma improves, the improvement typically progresses gradually throughout pregnancy (Schatz M., 1988).

In both cases the severity of asthma symptoms during the first pregnancy is often similar in subsequent pregnancies (Schatz M., 1988).

Asthma attacks occur in 20 to 36% of pregnant women with this disease. Attacks seem to be most likely during second trimester of gestation. This may happen because some women stop using asthma-controlling drugs when they realize they are pregnant, increasing their risk for attacks. Attacks are uncommon during labor and delivery, probably due to the rise of endogenous cortisol that occurs at the end of gestation, as mentioned before.

3.2. Effects of Asthma on Pregnancy

Asthma can negatively alter the normal development of the pregnancy, affecting the placenta, the mother or the fetus, although the reasons for this are still unknown.

The fetus presents a physiological state of hypoxemia, which is compensated by fetal haemoglobin and changes in the oxyhemoglobin dissociation curve.

However, maternal hypoxemia can produce an impact in the fetus by reducing the fetal oxygen supply. Even so, the fetus can activate compensating mechanisms to ensure an appropriated irrigation of vital organs, although this might affect fetal growth.

Polymorphisms in the beta2 adrenergic receptor have been proposed as an explanation for the link between asthma and preterm delivery, although the clinical relevance of these polymorphisms remains unclear.

In addition, several drugs used for asthma treatment may have adverse fetal effects, which will be discussed later on this chapter.

3.3. Complications during Pregnancy

Many studies have been published on the increase in maternal and fetal complications like abortion, perinatal mortality, preeclampsia, prematurity or low birth weight, presenting very heterogeneous data

A recent meta-analysis, analyzing maternal and fetal complications has found an increase in the risk of gestational diabetes (RR = 1.39, 95% CI = [1.17-1.66]), caesarean section (RR = 1.31, 95% CI = [1.22-1.39]), pre and postpartum hemorrhage (antepartum: RR = 1.25, 95% CI = [1.10-1.42]; postpartum: RR = 1.29, 95% CI = [1.18-1.41]), Placenta praevia (RR = 1.23, 95% CI = [1.07-1.40]) Placental abruption (RR = 1.29, 95% CI = [1.14-1.47]) and premature rupture of membranes (RR = 1.21, 95% CI = 1.07-1.37), being caesarean section and gestational diabetes far more frequent in moderate to severe than in mild asthma. (Wang et al., 2014).

A different meta-analysis found an increase in fetal malformations among patients with asthma that were not being treated (RR = 1.11, 95% CI = 1.02-1.21), although the level of evidence was not very strong since data was retrospectively analysed (Murphy V. E., 2013).

Other studies have found an increased rate of preeclampsia, perinatal mortality, preterm delivery and low birth weight, being all of them more frequent in severe asthma.

Although the results of the different studies are not completely homogeneous, a general increase in the risk of maternal and fetal complications can be clearly observed in patients with asthma, being this increase higher in patients with severe asthma.

The clinical relevance of an appropriated asthma treatment during pregnancy is still unclear, although it is very likely that the risk of maternal and fetal complications can be lowered.

3.4. Therapeutic Management

In the first place, therapeutic management must focus on controlling external factors like allergens exposure and giving up smoking.

The use of drugs against asthma during pregnancy is controversial because there are some studies that suggest different levels of teratogenicity. This makes difficult to reach an agreement on the best therapeutic option. It is necessary to evaluate the maternal and fetal risk of each patient, regarding the severity of the symptoms and the improvement that each drug may produce, in order to choose the less teratogenic drug at the lower possible dose for controlling the symptoms.

The most commonly used drugs during pregnancy are albuterol, metaproterenol, teophyline, cromolyn sodium, beclomethasone and budesonide, due to their lower fetal effects (National Heart, Lung, and Blood Institute; National Asthma Education and Prevention Program Asthma and Pregnancy Working, 2008).

3.4.1. Inhaled Beta-adrenergic Agonists

Short-acting beta2-adrenergic agonists, especially albuterol for being the oldest one, are in general considered to be safe to use during pregnancy. (National Heart, Lung, and Blood Institute; National Asthma Education and Prevention Program Asthma and Pregnancy Working, 2008) However, some recent studies in humans have shown an increase in cardiac defects, orofacial clefts and anal atresia (Källén & Otterblad Olausson, 2007).

There is not so much data about long-acting beta2-adrenergic agents in terms of fetal damage as they are relatively new drugs. However, no adverse fetal effects have been shown until now (Schatz & Dombrowski, Clinical practice. Asthma in pregnancy., 2009).

Perinatal outcomes do not seem to be modified by the use of beta2-adrnergic agonists during pregnancy (Schatz et al., 2004).

3.4.2. Oral Glucocorticoids

Oral glucocorticoids have been linked with several fetal malformations and adverse perinatal outcomes.

Specially during the first trimester, oral glucocorticoids are linked with cleft lip with or without cleft palate, although this increased risk is not very high (0,1% in general population versus 0,3% in patients treated whit oral glucocorticoids) (Park-Wyllei, et al., 2000).

Focusing on perinatal outcomes, oral glucocorticoids may be responsible for an increased risk of preterm delivery, low birth weight and preeclampsia.

However, this data should be considered carefully since the dose and duration of treatment are highly variable. In addition the effects of the drugs may be difficult to differentiate from the effects of the illness itself.

3.4.3. Inhaled Glucocorticoids

Budesonide is considered to be a safe drug to use during pregnancy. No teratogenicity or adverse perinatal outcomes has been shown (National Heart, Lung, and Blood Institute; National Asthma Education and Prevention Program Asthma and Pregnancy Working, 2008).

3.4.4. Leukotriene Receptor Antagonists

Montelukast and zaferlukast haven't shown an increase in major fetal malformations. However available studies have a sample size too small to detect rare malformations.

3.4.5. Other Agents

Other drugs are anticholinergic agents, methylxanthines and cromoglycates.

Among anticholinergic agents, inhaled ipratropium is the most studied one. It seems to be a safe drug to use during pregnancy, although it has a chronotropic effect over the fetal heart, it is unlikely to have any impact when taken by inhalation (National Heart, Lung, and Blood Institute; National Asthma Education and Prevention Program Asthma and Pregnancy Working, 2008).

Methylxanthines do not seem to have any teratogenic effects. However, due to their metabolism during pregnancy their blood level must be monitored, so they are not so useful.

There is very limited data available about the use of cromoglycates during pregnancy, although no increased risk of malformations has been shown (National Heart, Lung, and

Blood Institute; National Asthma Education and Prevention Program Asthma and Pregnancy Working, 2008).

3.5. Use of Prostaglandins

The use of prostaglandins for labor induction and for uterine atony has been classically contraindicated among asthma patients due to the risk of triggering bronchoconstriction (Kawikova, Barnes, Takahashi, Tadjkarimi, Yacoub, & Belvisi, 1996). However, recent studies show that prostaglandins E2 and E1 are not a cause of bronchoconstriction, so they can be used in asthma patients.

4. Pneumonias and Pregnancy

The incidence of pneumonia during pregnancy is estimated to be around 0.2 to 8.5 per 1000 deliveries (Lim, Macfarlane, & Colthorpe, 2003), similar to the nonpregnant population.

Pneumonias' treatment during pregnancy is quite similar to the standard one, although there are some issues that must be beared in mind.

Pneumonias can have viral or bacterial causes. H1N1 Influenza virus subtype is especially relevant as the cause of a recent outbreak with high maternal and fetal morbimortality.

4.1. Pneumonia: Maternal and Fetal Complications

Pregnancy involves several particular complications related to pneumonia.

In the first place, pregnant women have a higher susceptibility to the infection and an increased severity of the symptoms due to the immunosuppression that takes place during pregnancy (Dennis & Solnordal, 2012).

In addition, due to the physiological changes during pregnancy, the adaptation to acidosis is worse and there is a predisposition to suffer acute pulmonary edema and aspiration pneumonia, as the cardiamuscle tone is diminished (Lim, Macfarlane, & Colthorpe, 2001).

Pregnant patients are more likely to suffer other complications like pleural empyema, atelectasis, pulmonary abscess, parenchymal necrosis, pneumatocele, pneumothorax and bronchopleural fistula (Goodnight & Soper, 2005).

Regarding fetal complications, several studies have reported an increased risk of preterm birth and low birth weight. This may be caused by a decrease in uterine blood flow produced by metabolic alkalosis due to hypoxemia related tachypnea (Bánhidy, Acs, Puhó, & Czeizel, 2008) (Yost, Bloom, Richey, Ramin & Cunningham, 2000).

Consequently, pregnant patients have an increased risk of suffering more severe pneumonias. It is essential to make a correct diagnosis and perform a specific management to ensure maternal and fetalwell-being and reduce adverse perinatal complications.

4.2. Diagnosis

Diagnosis is based on clinical signs and on diagnostic tests.

Typical symptoms include temperature, cough productive of purulent sputum, shivering, dysnea and pleuritic chest pain. However, symptoms may not always be so evident. In addition dysnea is often present in healthy pregnants. This can delay the correct diagnose and increase maternal and fetal complications.

Blood tests and imaging techniques are the most useful diagnostic tests.

Chest x-ray is a fundamental diagnostic test. It is useful for assessing severity, detecting complications, providing hints about etiology and performing differential diagnosis whit other diseases like pulmonary edema or pulmonary metastatic choriocarcinoma. Radiation doses are low and there are no studies showing an increase in fetal malformations (Groen, Bae, & Lim, 2012).

However, there are some issues that must be considered in order to avoid unnecessary risks. Chest x-ray must be avoided during the first trimester, when central nervous system is developing. Fetal protection protocols must be optimized. Initially just the postero-anterior projection may be enough and lateral projection can be avoided. Sonography can replace x-ray for the initial study and monitoring of pleural collections and MRI may be useful for assessing etiological possibilities.

4.3. Treatment

As mentioned before in this chapter, pregnant women are more likely to suffer more severe pneumonia than general population, so it is essential to provide a proper therapeutic management with close vital signs monitoring and eventual ICU admission.

In the first place, an over 95% SpO2 must be granted in order to provide a proper fetal oxygenation. Arterial blood gas must be performed in order to measure PaO2, that must be over 70 mmHg.

Otherwise, it is important to perform daily fluid balance to assess the risk of developing acute pulmonary edema.

Regarding antipyretic treatment, paracetamol is safer than NSAIDs, as this last one may cause perinatal complications in preterm childbirth.

Finally, the best antibiotic treatment must be adjusted depending on whether we are dealing whit community acquired pneumonia, hospital acquired pneumonia or even pneumonia related to bronchoaspiration. The most commonly involved pathogens are Streptococcus pneumoniae, Haemophilus influenzae, Mycoplasma, Chlamydia, Legionella, Staphylococcus aureus and gram negative bacilli (Sheffield & Cunningham, 2009).

Doxyciclina, claritrhomycin and fluorquinolones must be avoided during pregnancy, since they belong to D, C and C FDA categories respectively.

One broadly accepted treatment for community acquired pneumonias is Azitrhomycin due to its good security profile and broad antibiotic spectrum. Other similar and safe drugs are beta-lactams, clindamycin and aminoglycosides.

Regarding hospital acquired pneumonias, drugs effective against Pseudomonas and Staphylococcus aureus Meticylin-resistent must be used.

At last, when brochoaspiration related pneumonia is suspected, effective drugs against gram-negative bacilli must be used.

4.4. Viral Pneumonias

Viral pneumonias are highly relevant during pregnancy due to their important mortality among these patients.

Influenza A virus produced pneumonias have been the cause of several outbreaks along the twentieth and twenty-first centuries. The last one, caused by the H1N1 virus had high mortality rates among general population and even a higher one among pregnant patients, as 5% of the total deaths caused by this virus were pregnant women.

Although all pregnant women present high mortality, the ones with a higher risk are the ones at the third trimester and first month after delivery (Mertz et al., 2013).

Vaccination with inactivated Influenza has shown up to 89% decrease in the odds of being infected among pregnant women (Jefferson, Di Pietrantonj, Rivetti, Bawazeer, Al-Ansary, & Ferroni, 2014).

In addition, early treatment with neuraminidase inhibitors (oseltamivir and zanamivir) has shown a decrease in morbidity and mortality (PRIDE Consortium Investigators, 2014), without increasing the risk of fetal malformations (Saito, Minakami, Nakai, Unno, Kubo, & Yoshimura, 2013), although those drugs belongs to C FDA category.

Another severe viral pneumonia, although much less frequent, is the one produced by Varicella-Zoster virus. 40% mortality has been reported (Duong & Munns, 1979), although more recent studies report much lower mortality rates (Zhang, Patenaude, & Abenhaim, 2014). Vaccination before pregnancy is effective, but it is contraindicated during pregnancy. Regarding treatment, acyclovir improves severity during pregnancy (Noce, Berger, & Pomeranz, 2013) (Daley, Thorpe, & Garland, 2008).

5. Bronchiectasis and Pregnancy

Bronchiectasis is the consequence of several respiratory illnesses that produce inflammation, bronchial hyper-reactivity, bronchial walls thinning and dilatation of the respiratory airway.

The most frequent symptom is chronic cough with mucopurulent sputum production. Etiology includes rheumatic illnesses, pulmonary infections, dyskinetic cilia or cystic fibrosis (McShane, Naureckas, & Strek, 2012).

Regarding diagnosis, chest computed tomography is very useful for detecting respiratory airway dilatations (Barker, 2002).

The behaviour of this illness during pregnancy is quite similar to the one previously described for asthma, as they are obstructive illnesses. However there are not recent and well designed studies on this topic. The ones that can be found are old and mostly based on cases report.

Regarding treatment, it is based on the use of bronchodilator and antibiotics during infectious exacerbations, considering the previously mentioned particularities of these drugs during pregnancy.

References

Bánhidy, F., Acs, N., Puhó, E., & Czeizel, A. (2008). Maternal acute respiratory infectious diseases during pregnancy and birth outcomes. *European journal of epidemiology.,* 23 (1), 29-35.

Bakhireva, L., Jones, K., Schatz, M., Klonoff-Cohen, H., Johnson, D., Slymen, D., et al. (2007). Safety of leukotriene receptor antagonists in pregnancy. *The Journal of allergy and clinical immunology.,* 119 (3), 618-625.

Barker, A. (2002). Bronchiectasis. *New England journal of medicine,* 346 (18), 1383-1393.

Daley, A., Thorpe, S., & Garland, S. (2008). Varicella and the pregnant woman: Prevention and management. *The Australian & New Zealand journal of obstetrics & gynaecology.,* 48 (1), 26-33.

Dennis, A., & Solnordal, C. (2012). Acute pulmonary edema in pregnant women. *Anaesthesia.,* 67 (6), 646-659.

Dombrowski, M., Schatz, M., Wise, R., Thom, E., Landon, M., Mabie, W., et al. (2004). Randomized trial of inhaled beclomethasone dipropionate versus theophylline for moderate asthma during pregnancy. *American journal of obstetrics and gynecology,* 190 (3), 737-744.

Duong, C., & Munns, R. (1979). Varicella pneumonia during pregnancy. *The Journal of family practice,* 8 (2), 277-280.

Goodnight, W., & Soper, D. (2005). Pneumonia in pregnancy. *Critical care medicine,* 33, 390-397.

Groen, R., Bae, J., & Lim, K. (2012). Fear of unknown ionizing radiation exposure during pregnancy. *American journal of obstetrics and gynecology.,* 206 (6), 456-462.

Jefferson, T., Di Pietrantonj, C., Rivetti, A., Bawazeer, G., Al-Ansary, L., & Ferroni, E. (2014). *Vaccines for preventing influenza in helathy adults.* Cochrane Database Systematic Review.

Källén B. R. H. (2000). Asthma during pregnancy: A population based study. *European journal of epidemiology,* 16 (2), 167-171.

Källén, B., & Otterblad Olausson, P. (2007). Use of anti-asthmatic drugs during pregnancy. 3. Congenital malformations in the infants. *European journal of clinical pharmacology.,* 63 (4), 383-388.

Kawikova, I., Barnes, P., Takahashi, T., Tadjkarimi, S., Yacoub, M., & Belvisi, M. (1996). 8-Epi-PGF2 alpha, a novel noncyclooxygenase-derived prostaglandin, constricts airways *in vitro. American journal of respiratory and critical care medicine.,* 153 (2), 590-596.

Kurincsuk, J., Parsons, D., Dawes V., & Burton, P. (1999). The relationship between asthma and smoking during pregnancy. *Women Health,* 29 (3), 31-47.

Laibl, V., & Sheffield, J. (2006). The management of respiratory infections during pregnancy. *Immunology and allergy clinics of North America,* 26 (1), 155-172.

Landau, R., Xie, H., Dishy, V., CM, S., AJ, W., CW, E. et al. (2002). beta2-Adrenergic receptor genotype and preterm delivery. *American journal of obstetrics and gynecology.*, 187 (5), 1294-1298.

Lim, W., Macfarlane, J., & Colthorpe, C. (2001). Pneumonia and pregnancy. *Thorax,* 56 (5), 398-405.

Lim, W., Macfarlane, J., & Colthorpe, C. (2003). Treatment of community-acquired lower respiratory tract infections during pregnancy. *American journal of respiratory medicine: Drugs, devices, and other interventions.*, 2 (3), 221-233.

M, S., RS, Z., KM, H., CP, H., AB, F., LM, C. et al. (1988). The safety of inhaled beta-agonist bronchodilators during pregnancy. *The Journal of allergy and clinical immunology.*, 82 (4), 686-695.

McShane, P., Naureckas, E., & Strek, M. (2012). Bronchiectasis in a diverse US population: Effects of ethnicity on etiology and sputum culture. *Chest,* 142 (1), 159-167.

Mertz, D., Kim, T., Johnstone, J., Lam, P., Science, M., Kuster, S., et al. (2013). Populations at risk for severe or complicated influenza illness: Systematic review and meta-analysis. *British medical journal,* 347, 1094.

Murphy V. E. W. G. (2013). The risk of congenital malformations, perinatal mortality and neonatal hospitalisation among pregnant women with asthma: A systematic review and meta-analysis. *British journal of obstetrics and gynaecology,* 120 (7), 812-822.

Murphy, V., Gibson P, Talbot, P., & Clifton, V. (2005). *Severe asthma exacerbetions during pregnancy.* 106 (5), 1046-1054.

Murphy, V., Gibson, P., Smith, R., & Clifton, V. (2005). Asthma during pregnancy: Mechanism and treatment implications. *European Respiratory Journal,* 25 (4), 731-750.

National Heart, Lung, and Blood Institute; Working, National Asthma Education and Prevention Program Asthma and Pregnancy. (2008). NAEPP expert panel report. Managing asthma during pregnancy: Recommendations for pharmacologic treatment-2004 update. *The Journal of allergy and clinical immunology.*, 115 (1), 34-46.

Noce, N., Berger, E., & Pomeranz, M. (2013). Management and prevention of varicella-zoster virus infection in pregnancy: A case report and review of the literature. *Cutis,* 92 (2), 88-90.

Park-Wyllei, L., Mazzotta, P., Pastuszak, A., Moretti, M., Beique, L., Hunniset, L., et al. (2000). Birth defects after maternal exposure to corticosteroids: Prospective cohort study and meta-analysis of epidemiological studies. *Teratology,* 62 (6), 385-392.

Powrie R. O. G. M. (2010). *de Swiet's Medical Disorders in Obstetric Practice.* Chichester, UK: Wiley-Blackwell.

PRIDE Consortium Investigators. (2014). Effectiveness of neuraminidase inhibitors in reducing mortality in patients admitted to hospital with influenza A H1N1pdm09 virus infection: A meta-analysis of individual participant data. *The Lancet. Respiratory medicine.*, 2 (5), 395-404.

Saito, S., Minakami, H., Nakai, A., Unno, N., Kubo, T., & Yoshimura, Y. (2013). Outcomes of infants exposed to oseltamivir or zanamivir in utero during pandemic (H1N1) 2009. *American journal of obstetrics and gynecology.*, 209 (2), 130.

Sarkar, M., Koren, G., Kalra, S., Ying, A., Smorlesi, C., De Santis, M., et al. (2009). Montelukast use during pregnancy: A multicentre, prospective, comparative study of infant outcomes. *European journal of clinical pharmacology.*, 65 (12), 1259-1264.

Schatz, M., H. K. (1988). The course of asthma during pregnancy, post partum, and with successive pregnancies: A prospective analysis. *The Journal of allergy and clinical immunology*, 509-17.

Schatz, M., & Dombrowski, M. (2009). Clinical practice. Asthma in pregnancy. *The New England journal of medicine.*, 360 (18), 1862-1869.

Schatz, M., Dombrowski, M., Wise, R., Momirova, V., Landon, M., Mabie, W., et al. (2004). *The relationship of asthma medication use to perinatal outcomes.* 113 (6), 1040-1045.

Sheffield, J., & Cunningham, F. (2009). Community-acquired pneumonia in pregnancy. *Obstetrics and gynecology.*, 114 (4), 915-222.

Siston, A., Rasmussen, S., Honein, M., Fry, A., Seib, K., Callaghan, W., et al. (2010). Pandemic 2009 influenza A (H1N1) virus ilness among pregnant woman in the United States. *JAMA: The journal of the American Medical Association.*, 303 (15), 1517-1525.

Tata L. J. L. S. (2007). A comprehensive analysis of adverse obstetric and pediatric complications in women with asthma. *American journal of respiratory and critical care medicine.*, 175 (10), 991-997.

Towers, C., Briggs, G., & Rojas, J. (2004). The use of prostaglandin E2 in pregnant patients with asthma. *American journal of obstetrics and gynecology.*, 190 (6), 1777-1780.

Wang, G., Murphy, V., Namazy, j., Powell, H., Schatz, M., Chambers, C., et al. (2014). The risk of maternal and placental complications in pregnant women with asthma: A systematic review and meta-analysis. *Journal of maternal-fetal and neonatal medicine*, 27 (9), 934-942.

Yost, N., Bloom, S., Richey, S., Ramin, S., & Cunningham, F. (2000). An appraisal of treatment guidelines for antepartum community-acquired pneumonia. *American journal of obstetrics and gynecology.*, 183 (1), 131-135.

Zhang, H., Patenaude, V., & Abenhaim, H. (2014). Maternal outcomes in pregnancies affected by varicella zoster virus infections. *Obstetrics and gynecology.*, 123 (Suppl 1), 86S-87S.

In: Handbook for High Risk Pregnancy: Clinical Management ISBN: 978-1-63482-299-2
Editors: E. González-Mesa and D. Abehsera

Chapter 16

MULTIPLE PREGNANCY

Ana Nieto Moreno**, MD, Yolanda Romero Espinar, MD, and Juan Francisco Gamonal Segura, MD
Obstetrics and Gynecology Department,
Quirón University Hospital, Málaga, Spain

INTRODUCTION

Multiple pregnancies are commonly associated with maternal-fetal complications; that is the reason why these cases have always been a highlight in classic perinatal medicine studies. Nevertheless, this area of knowledge has currently gained popularity because of an increase of its incidence and the further investigations on multiple pregnancies.

Factors that have predetermined an increase of the rate of twin gestation during the last years are quite diverse; however, it seems important to point out two of them that are also related.

Advanced maternal age: as for older women the probability of double ovulation increases by an increase in the secretion of follicle stimulating hormone (FSH).

Increased use of artificial reproductive technologies and fertility drugs. Approximately 30-35% of fertility treatments develop in a multiple pregnancy.

DIAGNOSIS AND TREATMENT

The early determination of chorionicity in twin gestations is a critical factor in the management of twin gestations. While twins and higher order multiple gestations have increased risks of almost any complication of pregnancy, those pregnancies involving a monochorionic twin pair are at an especially high risk.

* Corresponding author: ananm9@gmail.com.

The diagnosis of chorionicity performed at first trimester is the reference for the rest of the pregnancy. Indeed, further determination of the chorionicity at second or third trimester is less accurate and more difficult.

The presence of the 'lambda' or the 'T' sign in the presence of a single placenta, best determined in the first trimester, is the most reliable indicator of chorionicity, with measurements of the inter-twin membrane thickness and counting of the membrane layers being less reliable. During the first trimester, a "lambda sign" on ultrasound can differentiate between monozygotic twins and a separate fetus.

The reasons for ultrasound in twins include pregnancy dating, determination of chorionicity, nuchal translucency assessment, anatomical survey, placental evaluation, cervical length assessment, routine fetal growth, and serial surveillance of pregnancies complicated by anomalies, cervical shortening, fetal growth disturbances, and amniotic fluid abnormalities. Twins with monochorionic placentation require heightened scrutiny for monoamnionicity, conjoined twins, twin reversed arterial perfusion (TRAP) syndrome, twin-twin transfusion syndrome, unequal placental sharing with discordant twin growth or selective intrauterine fetal growth restriction (IUGR), twin anemia-polycythemia sequence (TAPS), and single fetal demise. Ultrasound is essential for the detection and management of conditions that can complicate dichorionic and monochorionic twin pregnancies.

Combined First Trimester Screening

We can find some differences depending on the chorionicity:

In dichorionic twins, patient-specific risks for trisomy 21 are calculated for each fetus based on maternal age and fetal nuchal translucency and the detection rate and false positive rate are similar to those in singleton pregnancies.

All monochorionic twins are monozygotic and they are invariably concordant for fetal karyotype. They are always monozygotic, the maternal age-related risk for chromosomal abnormalities is the same as in singleton pregnancies, and in the vast majority of cases both fetuses are affected. The false-positive rate of nuchal translucency screening (13% per pregnancy) is higher than in dichorionic twins, because increased nuchal translucency in at least one of the fetuses is an early manifestation of twin-to-twin transfusion syndrome.

To calculate the risk you can use the average of both nuchal translucencies or use the larger of the two. With the combined risk calculation must take into account that certain biochemical markers in blood as both fetuses contribute to the production of these and cannot calculate the specific risk for each twin. Thus, the sensitivity of first-trimester screening for twin pregnancies is 75% compared to 90% of singleton pregnancies. The false positive rate is 5%. There are also specific chromosomal markers of twin pregnancy like the size disparity between the two fetuses. One major difference of 10% in the CRL was significantly associated with a high incidence of structural and chromosomal abnormalities.

Regarding invasive diagnostic techniques is noted that are technically more difficult with increased fetal loss rate. However, the complication rate is very dependent on operator experience. In most cases combined risk 1:50 is advised as chorionic villus sampling has the advantage of an earlier result and the possibility of selective feticide at an earlier stage of pregnancy in the case to be stated, with a minor risk of loss of another fetus. For lower risk 1/50 amniocentesis is advised for ease of technique.

Cervical Length

Although current obstetric practice guidelines suggest cervical length assessment for preterm birth risk, transvaginal ultrasonography has availability limitations.

None of the existing preventive or intervention has proven to be useful in twin pregnancy (Berghella et al. 2013).

Complications Associated with Multiple Pregnancy

Multiple gestation is associated with higher rates of any of the possible maternal and fetal complications of pregnancy, except post-term pregnancy and macrosomia. There are also other complications that are unique to the twin pregnancy, even specific to the type. The twins have a perinatal mortality rate of 3-11 times that of singletons due to a higher incidence of complications.

Thus there are a higher incidence of vomiting in the first quarter, gastro esophageal reflux, urinary frequency, anemia, increased cardiac output, increased body weight and increased incidence of hypertensive problems from the second trimester, all related to the mother's body changes that occur in singleton pregnancies when we find multiple gestations are more pronounced.

From the point of view of the fetal complications we found increased incidence of abortion and stillbirth, Polihydramnios, prematurity, low birth weight, intrauterine growth restricted, twin-twin transfusion syndrome and higher frequency of congenital malformations.

Preterm Birth

Preterm birth is a major health problem and contributes to more than 50% of the overall perinatal mortality. Preterm birth has multiple risk factors including cervical incompetence and multiple pregnancy.

In multiple gestations cervical length experiences a very marked decrease compared to singleton pregnancies especially after 24 weeks. Although a cervical length less than 25 mm at 20-24 weeks increased almost 6 times the risk of preterm delivery before 32 weeks, none of the existing preventive or intervention has proven to be useful in twin pregnancy.

Different management strategies have been tried to prevent preterm birth, including cervical cerclage.

Cervical cerclage is an invasive technique that needs anesthesia and may be associated with complications. Moreover, there is still controversy regarding the efficacy and the group of patients that could benefit from this operation.

Cervical pessary has been tried as a simple, non-invasive alternative that might replace the above invasive cervical stitch operation to prevent preterm birth.

There is evidence from one randomized controlled trial that using cervical pessary is superior to expectant management in prevention of preterm birth in women with a singleton pregnancy and a short cervix. Evidence for its beneficial effect in other settings and for other groups of patients is not yet documented.

There is a need for more well-designed randomized controlled trials to confirm the beneficial effect of cervical pessary in reducing preterm birth in women with a short cervix in different settings and in women with other risk factors for preterm birth including multiple pregnancy.

Specific Complications Monochorionic Gestations

While twins and higher order multiple gestations have increased risks of almost any complication of pregnancy, those pregnancies involving a monochorionic twin pair are at an especially high risk. The presence of vascular anastomoses within a monochorionic placenta creates risk for discordant malformations; twin reversed arterial perfusion sequence, twin-to-twin transfusion syndrome, or severe selective intrauterine growth restriction.

Twin to Twin Transfusion Syndrome

Exclusive complication of monochorionic twin pregnancies with a prevalence of 15%. It´s characterized by a gradual shift of blood volume from the donor twin to the recipient twin through placental vascular connections

This syndrome is a severe hemodynamic disorder which leads to a progressive sequence characterized by hypovolemia, oliguria, and oligohydramnios in the donor, and hypervolemia, polyuria, and polyhydramnios in the recipient (Quintero et al., 1999):

- Diagnostic criteria:
  - ✓ Confirmed monochorionic pregnancy.
  - ✓ Polihydramnios in the recipient with deepest vertical pocket most of 8cm.
  - ✓ Oligohydramnios in the donor with a deepest vertical pocket less of 2cm.
  - ✓ This syndrome must to begin before 26 weeks.
- Quintero staging system:
  - ✓ I: the bladder is still visible in the donor twin.
  - ✓ II: the bladder is no longer visible in the donor twin.
  - ✓ III: critically abnormal Doppler in either twin: absent/reverse diastolic flow in the umbilical artery of the donor or recipient and/or reverse flow in the ductus venous or pulsatile in the umbilical vein of the recipient.
  - ✓ IV: hydrops in either fetus.
  - ✓ V: demise of one or both twins.

It´s important to do differential diagnosis with Inconsistency of amniotic fluid: oligoanhidramnios-polyhydramnios sequence without other diagnostics criteria.

Should be performed to rule out weekly monitoring progress towards twin to twin transfusion syndrome. Presents good prognosis and do not require treatment.

Selective intrauterine growth restriction. One of the fetuses has a lower 10th percentile estimated fetal weight. However there is polihydramnios-oligohydramnios sequence or mismatch between bladders.

- Treatment:

The perinatal mortality due to twin to twin transfusion syndrome without treatment is 80-100% with associated neurological morbidity 15-50%.

Fetoscopyc laser coagulation has been shown to improve survival and reduce neurological morbidity in twin to twin transfusion syndrome. It´s has been shown to be the treatment of choice in gestations under 26 weeks, with a survival of at least one fetus between 75-85% and an associated neurological morbidity between 4 and 6% (Akkermans et al., 2014).

Fetoscopyc laser photocoagulation of placental anastomoses is an effective treatment addressing the underlying pathophysiology.

Sonographic signs of resolution of symptoms usually appear several days after making it necessary to monitor weekly amniotic fluid, urinary bladders of both fetuses and Doppler normalizaicón when there have been previous alterations.

Maternal complications associated with fetoscopic: ascites by amniotic fluid, mirror syndrome, chorioamnionitis or abruption.

Altouht fetoscopyc laser photocoagulation is the best treatment there are others options: amniotic fluid extraction to reduce symptomatic polihydramnios and reduce the risk of prematurity treatment.

Another choice of treatment is fetal reduction. Selective termination in complex monochorionic pregnancies can be lifesaving for the co-twin by preventing intrauterine demise or extreme prematurity.

- Clinical management of twin to twin transfusion syndrome:

Once the diagnosis is established, treatment of choice is fetoscopy except:

- Fetal reduction: exist neurological injury or preterminal stage of a fetu, existence of congenital defect associated or technical impossibilities
- Amniotic fluid extraction: when gestations is more than 26 weeks.
- End of gestation if the diagnosis is more than 32 weeks.

Selective Intrauterine Growth Restriction

There is an intrauterine growth restriction in one fetus having an estimated fetal weight below the percentile 10 and after exclusion of twin to twin transfusion syndrome.

There are several factors involved in: asymmetric distribution placental, vascular anastomosis and the possibility of abnormal cord insertion.

Diagnosis criteria are: estimated fetal weight of a fetus below the 10th percentile and biometric unconformity above 25% (EFW1-EFW2/EFW1 x 100).

Staging system:

- Type I: Umbilical artery Doppler normal. They have good prognosis. No treatment. Ultrasound each week.

End of gestation when have been an arrest of fetal growth or evolution to type II or III.

- Type II: absent or reverse diastolic flow in the umbilical artery.

They have a poor prognosis but predictable. The test of fetal wellbeing are useful and allow monitoring of pregnancy, fetal impairment diagnose and determine the appropriate date to end the pregnancy.

Should be performed weekly monitoring of fetal wellbeing.

- Before 28 weeks if there are reviews of umbilical Doppler abnormalities can raise the cord occlusion or laser photocoagulation of vascular anastomosis.
- Between 28-32 weeks, end of pregnancy after induction of fetal lung maturation with corticosteroids.
- Type III: absente or reverse diastolic flow in the umbilical artery intermittently. The clinical course is atypical and unpredictable so that clinical management is complicated. End of pregnancy between 30-32 weeks, after induction of fetal lung maturation with corticosteroids.

Twin Reversed Arterial Perfusion (TRAP) Sequence

It is a rare malformation occurring in monozygotic multiple gestations. One well-developed normal (pump) twin and the other twin with absent cardiac structure (acardiac), who is hemodynamically dependent on the normal (pump) twin are characteristic of this syndrome. The acardiac twin develops multiple anomalies that make survival difficult.

The prognosis of the pump twin is variable with mortality rate ranging from 50% to 70%. Complications that affect the prognosis of the pump twin include complications of congestive cardiac failure due to increased cardiac demand, prematurity secondary to preterm delivery, and polihydramnios. Because of these complications prompt detection, follow-up, and treatment of this condition is very important.

Adequate follow-up and management of monochorionics twins can be accomplished by means of an integrated view of the main groups of complications and should be guided by very basic principles. The complexity and the uncountable number of combined complications that monochorionics twin pregnancies can present may often blur clinical decisions in a way that such basic principles are forgotten. Gratacós et al., propose a simplified (but clinically useful) approach to follow-up and management of monochorionic twins, which in essence contains the obvious principles of early diagnosis, proper follow-up, and timely intervention.

The rules proposed here might look too simplistic to condense the vast knowledge behind monochorionic twin pregnancy. Of course, there will always be exceptional cases of high difficulty which are not covered by these rules. However, clinical experience of more than 15 years demonstrates that, still today, most instances of poor or suboptimal management derive from failure to comply with one or more of this basic set of principles. (Gratacos et al., 2012)

1. Early diagnosis (at 11 to 14 week scan) and ruling out malformations.
2. Follow up every two weeks (EFW, AF, and MCA) by a fetal medicine specialist.
3. If suspicious: weekly follow up.
4. If polyhydramnios/oligohydramnios sequence and diagnostic criteria are met: twin to twin transfusion syndrome, inmediate treatment.
5. If EFW <10th percentile in one fetus: selective intrauterine growth restriction, umbilical artery Doppler:
    - Normal: expectant management.
    - Abnormal: discuss opinions with parents.
    - If no complications: elective delivery at 36-37 weeks of gestation.

FETAL GROWTH CONTROL

The intrauterine growth retardation with prematurity is the leading cause of perinatal morbidity and mortality in twin gestations. It is therefore very important ultrasound monitoring of fetal growth. Through week 28 to 30 the weight of the twins is similar that of singletons.

From there the differences are progressively increased with the duration of pregnanc. The frequency of ultrasound depends on the type of twin pregnancy question, week of gestation and associated pathology in the event of any.

Test of Fetal Weelbeing

Twin pregnancy is considered high risk pregnancy high maternal and fetal morbidity and mortality for this reason, the antepartum fetal monitoring twin pregnancies should be stricter than in singleton pregnancies. In high-risk pregnancies monitoring fetal wellbeing starts between week 32 and 34 of gestation. In the case of any complications will occur this that indicate the onset and frequency of tests to be carried out.

- Non stress test: Provides a margin of safety of fetal wellbeing than a week but the period of maximum reliability corresponds to the first 48 hours.
- Index of amniotic fluid: early finding of oligohydramnios may indicate a redistribution of fetal blood flow level.
- Fetal biophysical profile: report on the integrity of the fetal brain function and therefore the absence of systemic hypoxia.
- Doppler: noninvasive method for the study of blood flow in the fetal vessels.

Embryo Reduction

First-trimester transvaginal embryo reduction is an effective alternative for the management of multifetal pregnancy in assisted reproduction, when there are three or more embryos (Drugan et al., 2013).

Assistance Twin Births

The twin birth is considered a high-risk birth. As a result multiple pregnancies account for 11% of early neonatal deaths, 3.4% of neonatal deaths and later 10% of cerebral palsy.

The management of twin delivery will depend on the type of presentation, estimated fetal weight, weeks of gestation as well as the surgeon's experience.

Optimal timing of birth twin pregnancy

A twin pregnancy is considered post-term when it goes beyond 40 weeks of gestation.

The optimal timing of birth for women with a twin pregnancy is uncertain, with clinical support for both elective delivery at 37weeks'gestation (either by induction of labour or caesarean birth), and for waiting for labour to start spontaneously (expectant management).

Two randomised controlled trials were included in this review involving a total of 271 women with twin pregnancies at 37 weeks' gestation. One of the two trials (involving 235 women) was of high quality, and the quality of the second trial (involving 36 women) was unclear. There were no differences shown between the group of women who had an elective birth at 37 weeks' gestation and the group of women who waited for labour to start spontaneously for the outcomes: birth by caesarean section, perinatal (fetal or neonatal) death or serious perinatal morbidity, or maternal death or serious maternal morbidity. No other differences between the two groups of women were shown for other pregnancy and birth complications or for complications for the infant.

Elective birth at 37 weeks' gestation compared with ongoing expectant management for women with uncomplicated twin pregnancies does not appear be associated with an increased risk of harms.

Mode of delivery in twin pregnancies

In daily clinical practice, decisions regarding the mode of delivery of a twin pregnancy rely on several factors including gestational age, fetal presentation, underlying severe maternal and fetal complications, past obstetric history, parental wishes and beliefs, and the obstetrician's skill, confidence, and ability to deliver a non-vertex second twin.

The indications for cesarean delivery in twin pregnancies include first twin non-vertex, second twin with an estimated weight that is 500g greater than that of the presenting twin, both fetuses estimated to weigh <1500g, monoamniotic twins and the usual obstetric indications for singleton pregnancies.

We can classify the presentation of the twins into three groups, each of which will condition obstetric behavior:

- Both twins in vertex position. Vaginal delivery would be indicated unless excite contraindications for vaginal it.
- After the birth of the first twin events can occur cesarean practice for the second twin as necessitating: cord prolapse, fetal distress, abruptio placentae or fetal malposition.
- Recommendations:
- Continuous and simultaneous monitoring of both twins.
- After the birth of the first twin must be confirmed by submission of the second touch being able to use vaginal ultrasound.
- Start or increase the dose of oxytocin after the birth of the first twin.
- Amniorrhexis second bag when the presentation of the second twin is in the pelvis.
- Twin A in vertex position an twin B in different position:
- While the safety of a vaginal delivery for vertex/vertex twins is well documented, the ideal management when the second twin is non-vertex is still controversial.
- There is clear evidence of adverse perinatal outcome after breech delivery of the second twin when the estimated fetal weight less than 1,500g. So just try vaginal delivery in breech presentation when the calculated weight greater than 1,500g. (Adam, 1991).
    - ✓ Elective caesarean: there is no scientific evidence of benefit on some parameter of perinatal morbidity and mortality.
    - ✓ Twin A vaginal delivery and twin B vaginal delivery after external cephalic version. There is work in which a significantly lower incidence of fetal distress in the breech birth of twin B with respect to the external version of this twin is appreciated.
    - ✓ Twin A vaginal delivery and breech extraction twin B:
    - ✓ Adequate anesthesia and adequate experience is required. In the absence of an operator experienced in vaginal breech delivery, cesarean delivery is prudent.
    - ✓ Introduce one hand into the uterus and grasp the feet through the intact membranes. Palpation of the malleolus at a perpendicular angle with the distal tibia and fibula confirms that the lower extremities are being grasped. Gentle continuous axis traction toward the birth canal should then be applied. The other hand should be used to guide the fetal head upward. Gently perform continuous axis traction toward the birth canal. Encourage the mother to push. Once the presenting part is engaged, rupture the membranes. Then we will proceed to breech second twin.
    - ✓ Twin A vaginal delivery and twin B breech delivery.
    - ✓ Twin A vaginal delivery and twin B caesarean.
    - ✓ Twin A no vertex: caesarean section is the safest way of completion.

Birth interval between twins

The second twin is at greatest risk at the time of delivery. The delay in the birth of twin B could condition moderate respiratory acidosis.

The increase in birth interval is associated with a higher rate of caesarean sections and maternal morbidity.

Vaginal birth after cesarean section is safe in twin pregnancies without having detected increased morbidity labor (Miller, 1991).

Postpartum Complications

Maternal postpartum complications occur in approximately 7% of twin deliveries. These complications are associated with pregnancies with concomitant clinical or obstetrical complications, earlier gestational age at delivery and emergency cesarean deliveries.

Twin pregnancies have an associated morbidity and mortality significantly higher than that of single-fetus pregnancies; behave as an exacerbation of the signs and symptoms of pregnancy so pose a risk for both mother and fetus.

Complications mainly include increased risk of bleeding, retained placenta, thromboembolic events, endometritis, preeclampsia and higher incidence of depressive symptoms. There is also an increase in caesarean section; it also increases morbidity and mortality.

Obstetric hemorrhage: early postpartum hemorrhage complicates 5 to 15% of all births. It is the most important cause of maternal mortality.

In the twin pregnancy have an increased incidence of postpartum hemorrhage due to uterine distension, increased risk of retained placental tissue and the highest rate of caesarean sections.

The best treatment for postpartum hemorrhage is early prevention.

It is demonstrated that the routine use of oxytocin reduces the risk of postpartum hemorrhage. After, we may to use oxytocin or other uterotonic for 4-6 hours. In the case of delivery by cesarean section in twin and under epidural or spinal anesthesia is indicated Carbetocin instead of oxytocin, synthetic analogue of oxytocin with a longer shelf life.

REFERENCES

Adam C, Allen AC, Baskett TF. (1991)Twin delivery: Influence of the presentation and method of delivery on the second twin. *American journal of obstetrics and gynecology*; 165:23-7.

Akkermans J, Peeters SH, Klumper FJ, Middeldorp JM, Lopriore E, et al. (2014) Is the Sequential Laser Technique for Twin-to-Twin Transfusion Syndrome Truly Superior to the Standard Selective Technique A Meta-Analysis. *Fetal diagnosis and therapy.*

Berghella V, Baxter JK, Hendrix NW. (2013) Cervical assessment by ultrasound for preventing preterm delivery. NW. *Cochrane Database System Review*. DOI 10.1002/14651858. CD007235.pub3.

Clery-Golman J, Berkowitz RL. (2005) First trimester screening for Down syndrome in multiple pregnancy. *Seminars in perinatology*. 29:395-400.

Drugan A, Ulanovsky I, Burke Y, Blazer S, Weissman A. (2013) Fetal reduction in triplet gestations: twins still fare better. *The Israel Medical Association journal*.15(12):745-7.

Gratacós E, Ortiz JU, Martinez JM. (2012). A Systematic Approach to the Differential Diagnosis and Management of the Complications of Monochorionic Twin Pregnancies. *Fetal diagnosis and therapy*. November; 32:145–155.

Huertas MA, Martinez L. (2010). *Gestación gemelar. Manejo y tratamiento.*

Miller DA, Mullin P, Hou D, Paul RH. (1996) Vaginal birth after cesarean section in twin gestation. *American journal of obstetrics and gynecology*. July; 175(1)194-8.

Quintero RA, Morales WJ, Allen MH, Bornick PW, Joheson PK et al.(1999) Staging of twin-twin transfusion syndrome. *Journal of Perinatology*. 19:550-5.

Smithz T, Azria E, Cabrol D, Goffinet F. (2009) Is vaginal delivery in twin pregnancy still an option? An analysis of the literature data. *Journal of gynecology, obstetric and biology reproduction* (Paris). 38:367-76.

EDITORS' CONTACT INFORMATION

Dr. Ernesto González-Mesa, PhD
Professor
School of Medicine
Obstetrics and Gynecology Department
University Malaga Hospital
Arroyo de los Angeles Av.
29011 Málaga, Spain
Email: egonzalezmesa@gmail.com

Dr. D. Abehsera
Obstetrics and Gynecology Department
Quirón University Hospital
Málaga, Spain
Email: danielabehsera@hotmail.com.

INDEX

A

B

C

D

E

G

H

I

J

K

L

M

N

O

P

T

U

V

W

Y